Platelet Rich Fibrin in
Regenerative Dentistry

Platelet Rich Fibrin in Regenerative Dentistry

Biological Background and Clinical Indications

Edited by

Richard J. Miron, Dr. med. dent., DDS, BMSC, MSc, PhD
Department of Periodontology
College of Dental Medicine
Nova Southeastern University
Fort Lauderdale, Florida, USA

Joseph Choukroun, MD
Private practice, Pain Therapy Center
Nice, France

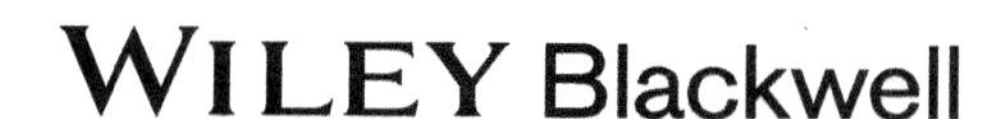

This edition first published 2017

Registered Offices
John Wiley & Sons, Inc., 111 River Street, Hoboken, NJ 07030, USA
John Wiley & Sons Ltd, The Atrium, Southern Gate, Chichester, West Sussex, PO19 8SQ, UK

Editorial Office
9600 Garsington Road, Oxford, OX4 2DQ, UK

For details of our global editorial offices, customer services, and more information about Wiley products visit us at www.wiley.com.

Wiley also publishes its books in a variety of electronic formats and by print-on-demand. Some content that appears in standard print versions of this book may not be available in other formats.

Library of Congress Cataloging-in-Publication Data

Names: Miron, Richard J. (Richard John), 1983– editor. | Choukroun, Joseph, 1952– editor.
Title: Platelet rich fibrin in regenerative dentistry : biological background and clinical indications / edited by Richard J. Miron, Joseph Choukroun.
Description: Hoboken, NJ : Wiley, 2017. | Includes bibliographical references and index. |
Identifiers: LCCN 2017017750 (print) | LCCN 2017018765 (ebook) | ISBN 9781119406891 (pdf) | ISBN 9781119406808 (epub) | ISBN 9781119406815 (cloth)
Subjects: | MESH: Oral Surgical Procedures | Fibrin–therapeutic use | Platelet-Rich Plasma | Tissue Engineering | Bone Regeneration
Classification: LCC RK307 (ebook) | LCC RK307 (print) | NLM WU 600 | DDC 617.522–dc23
LC record available at https://lccn.loc.gov/2017017750

Cover Design: Wiley
Cover Images: (Foreground, PRF clot & instruments) Courtesy of Jonathan Du Toit; (Background, centrifuge image) Courtesy of Joseph Choukroun

Set in 10/12pt WarnockPro by Aptara Inc., New Delhi, India

Printed in the United States of America

V008670_013119

To my parents, family, and friends who have all sacrificed far too often in my pursuit of a career in academic dentistry

To my classmates, colleagues, and mentors who constantly raised the bar and strived for better

To the team at Advanced PRF Education who made excellence in teaching a top priority

In gratitude to my Mentors and Professors at the University of Montpellier and Strasbourg, France. Your education and mentorship has given me the means to innovate in the treatment of pain and wound healing.

Contents

About the Authors

Editor, *Richard J. Miron, Dr. med. dent., DDS, BMSC, MSc, PhD*
Adjunct Professor
Department of Periodontology
College of Dental Medicine
Nova Southeastern University
Fort Lauderdale, Florida, USA

Co-Editor, *Joseph Choukroun, MD*
Private practice, Pain Therapy Center,
Nice, France

Alain Simonpieri, DDS
Professor
Department of Oral surgery
University Federico II Naples
Naples, Italy

Alberto Monje, DDS, MS, PhD
Research Associate
Department of Periodontics and Oral Medicine
The University of Michigan, School of Dentistry
Ann Arbor, Michigan, USA

Alexandre-Amir Aalam, DDS, MSc
Diplomate, American Academy Board of Periodontology
Diplomate, American Board of Oral Implantology
Clinical Assistant Professor, Herman Ostrow School of Dentistry of USC

Alina Krivitsky Aalam, DDS, MSc
Diplomate, American Academy Board of Periodontology
Diplomate, American Board of Oral Implantology
Private Office, Center for Advanced Periodontal and Implant Therapy
Los Angeles, California, USA

Anton Sculean, Dr. med. dent., Dr. h.c., M.S.
Professor, Executive Director and Chairman
Department of Periodontology
University of Bern
Bern, Switzerland

Brian L. Mealey, DDS, MS
Professor and Graduate Program Director
Department of Periodontics
UT Health Science Center at San Antonio
San Antonio, Texas, USA

Cleopatra Nacopoulos, DDS, PhD
Research Associate
Laboratory for Research of the Musculoskeletal System
KAT Hospital, School of Medicine, National and Kapodistrian
University of Athens
Athens, Greece

Giovanni Zuchelli, DDS, PhD
Professor
Department of Biomedical and Neuromotor Sciences
University of Bologna
Bologna, Italy

Hom-Lay Wang, DDS, MS, PhD
Collegiate Professor of Periodontics
Professor and Director of Graduate Periodontics
Department of Periodontics and Oral Medicine
The University of Michigan, School of Dentistry
Ann Arbor, Michigan, USA

Howard Gluckman, BDS, MChD (OMP)
Specialist in Periodontics, Implantology and Oral Medicine
Director of Implant & Aesthetics Academy
Cape Town, South Africa

Jonathan Du Toit, DDS
Research Associate
Department of Periodontics and Oral Medicine
Faculty of Health Sciences
University of Pretoria
Pretoria, South Africa

Masako Fujioka-Kobayashi, DDS, PhD
Assistant Professor
Department of Oral Maxillofacial Surgery
Tokushima University
Tokushima, Japan

Michael A. Pikos, DDS, MD, MS
Director, Pikos Institute
Tampa, Florida, USA

Shahram Ghanaati, MD, DMD, PhD
Professor
Department for Oral, Cranio-Maxillofacial and Facial Plastic Surgery
FORM-Lab (Frankfurt Orofacial Regenerative Medicine)
University Hospital Frankfurt Goethe University
Frankfurt am Main, Germany

Tobias Fretwurst, DDS
Department of Oral and Maxillofacial Surgery
University of Freiburg
Freiburg, Germany

Yufeng Zhang, DDS, MD, PhD
Professor
Department of Oral Implantology
University of Wuhan
Wuhan, China

Foreword

It brings great pleasure to write the foreword for this first textbook on platelet rich fibrin (PRF) by Drs. Richard Miron and Joseph Choukroun. The book covers many aspects of tissue regeneration in an evidence-based and clinically relevant manner and includes all the key leaders in this field in what has now been over 15 years since the first use of PRF. Virtually all topics and areas involving hard- and soft-tissue regeneration with PRF are covered with many photos that complement the text. The subject matter is presented with a focus and depth consistent with a rigorous scientific periodical. Importantly, information is presented in a way that fits the clinician's needs to better understand the biological rationale for utilizing PRF, as well as when and where to use various protocols with PRF in regenerative dentistry in an evidence-based manner.

Drs. Miron and Choukroun have gathered 17 authors from 10 different countries into 15 chapters that cover all the relevant aspects centered around PRF. The first chapters deal with the basic biological concepts of PRF with the later chapters dedicated to the clinical indications and applications for PRF in regenerative dentistry. Numerous clinical illustrations are given from many international experts and leaders in the field of bone and periodontal regeneration. A wide audience will benefit immensely from the content of this book, including all practicing dentists and dental residents who currently frequently utilize PRF in everyday practice, as well as new clinicians wishing to better understand and implement this technology within their practice in the near future. I fully anticipate that this textbook will represent a landmark contribution to the dental field and sets a new standard for the years to come.

Prof. Dr. med. dent. Anton Sculean, Dr. h.c., M.S.
Executive Director and Chairman
Department of Periodontology
School of Dental Medicine
University of Bern, Switzerland

Preface

When the concept of platelet rich fibrin was established almost 20 years ago, it was simply a means to provide a more natural way to bring blood-derived growth factors and vascularization to human tissues. Advancements in platelet rich plasma (PRP) and platelet rich growth factors (PRGF) had pioneered the influence of supplying blood-derived plasma proteins to tissues. By developing new protocols utilizing 100% natural methods (anti-coagulant removal) while simultaneously providing a three-dimensional scaffold made of autologous fibrin, an array of possibilities was created in regenerative medicine. This new field, now known as Platelet Rich Fibrin or PRF, forms the basis of this academic textbook aimed at providing an in-depth summary of its regenerative possibilities in dentistry.

Much advancement on PRF has been made since my first publication in 2001 not only in dentistry, but across many fields of medicine. While initially it became clear that the potential of PRF could serve a means to augment soft tissue regeneration, it was not until the past decade that a rapid and exponential increase in popularity had resulted from its use. This has been simultaneously paralleled with a large increase in scholarly activity and scientific publication supporting its regenerative potential. Thousands of dentists now use PRF and this number is only expected to continue to rise.

My passion for PRF began in my Pain Clinic in Nice, France when I was faced daily with large necrotizing leg ulcers in my private clinic. These patients were often later referred for amputation. In the late 1990s it became clear that infection was a secondary problem to low blood flow and by introducing a regenerative therapy focused specifically on improving vascularization to tissues, wound healing could be achieved. We have now learned a tremendous amount with respect to the impact of not only blood-derived growth factors, but also the marked impact of leukocytes and their implications in wound healing, as well as the specific role of fibrin in regenerative biology. These concepts have been studied by some of the top international biologists from around the world.

This book is a first of its kind. As we continue to learn more about PRF and its use, it becomes increasingly clear that several editions will follow in the years to come. We continue to gather new knowledge about the PRF concept and what factors help support its regenerative potential. Expert clinicians have further developed new surgical protocols that additionally improve the regenerative outcomes with PRF in every day clinical practice. I am grateful for their encouraging teamwork and mindset, as many of them have contributed entire chapters in this textbook supporting its use.

As we reach new goals and heights, let us not forget that PRF is not a miracle product, or a treat-all scaffold that can be utilized for every clinical application. It follows biological principles and guidelines that have been outlined in this book and more importantly documented over many years. I am thrilled at having this opportunity to share with you these discoveries, learned and unlearned protocols, gathered by whom I consider to be top experts from around the world to help present PRF in an academic manner.

I sincerely hope you enjoy what we have learned together over the past 15 years,

Joseph Choukroun, MD
Inventor of PRF, Nice, France

Around the year 2010, my lab was heavily involved in numerous projects investigating the regenerative potential of many growth factors and biomaterials. Many products were being investigated pre-clinically in both cell culture systems and animal models prior to their FDA approval and commercialization. From this respect, I was aware of many biomaterials even years before they became commercially available and marketed to dentists and doctors.

PRF came to our research group as a bit of a surprise. It was quite rare that a growing biomaterial had already been popularized without having been fully investigated intensively throughout the common international university research labs. It was difficult to assess its regenerative potential and many research groups became increasingly interested in this new phenomenon of utilizing naturally derived growth factors without anticoagulants. From a scientific standpoint, it offered many advantages over previous platelet formulations, namely being 100% natural and providing a three-dimensional scaffold containing living host cells at relatively no cost.

Over the past 5 years, a marked and substantial increase in scientific publications related to its use was seen, further forcing not only my research group, but many others in medicine, to investigate its potential. By the year 2012, we began a series of studies investigating PRF, as the demand for its use continued to rise. Many of the top researchers and expert clinicians presented in this book have learned so much with respect to PRF, and this trend will only continue.

It became clear that an academic textbook on this topic was needed. This enormous project focused on the revision of hundreds of written pages and illustrations and I thank Jessica Evans and the rest of the team at Wiley for their continuous support and guidance throughout this project. The work presented is meant to gather the current knowledge on PRF from an academic perspective, gathering the latest research on the topic in an evidenced-based manner. For these reasons, the use of company names or commercial partners were duly excluded from this textbook. Preference in all chapters was given to clinical studies of high quality, utilizing randomized methods conducted with appropriate protocols/controls. From this point of view, this book hopes not only to be a first of its kind, but one that will stand for the years to come based on the reputation of its contributing authors and quality of its content.

I, therefore, am very pleased to present to you the first edition of our textbook, Platelet Rich Fibrin in Regenerative Dentistry: Biological Background and Clinical Indications, and hope you enjoy learning the many aspects centered around the use of PRF in regenerative dentistry.

Sincerely,

Richard J. Miron, DDS, BMSC, MSc, PhD, dr. med. dent.
Department of Periodontology
Nova Southeastern University, Florida

1

Platelet Rich Fibrin: A Second-Generation Platelet Concentrate

Joseph Choukroun and Richard J. Miron

Abstract

Almost two decades have passed since platelet rich fibrin (PRF) was first introduced. Initially, the primary objective was to develop a therapy where platelet concentrates could be introduced into wounds by effectively utilizing the body's natural healing capacity. This was achieved by collecting growth factors derived from blood in a natural way. Platelet rich plasma (PRP) and platelet rich growth factor (PRGF) had been commercialized, yet both contained secondary byproducts that were both unnatural and known inhibitors of wound healing. By removing these anti-coagulants and modifying centrifugation protocols, PRF was introduced some years later with the potential to markedly impact many fields of medicine including dentistry. Many aspects important for tissue regeneration have since been revealed including the important role of fibrin as well as the preferential release of growth factors over longer periods of time from PRF. Furthermore, by introducing a new set of cells into platelet concentrates (namely leukocytes), a marked impact on tissue regeneration and wound healing was observed. Over the past 5 years, further modifications to centrifugation speed and time have additionally improved PRF into a concept now known as the "low-speed centrifugation concept." Investigators began to modify surgical techniques to favorably treat patients with PRF with improved clinical outcomes. Together, many key opinion leaders from around the globe have been gathered to share their experiences and knowledge in many educational courses and seminars in what we now know as platelet rich fibrin. In this first chapter, we highlight the discovery of PRF and the studies leading to its first use in regenerative medicine. We focus specifically on its properties for wound healing and how its presented advantages over previous versions of platelet concentrates have favorably enhanced the regenerative potential of platelet concentrates in dentistry.

Highlights

- Introduction of Platelet Rich Fibrin
- Reasons for its invention two decades ago
- Its variations from the formally known platelet concentrate "platelet rich plasma" or "PRP"
- The first case treated with PRF
- Properties important for wound healing

1.1 Introduction

Wound healing is a complex biological process where many cellular events taking place simultaneously leading to the repair or regeneration of damaged tissues [1–4]. Many attempts have been made in the field of tissue regeneration with the aim of predictably repairing, regenerating, or restoring

Platelet Rich Fibrin in Regenerative Dentistry: Biological Background and Clinical Indications, First Edition.
Edited by Richard J. Miron and Joseph Choukroun.

damaged and diseased tissues [1–4]. These include strategies with foreign materials often derived from allografts, xenografts, or synthetically produced alloplasts to regenerate host tissues [1–4]. While many of these materials have shown promise in various aspects of regenerative medicine, it is important to note that all create a "foreign body reaction," whereby a foreign material is introduced into human host tissues.

Platelet concentrates collected from whole blood was first introduced over 20 years ago. The concept was developed with the aim of utilizing human blood proteins as a source of growth factors capable of supporting angiogenesis and tissue ingrowth based on the notion that blood supply is a prerequisite for tissue regeneration [5]. Four aspects of wound healing have since been described as key components for the successful regeneration of human tissues (Figure 1.1). These include 1) hemostasis, 2) inflammation, 3) proliferation, and 4) maturation. Each phase encompasses various cell types. One of the main disadvantages of currently utilized biomaterials in the field of tissue engineering is that the great majority are typically avascular by nature, and therefore do not provide the necessary vascular supply to fully obtain successful regeneration of either soft or hard tissues [5].

It must further be noted that in general, wound healing demands the complex interaction of various cell types with a three-dimensional extracellular matrix as well as soluble growth factors capable of facilitating regeneration [6]. Certainly, one area of research in dentistry that has gained tremendous momentum in recent years is that of recombinant growth factors where a number have been used to successfully regenerate either soft or hard tissues [7–9]. Table 1.1 provides a list of currently approved growth factors along with their individual roles in tissue regeneration and clinical indications supporting their use. Similarly, a number of barrier membranes with various functions and resorption properties have also been commonly utilized in regenerative dentistry formulated from either synthetic or animal-derived materials [10]. Lastly, many bone-grafting materials are brought to market every year, all characterized by their specific advantages and disadvantages during tissue regeneration. While each of the above-mentioned biomaterials have been shown to

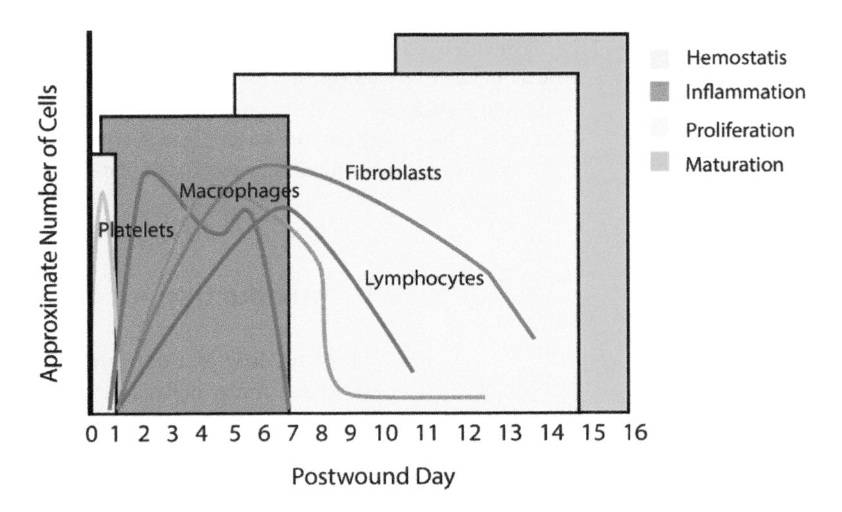

Figure 1.1 Four phases of wound healing including 1) hemostasis, 2) inflammation, 3) proliferation, and 4) maturation. Noteworthy are the overlaps between each of the phases and the population of cells found in each category. Whereas lymphocytes typically arise at 7 days, the ability for PRF to introduce a high number at day 0 acts to speed the regenerative phase during this process.

Table 1.1 List of growth factors used for the regeneration of periodontal intrabony defects with listed advantages and disadvantages.

Growth factor	Advantages	Disadvantages
Enamel Matrix Derivative	– Mimics the formation of root development – Amelogenin proteins improves PDL cell adhesion, proliferation and differentiation – Adsorbs to the root surface up to 4 weeks post-surgery – Histologically demonstrated as "true" periodontal regeneration with formation of Sharpey's fibers	– Gel formulation unable to prevent flap collapse – Adsorption to other materials uncertain
Platelet-Derived Growth Factor	– Growth factor with the strongest potential to recruit progenitor cells – Strong proliferative potential	– Necessitates a carrier system – No specific function in periodontal regeneration
Bone Morphogenetic Proteins	– Growth factor with the strongest potential to regenerate alveolar bone – Also some potential to recruit mesenchymal progenitor cells and induce cell proliferation	– Strong tendency to cause ankylosis – Lack of clinical trials demonstrating any use in periodontal regeneration
Platelet Rich Plasma and Fibrin	– Supernatural concentration of growth factors – Autologous source – Used for a variety of procedures and easily obtainable	– PRP contains anticoagulants – Typically requires the use of a bone grafting material to maintain volume
Growth and Differentiation Factor-5	– Recently demonstrated clinical safety and efficacy – Histologically shown to improve periodontal regeneration	– Less known about its mode of action – Need for more clinical trials demonstrating its validity

carry properties necessary for the repair and regeneration of various tissues found in the oral cavity, very few possess the potential to promote blood supply/angiogenesis directly to damaged tissues.

Wound healing has therefore previously been characterized as a four-stage process with overlapping phases [7–9]. What is noteworthy is the fact that platelets have been described as key components affecting the early phases of tissue regeneration important during hemostasis and fibrin clot formation [6]. Platelets have also been shown to secrete a number of important growth factors including platelet-derived growth factor (PDGF), vascular endothelial growth factor (VEGF), coagulation factors, adhesion molecules, cytokines/chemokines, and a variety of other angiogenic factors capable of stimulating the proliferation and activation of cells involved in the wound healing process including fibroblasts, neutrophils, macrophages, and mesenchymal stem cells (MSCs) [11].

Interestingly, in the mid- to late 1990s, two separate strategies were adopted to regenerate human tissues based on these concepts. First, the main growth factor secreted from platelets (PDGF) was commercialized into a recombinant growth factor (rhPDGF-BB). This has since been FDA-approved for the regeneration of numerous tissues in the human body including intrabony defects in the field of periodontology. A second strategy was proposed around the same time to collect supra-physiological doses of platelets by utilizing centrifugation. Since blood is naturally known to coagulate within minutes, the additional use of anti-coagulants was added to this process to maintain a liquid consistency of blood throughout this procedure. A positive correlation between platelet count and the regenerative phase was therefore observed for tissue wound healing. In fact, it has also been shown that the simple combination of bone grafting materials with blood alone is known to enhance angiogenesis and new bone formation of bone grafts when compared to implanted bone grafts alone that are not pre-coated [12]. Based on these findings, several research groups across many fields of medicine began in the 1990s to study the effects of various platelet concentrates for tissue wound healing by adapting various centrifugation techniques and protocols with the aim of improving tissue regeneration.

1.2 Brief history of platelet concentrates

It is interesting to point out that the use of platelet concentrates have dramatically increased in popularity over the past decade since the discovery of PRF. Despite this, it is important to understand that growth factors derived from blood had been used in medicine for over two decades [13]. These first attempts to use concentrated platelet growth factors was derived from the fact that supra-physiological doses could be obtained from platelets to promote wound healing during and following surgery [14,15]. These concepts were later established into what is now known as "platelet rich plasma" (PRP), which was later introduced in the 1990s in dentistry with leading clinician-scientists such as Whitman and Marx [16,17]. The main goal of PRP was to isolate the highest quantity of platelets and ultimately growth factors associated with their collection and re-use them during surgery. Typical protocols ranged in time from 30 minutes to more than 1 hour based on their respective collection methods. It has been well documented that their formulation contains over 95% platelets; cells having a direct effect on osteoblasts, connective tissue cells, periodontal ligament cells and epithelial cells [18,19].

Despite the growing success and use of PRP in the initial years following its launch, there were several reported limitations that prevented its full potential. The technique itself was lengthy and therefore required the additional use of anti-coagulant factors to prevent clotting using bovine thrombin or CaCl2, both known inhibitors of wound healing. These drawbacks in combination with the lengthy harvesting/centrifugation preparation times were then frequently being utilized in large maxillofacial surgeries, whereas the typical dental or medical practitioner was resistant to its use due to lengthy preparation times.

One of the other drawbacks of PRP was the fact that it was liquid by nature, and therefore required its combination with other biomaterials including bone grafts derived from human cadavers (allografts) or animal products (xenografts), thereby further combining its use with other "unnatural" products. Interestingly, very recent data from within our laboratories has pointed to the quick "burst" release of growth factors from PRP (Figure 1.2) [20]. It has since been suggested that a preferential release of growth factors may be obtained by a more slowly-releasing curve over time as opposed to a quick and short burst as found using PRP [20–22].

In summary, the combination of several of these limitations has forced others to investigate new modalities for successful regeneration. From this perspective, a second-generation platelet concentrate, without the use of anti-coagulants, was therefore developed with shorter preparation times termed platelet rich fibrin (PRF) [23]. During this harvesting procedure, many of the cells

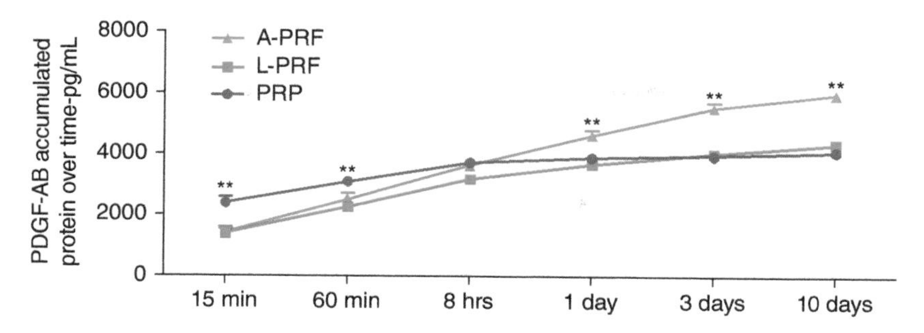

Figure 1.2 Growth factor release of PDGF-AB from A-PRF, L-PRF, and PRP. Notice the initial burst of growth factor increase from PRP; however, after a 10-day period, significantly higher growth factors are released from A-PRF. (** signifies $p<0.01$). Source: Kobayashi *et al.* 2016 [20]. Reproduced with permission of Springer.

(which now include additional leukocytes) were trapped within the fibrin matrix along with growth factors [24]. PRF (which was later renamed leukocyte PRF or L-PRF due to its additional leukocyte content) contains a variety of cells, which have individually been studied for their role in the regeneration process later described throughout this book.

1.3 The development of PRF from PRP

In the early 2000s, the focus of research in the Pain Clinic in Nice, France was to try and solve blood-flow–related issues to large ulcers often leaving patients with large chronic wounds that potentially resulted in amputation. At the time, certain research groups were suggesting that PRP, which was mainly utilized as a supra-physiological dose of blood-derived growth factors, could enhance wound healing. Despite this, a desire to develop a new platelet concentrate without the use of anti-coagulants (known inhibitors of wound healing) was a primary objective. With these concepts in mind, further research in the early 2000s was undertaken to develop what is now known as a second-generation platelet concentrate without utilizing anti-coagulation factors [23]. The protocol was developed using a simpler centrifugation protocol requiring only 1 cycle of 12 minutes at 2700 rpm (750 g). The original objective was to spin at high centrifugation speeds in order to phase separate the layers between the red corpuscle base and the overlaying clear liquid containing leukocytes and plasma. As no anti-coagulants were utilized, the resultant formulation came with a three-dimensional fibrin scaffold termed PRF [25–27]. PRF has now been highly researched with over 500 publications on its topic, many of which are discussed within this textbook.

Additional research from various groups around the world have since shown the marked impact of white blood cells found within the fibrin matrix and their involvement in the wound healing process. For these reasons, an improved defense to foreign pathogens has been observed when surgery is performed with PRF leading to the more favorable clinical results resulting in lower infection rates [28–33]. Additionally, macrophages and neutrophils contained within PRF are naturally one of the first cells found within infected wounds. For these reasons, the use of PRF during surgery increases their numbers at the initial stages of healing thereby playing a central role in the phagocytosis of debris, microbes and necrotic tissues, as well as directing the future regeneration of these tissues through release of cytokines and growth factors.

Three main components of PRF have been noted as being key components assisting in tissue regeneration. As illustrated in Figure 1.3, PRF not only contains host cells,

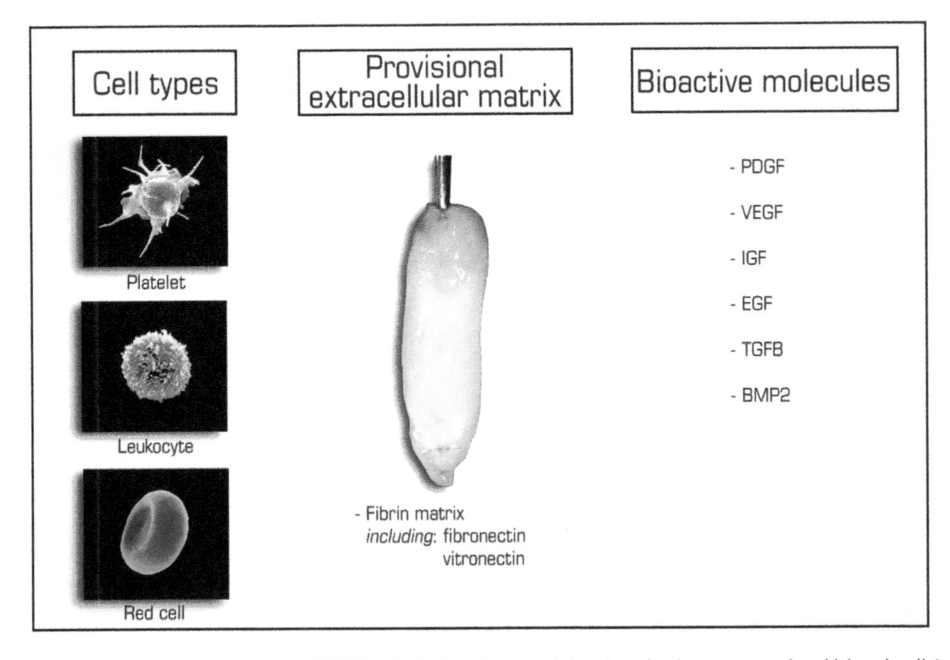

Figure 1.3 Three main components of PRF include 1) cell types (platelets, leukocytes, and red blood cells), 2) a provisional extracellular matrix three-dimensional scaffold fabricated from autologous fibrin (including fibronectin and vitronectin) and 3) a wide array of over 100 bioactive molecules including most notably PDGF, VEGF, IGF, EGF, TGF-beta, and BMP2. Source: Miron *et al.* 2016 [54]. Reproduced with permission of Elsevier.

but also contains a three-dimensional fibrin matrix containing various growth factors. These include transforming growth factor beta (TGF-beta), PDGF and VEGF, insulin growth factor (IGF), and epidermal growth factor (EGF). Recent research has more specifically shown how leukocytes (as opposed to platelets) are the main implicators in the tissue wound healing process capable of further enhancing new blood vessel formation (angiogenesis) and tissue formation [25–27, 30, 34].

It is also important to note that PRF has not solely been utilized in dentistry and much research has been dedicated to its use in various other fields of medicine. Recently, PRF has shown effectiveness for the clinical management of hard-to-heal leg ulcers including diabetic foot ulcers, venous leg ulcers, and chronic leg ulcers [35–39]. Furthermore, PRF has had positive outcomes for hand ulcers [40], facial soft tissue defects [41], laparoscopic cholecystectomy [42], deep nasolabial folds, volume-depleted midfacial regions, facial defects, superficial rhytids, and acne scars [43]. Its use has also been extended toward the induction of dermal collagenesis [44], vaginal prolapse repair [45], urethracutaneous fistula repair [46,47], lipostructure surgical procedures [48], chronic rotator cuff repair [49], and acute traumatic ear drum perforation healing [50]. It goes without further mention that by increasing blood flow to defect sites from various etiology, favorable wound healing and tissue regeneration may take place. We now know that PRF serves all three important criteria for tissue regeneration including 1) serving as a three-dimensional fibrin scaffold, 2) includes autologous cells such as leukocytes, macrophages, neutrophils, and platelets, and 3) serves as a reservoir of natural growth factors that may be released over a 10- to 14-day period. Research has now demonstrated that each of these three individual components of tissue regeneration are important during wound healing with PRF.

1. **Major cell types in PRF**
   The aim of this introductory chapter is not to introduce the important cell-types found in PRF. This will be described later in Chapter 2. However, it is important to note that PRF contains a number of cells including platelets, leukocytes, macrophages, granulocytes, and neutrophils. Following the centrifugation cycle, the majority of these cells are trapped within the three-dimensional fibrin matrix. As stated previously, the addition of blood alone to bone biomaterials has been shown to drastically improve wound angiogenesis [12]. One of the main differences between PRF and previously utilized PRP is the incorporation of leukocytes in PRF. Several studies have shown their key importance during anti-infectious pathogen resistance as well as their implications in immune regulation [51–53]. Furthermore, they play a significant role during host tissue-to-biomaterial integration [31,33,54]. Due to the added benefits of leukocytes, it is not surprising to learn that extraction of third molars have specifically shown up to a 10-fold decrease in osteomyelitis infections as well as greater wound healing following simple placement of PRF into extraction sockets [55]. Therefore, the influence of autologous cells contained within PRF, most noteworthy leukocytes, should be considered a major advantage during regenerative therapy.
2. **A natural fibrin matrix and its biological properties**
   A second major difference between PRF and PRP as previously mentioned is the lack of anti-coagulants thus resulting in a fibrin matrix (Figure 1.4). Naturally without anti-coagulants blood will clot and for these reasons, centrifugation *must* take place immediately following blood collection. Initial protocols were established whereby 10-mL of blood was collected and centrifuged for 12 minutes at 2700 rpm (750g). In Chapter 3, the biological concept of utilizing lower centrifugation speeds and time will be discussed.

   Nevertheless, what was once thought to be simply a carrier for growth factors and cells, the fibrin matrix has since been shown to be a main feature of PRF. The PRF matrix acts as a key component of tissue wound healing as highlighted in more scientific detail in Chapter 2.
3. **Cytokines contained within PRF**
   The third primary advantage of PRF is the fact it contains natural growth factors found in blood. While their individual biological roles will be explained in the

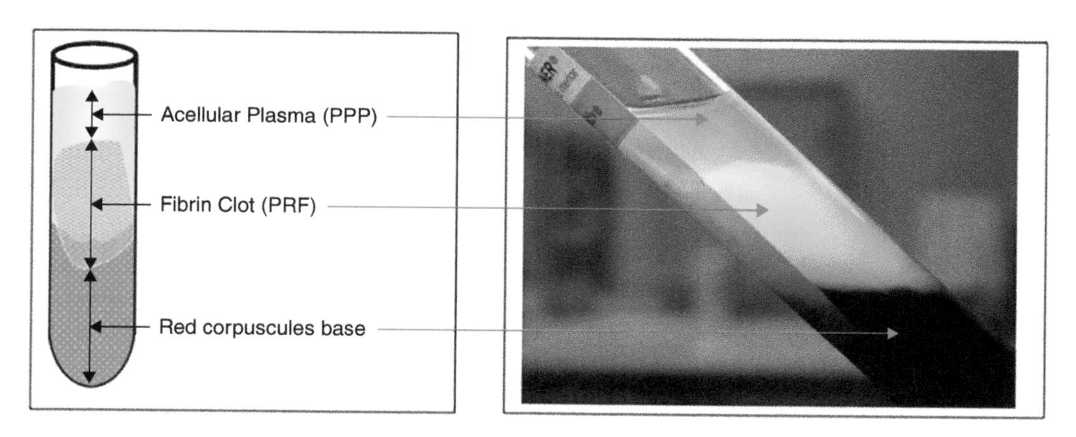

Figure 1.4 Platelet Rich Fibrin (PRF) clot formed in the upper third of glass tubes after centrifugation.

following chapter, PRF contains TGF-beta, a known agent responsible for the rapid proliferation of various cell types found in the oral cavity [56,57]. Its other major growth factor is PDGF, an essential regulator for the migration, proliferation, and survival of mesenchymal cells. A third important growth factor in PRF is VEGF responsible for angiogenesis and future blood flow to damaged tissues [58]. Other growth factors are epidermal growth factor and insulin-like growth factor, both regulators of the proliferation and differentiation of many cells types later described in Chapter 2.

The combination of 1) host cells, 2) a three-dimensional fibrin matrix and 3) growth factors contained within PRF act to synergistically enhance faster and more potent tissue wound healing and regeneration.

1.4 Effect of PRF on periosteum behavior

Following years of practice with the use of PRF, one biological property observed with almost every surgical technique has been its stimulation of the capacity of blood supply within the periosteum. From this point of view, direct contact of PRF with periosteum substantially improves the blood supply to the keratinized soft tissue favoring its thickness, as well as improves blood supply to the underlying bone tissues. This has been one of the key activities of PRF, whereby stimulation with growth factors over a long period of release.

1.5 The first case treated with PRF

The most appropriate way to conclude this first chapter is by introducing the concept of PRF utilized in regenerative medicine in the first years. Leg ulcers are a common reported problem in diabetic patients often resulting in amputation. In my pain clinic, a patient with obvious skin necrosis caused by Lyell syndrome with repeated failed antibiotic treatment was referred to me (Figure 1.5). From this perspective, patients were often directed to my pain clinic in Nice, France to receive treatment for pain. Over the years, science has shown that infection was often a secondary problem to poor blood supply. Therefore, to improve treatment outcomes, attempts were being made to see if PRF fibrin clots could be utilized to regenerate these defects (Figure 1.6). The idea was that by introducing supra-physiological doses of growth factors from blood, one could potentially re-introduce blood flow into these tissues. To our great interest, wounds that were initially covered with PRF and plastic "Saran" wrap began to heal in as early as 10 days, and infection had disappeared. By 30 days, great clinical improvements could be visualized and this was achieved utilizing PRF alone even in the absence of antibiotics (Figure 1.7). Similar clinical outcomes could also be observed following foot amputation where resulting wounds were extremely difficult to heal. The application of PRF alone could re-introduce blood flow into these defects, improving significantly tissue regeneration (Figures 1.8 and 1.9). Most interesting is at which point the body's natural ability proves to treat these defects in a physiological way with 100% naturally derived human blood.

Following these early treatments, it was obvious that the potential for PRF to be utilized across many fields of medicine was clear. The concept was later introduced to the dental field where a much larger number of regenerative procedures could be performed on a yearly basis. From there, expert clinicians have attempted to use PRF in various regenerative procedures in dentistry later discussed in this textbook and the field has been expanding ever since.

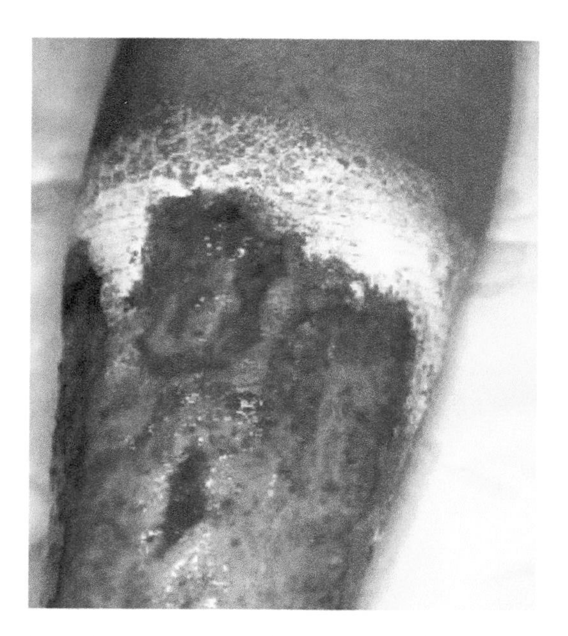

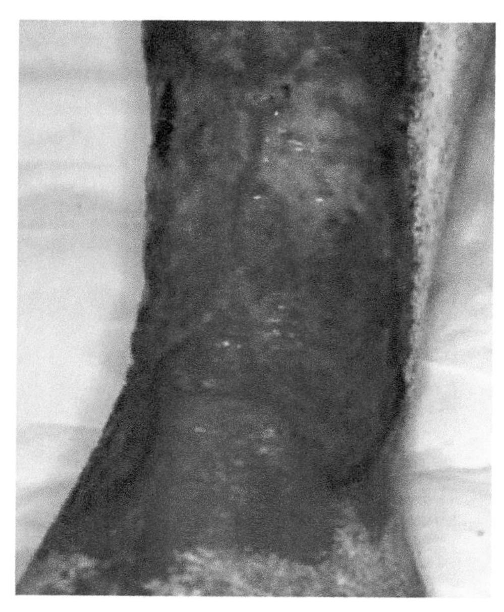

Figure 1.5 Patient presenting to the Pain Clinic in Nice, France with Lyell syndrome. Antibiotic therapy in such cases is not always effective (Case performed by Dr. Joseph Choukroun).

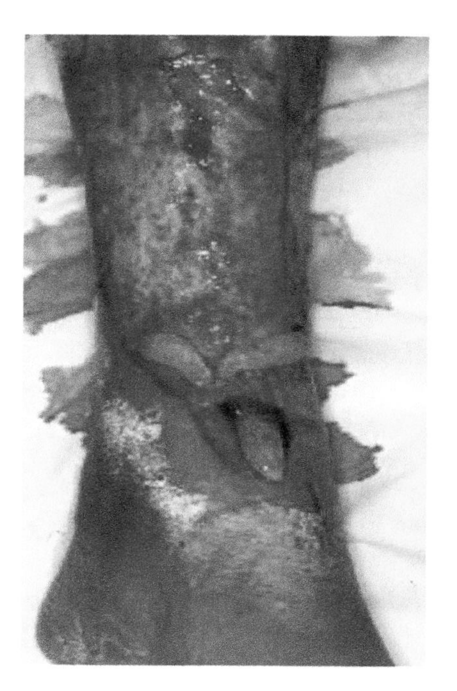

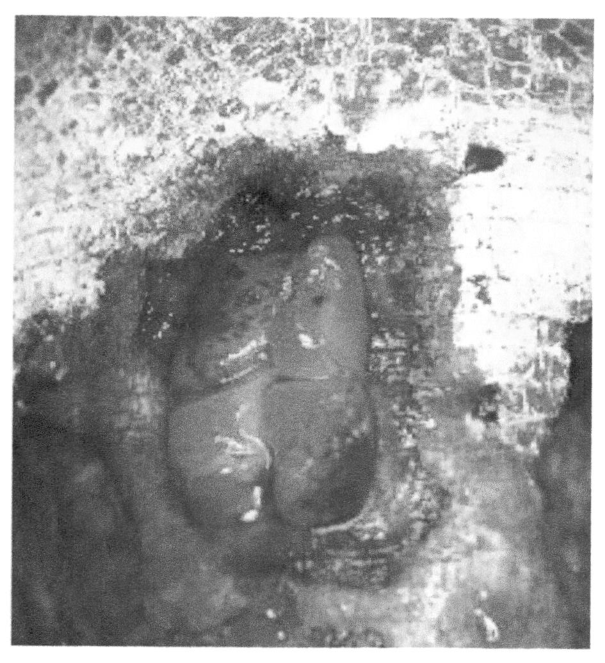

Figure 1.6 Patient from Figure 1.5 with Lyell syndrome treated with PRF. PRF membranes were placed on the defects, wrapped in a plastic wrap, and allowed to heal without use of antibiotic therapy (Case performed by Dr. Joseph Choukroun).

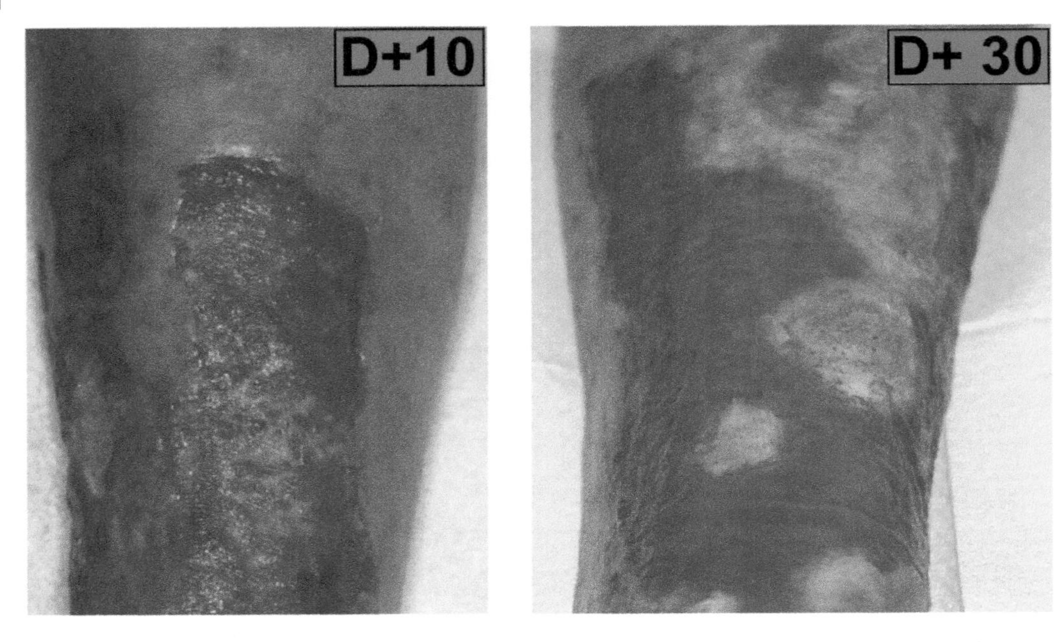

Figure 1.7 Patient from Figures 1.5 and 1.6 with Lyell syndrome treated with PRF. After 10 and 30 days of healing, notice the marked improvement in tissue revascularization and wound healing (Case performed by Dr. Joseph Choukroun).

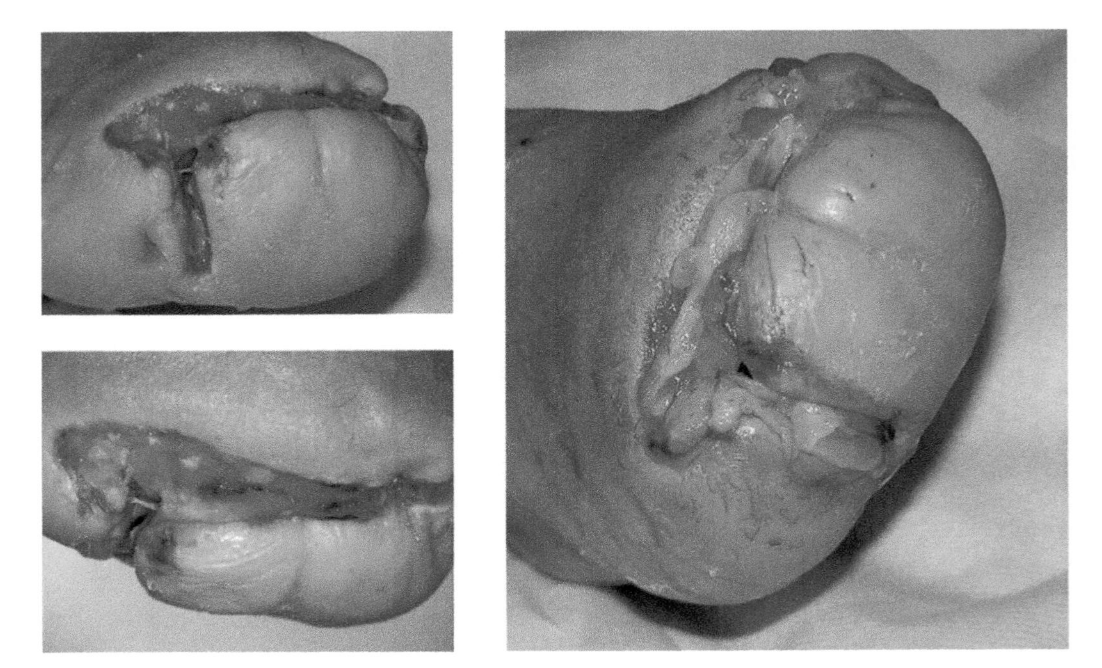

Figure 1.8 Diabetic foot amputation with infection after 15 days. Right photo demonstrates PRF clots that are applied to the wound (Case performed by Dr. Joseph Choukroun).

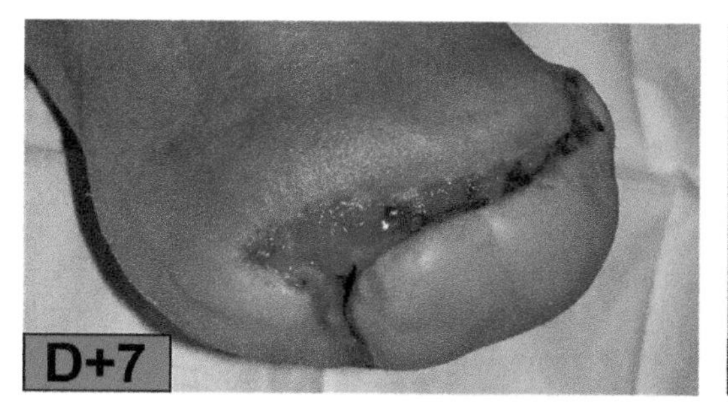

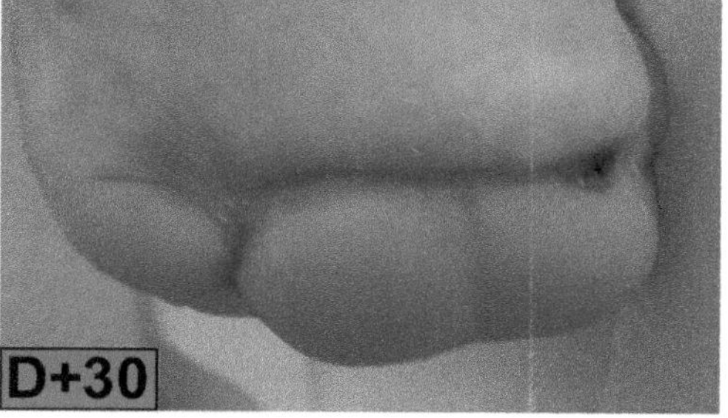

Figure 1.9 Diabetic foot amputation (patient from Figure 1.8) following 7 and 30 days of healing (Case performed by Dr. Joseph Choukroun).

1.6 Conclusion

The use of PRF has seen a large and steady increase in popularity since it was first introduced in medicine for the treatment of hard-to-heal leg ulcers and wounds. While described as a second-generation platelet concentrate, one of the main advantages of PRF is the fact that it is produces without use of anti-coagulants or other unnatural by-products that prevent the coagulation cascade and is therefore considered 100% autologous and natural. While PRF contains three important aspects for tissue wound healing, including 1) host cells, 2) a three-dimensional fibrin matrix, and 3) accumulation of growth factors, its synergistic effects has frequently been recognized in dentistry most notably for the healing of soft tissues. Future strategies to improve PRF formulations and techniques are continuously being investigated to further enhance the clinical outcomes following regenerative procedures utilizing this technology.

References

1 Coury AJ. Expediting the transition from replacement medicine to tissue engineering. Regenerative biomaterials. 2016;3(2):111–3.
2 Dai R, Wang Z, Samanipour R, Koo KI, Kim K. Adipose-Derived Stem Cells for Tissue Engineering and Regenerative Medicine Applications. Stem cells international. 2016;2016:6737345.
3 Rouwkema J, Khademhosseini A. Vascularization and Angiogenesis in Tissue Engineering: Beyond Creating Static Networks. Trends Biotechnol. 2016.
4 Zhu W, Ma X, Gou M, Mei D, Zhang K, Chen S. 3D printing of functional biomaterials for tissue engineering. Current opinion in biotechnology. 2016;40:103–12.
5 Upputuri PK, Sivasubramanian K, Mark CS, Pramanik M. Recent developments in vascular imaging techniques in tissue engineering and regenerative medicine. BioMed research international. 2015; 2015:783983.
6 Guo S, Dipietro LA. Factors affecting wound healing. J Dent Res. 2010;89(3): 219–29.
7 Gosain A, DiPietro LA. Aging and wound healing. World journal of surgery. 2004;28(3):321–6.
8 Eming SA, Brachvogel B, Odorisio T, Koch M. Regulation of angiogenesis: wound healing as a model. Progress in histochemistry and cytochemistry. 2007;42(3):115–70.
9 Eming SA, Kaufmann J, Lohrer R, Krieg T. [Chronic wounds. Novel approaches in

research and therapy]. Der Hautarzt; Zeitschrift fur Dermatologie, Venerologie, und verwandte Gebiete. 2007;58(11): 939–44.
10 Zhang Y, Zhang X, Shi B, Miron R. Membranes for guided tissue and bone regeneration. Annals of Oral & Maxillofacial Surgery. 2013;1(1):10.
11 Nurden AT. Platelets, inflammation and tissue regeneration. Thrombosis and haemostasis. 2011;105 Suppl 1:S13–33.
12 Barbeck M, Najman S, Stojanovic S, Mitic Z, Zivkovic JM, Choukroun J, et al. Addition of blood to a phycogenic bone substitute leads to increased in vivo vascularization. Biomedical materials (Bristol, England). 2015;10(5):055007.
13 de Vries RA, de Bruin M, Marx JJ, Hart HC, Van de Wiel A. Viability of platelets collected by apheresis versus the platelet-rich plasma technique: a direct comparison. Transfusion science. 1993; 14(4):391–8.
14 Anfossi G, Trovati M, Mularoni E, Massucco P, Calcamuggi G, Emanuelli G. Influence of propranolol on platelet aggregation and thromboxane B2 production from platelet-rich plasma and whole blood. Prostaglandins, leukotrienes, and essential fatty acids. 1989;36(1):1–7.
15 Fijnheer R, Pietersz RN, de Korte D, Gouwerok CW, Dekker WJ, Reesink HW, et al. Platelet activation during preparation of platelet concentrates: a comparison of the platelet-rich plasma and the buffy coat methods. Transfusion. 1990;30(7):634–8.
16 Whitman DH, Berry RL, Green DM. Platelet gel: an autologous alternative to fibrin glue with applications in oral and maxillofacial surgery. Journal of oral and maxillofacial surgery. 1997;55(11): 1294–9.
17 Marx RE, Carlson ER, Eichstaedt RM, Schimmele SR, Strauss JE, Georgeff KR. Platelet-rich plasma: growth factor enhancement for bone grafts. Oral Surgery, Oral Medicine, Oral Pathology, Oral Radiology, and Endodontology. 1998;85(6): 638–46.
18 Jameson C. Autologous platelet concentrate for the production of platelet gel. Lab Med. 2007;38:39–42.
19 Marx RE. Platelet-rich plasma: evidence to support its use. Journal of oral and maxillofacial surgery : official journal of the American Association of Oral and Maxillofacial Surgeons. 2004;62(4):489–96.
20 Kobayashi E, Fluckiger L, Fujioka-Kobayashi M, Sawada K, Sculean A, Schaller B, et al. Comparative release of growth factors from PRP, PRF, and advanced-PRF. Clinical oral investigations. 2016.
21 Lucarelli E, Beretta R, Dozza B, Tazzari PL, O'Connel SM, Ricci F, et al. A recently developed bifacial platelet-rich fibrin matrix. European cells & materials. 2010; 20:13–23.
22 Saluja H, Dehane V, Mahindra U. Platelet Rich fibrin: A second generation platelet concentrate and a new friend of oral and maxillofacial surgeons. Annals of maxillofacial surgery. 2011;1(1):53–7.
23 Choukroun J, Adda F, Schoeffler C, Vervelle A. Une opportunité en paro-implantologie: le PRF. Implantodontie. 2001;42(55):e62.
24 Dohan Ehrenfest DM, Del Corso M, Diss A, Mouhyi J, Charrier JB. Three-dimensional architecture and cell composition of a Choukroun's platelet-rich fibrin clot and membrane. Journal of periodontology. 2010;81(4):546–55.
25 Choukroun J, Diss A, Simonpieri A, Girard MO, Schoeffler C, Dohan SL, et al. Platelet-rich fibrin (PRF): a second-generation platelet concentrate. Part IV: clinical effects on tissue healing. Oral surgery, oral medicine, oral pathology, oral radiology, and endodontics. 2006; 101(3):e56–60.
26 Dohan DM, Choukroun J, Diss A, Dohan SL, Dohan AJ, Mouhyi J, et al. Platelet-rich fibrin (PRF): a second-generation platelet concentrate. Part I: technological concepts and evolution. Oral surgery, oral medicine, oral pathology, oral radiology, and endodontics. 2006;101(3):e37–44.

27 Dohan DM, Choukroun J, Diss A, Dohan SL, Dohan AJ, Mouhyi J, et al. Platelet-rich fibrin (PRF): a second-generation platelet concentrate. Part II: platelet-related biologic features. Oral surgery, oral medicine, oral pathology, oral radiology, and endodontics. 2006;101(3):e45–50.

28 Martin P, Leibovich SJ. Inflammatory cells during wound repair: the good, the bad and the ugly. Trends in cell biology. 2005; 15(11):599–607.

29 Tsirogianni AK, Moutsopoulos NM, Moutsopoulos HM. Wound healing: immunological aspects. Injury. 2006;37 Suppl 1:S5–12.

30 Adamson R. Role of macrophages in normal wound healing: an overview. Journal of wound care. 2009;18(8):349–51.

31 Davis VL, Abukabda AB, Radio NM, Witt-Enderby PA, Clafshenkel WP, Cairone JV, et al. Platelet-rich preparations to improve healing. Part I: workable options for every size practice. The Journal of oral implantology. 2014;40(4):500–10.

32 Davis VL, Abukabda AB, Radio NM, Witt-Enderby PA, Clafshenkel WP, Cairone JV, et al. Platelet-rich preparations to improve healing. Part II: platelet activation and enrichment, leukocyte inclusion, and other selection criteria. The Journal of oral implantology. 2014;40(4):511–21.

33 Ghasemzadeh M, Hosseini E. Intravascular leukocyte migration through platelet thrombi: directing leukocytes to sites of vascular injury. Thrombosis and haemostasis. 2015;113(6):1224–35.

34 Dohan DM, Choukroun J, Diss A, Dohan SL, Dohan AJ, Mouhyi J, et al. Platelet-rich fibrin (PRF): a second-generation platelet concentrate. Part III: leucocyte activation: a new feature for platelet concentrates? Oral surgery, oral medicine, oral pathology, oral radiology, and endodontics. 2006;101(3): e51–5.

35 Danielsen P, Jorgensen B, Karlsmark T, Jorgensen LN, Agren MS. Effect of topical autologous platelet-rich fibrin versus no intervention on epithelialization of donor sites and meshed split-thickness skin autografts: a randomized clinical trial. Plastic and reconstructive surgery. 2008;122(5):1431–40.

36 O'Connell SM, Impeduglia T, Hessler K, Wang XJ, Carroll RJ, Dardik H. Autologous platelet-rich fibrin matrix as cell therapy in the healing of chronic lower-extremity ulcers. Wound repair and regeneration : official publication of the Wound Healing Society [and] the European Tissue Repair Society. 2008;16(6):749–56.

37 Steenvoorde P, van Doorn LP, Naves C, Oskam J. Use of autologous platelet-rich fibrin on hard-to-heal wounds. Journal of wound care. 2008;17(2):60–3.

38 Jorgensen B, Karlsmark T, Vogensen H, Haase L, Lundquist R. A pilot study to evaluate the safety and clinical performance of Leucopatch, an autologous, additive-free, platelet-rich fibrin for the treatment of recalcitrant chronic wounds. The international journal of lower extremity wounds. 2011;10(4):218–23.

39 Londahl M, Tarnow L, Karlsmark T, Lundquist R, Nielsen AM, Michelsen M, et al. Use of an autologous leucocyte and platelet-rich fibrin patch on hard-to-heal DFUs: a pilot study. Journal of wound care. 2015;24(4):172–4, 6–8.

40 Chignon-Sicard B, Georgiou CA, Fontas E, David S, Dumas P, Ihrai T, et al. Efficacy of leukocyte- and platelet-rich fibrin in wound healing: a randomized controlled clinical trial. Plastic and reconstructive surgery. 2012;130(6):819e–29e.

41 Desai CB, Mahindra UR, Kini YK, Bakshi MK. Use of Platelet-Rich Fibrin over Skin Wounds: Modified Secondary Intention Healing. Journal of cutaneous and aesthetic surgery. 2013;6(1):35–7.

42 Danielsen PL, Agren MS, Jorgensen LN. Platelet-rich fibrin versus albumin in surgical wound repair: a randomized trial with paired design. Annals of surgery. 2010;251(5):825–31.

43 Sclafani AP. Safety, efficacy, and utility of platelet-rich fibrin matrix in facial plastic surgery. Archives of facial plastic surgery. 2011;13(4):247–51.

44 Sclafani AP, McCormick SA. Induction of dermal collagenesis, angiogenesis, and adipogenesis in human skin by injection of platelet-rich fibrin matrix. Archives of facial plastic surgery. 2012;14(2):132–6.

45 Gorlero F, Glorio M, Lorenzi P, Bruno-Franco M, Mazzei C. New approach in vaginal prolapse repair: mini-invasive surgery associated with application of platelet-rich fibrin. International urogynecology journal. 2012;23(6):715–22.

46 Soyer T, Cakmak M, Aslan MK, Senyucel MF, Kisa U. Use of autologous platelet rich fibrin in urethracutaneous fistula repair: preliminary report. International wound journal. 2013;10(3):345–7.

47 Guinot A, Arnaud A, Azzis O, Habonimana E, Jasienski S, Fremond B. Preliminary experience with the use of an autologous platelet-rich fibrin membrane for urethroplasty coverage in distal hypospadias surgery. Journal of pediatric urology. 2014;10(2):300–5.

48 Braccini F, Chignon-Sicard B, Volpei C, Choukroun J. Modern lipostructure: the use of platelet rich fibrin (PRF). Revue de laryngologie-otologie-rhinologie. 2013;134(4-5):231–5.

49 Zumstein MA, Rumian A, Lesbats V, Schaer M, Boileau P. Increased vascularization during early healing after biologic augmentation in repair of chronic rotator cuff tears using autologous leukocyte- and platelet-rich fibrin (L-PRF): a prospective randomized controlled pilot trial. Journal of shoulder and elbow surgery/American Shoulder and Elbow Surgeons [et al]. 2014;23(1):3–12.

50 Habesoglu M, Oysu C, Sahin S, Sahin-Yilmaz A, Korkmaz D, Tosun A, et al. Platelet-rich fibrin plays a role on healing of acute-traumatic ear drum perforation. The Journal of craniofacial surgery. 2014;25(6): 2056–8.

51 Kawazoe T, Kim HH. Tissue augmentation by white blood cell-containing platelet-rich plasma. Cell transplantation. 2012;21(2-3): 601–7.

52 Perut F, Filardo G, Mariani E, Cenacchi A, Pratelli L, Devescovi V, et al. Preparation method and growth factor content of platelet concentrate influence the osteogenic differentiation of bone marrow stromal cells. Cytotherapy. 2013;15(7): 830–9.

53 Pirraco RP, Reis RL, Marques AP. Effect of monocytes/macrophages on the early osteogenic differentiation of hBMSCs. Journal of tissue engineering and regenerative medicine. 2013;7(5):392–400.

54 Miron RJ, Bosshardt DD. OsteoMacs: Key players around bone biomaterials. Biomaterials. 2016;82:1–19.

55 Hoaglin DR, Lines GK. Prevention of localized osteitis in mandibular third-molar sites using platelet-rich fibrin. International journal of dentistry. 2013;2013:875380.

56 Border WA, Noble NA. Transforming growth factor beta in tissue fibrosis. The New England journal of medicine. 1994; 331(19):1286–92.

57 Bowen T, Jenkins RH, Fraser DJ. MicroRNAs, transforming growth factor beta-1, and tissue fibrosis. The Journal of pathology. 2013;229(2):274–85.

58 Shamloo A, Xu H, Heilshorn S. Mechanisms of vascular endothelial growth factor-induced pathfinding by endothelial sprouts in biomaterials. Tissue engineering Part A. 2012;18(3-4): 320–30.

2

Biological Components of Platelet Rich Fibrin: Growth Factor Release and Cellular Activity

Masako Fujioka-Kobayashi and Richard J. Miron

Abstract

During the natural wound healing process, blood plays a major role in accelerating tissue regeneration by providing various cells, growth factors, cytokines, and coagulation factors. Supraphysiological doses of platelets (platelet rich plasma) were initially developed to increase platelet numbers at defect sites, however, the additional use of additives were necessary, even though healing was deemed sub-optimal. A second-generation concentrate called platelet rich fibrin (PRF) was therefore developed being 100% natural and providing three fundamental keys for tissue engineering, namely cells, growth factors, and scaffold. Like PRP, PRF contains many platelets, and modifications to centrifugation speed and time have been shown to increase the number of macrophages and leukocytes, important cells for host defense and wound healing. Furthermore, they secrete a large number of growth factors including transforming growth factor-β1 (TGF-β1), platelet-derived growth factor (PDGF), vascular endothelial growth factor (VEGF), and insulin-like growth factor-I (IGF-1) capable of further promoting cell migration, proliferation, and differentiation. Lastly, since anti-coagulants are not utilized for PRF preparation, a three-dimensional fibrin scaffold is formed fulfilling the three main criteria of tissue engineering in an entirely biological and natural way. Over the years, many discoveries have been made including the understanding that fibrin simultaneously acts to hold various cell types but more importantly allows a slow and gradual release of growth factors over time. This release profile has been shown to enhance angiogenesis, cell behavior, and ultimately, tissue regeneration. This chapter aims to describe the main components of PRF. Thereafter, a biological understanding of the main growth factors found in PRF, as well as their release profiles from various formulations of PRF is discussed. We then compare the advantages of PRF over PRP and describe potential future research aimed at increasing our understanding of the biological properties of platelet concentrates.

Highlights

- What is platelet rich fibrin?
- How is PRF different from PRP?
- What are the roles of each of the cell types found in PRF?
- What are the roles of each of the growth factors in PRF?
- What is the role of fibrin in tissue wound healing and regeneration?
- How does centrifugation speed affect PRF and growth factor release?

Platelet Rich Fibrin in Regenerative Dentistry: Biological Background and Clinical Indications, First Edition.
Edited by Richard J. Miron and Joseph Choukroun.

2.1 Introduction

Wound healing is generally divided into a three-stage process—namely the inflammatory phase, proliferative phase, and remodeling phase. The inflammatory phase begins at the time of wounding and lasts between 24 and 48 hours. During this process, a dynamic interaction occurs among endothelial cells, angiogenic cytokines, and extracellular matrix (ECM), where the delivery of multiple growth factors in a well-controlled fashion aims to accelerate wound healing [1]. In general, blood provides essential therapeutic products that comprise both cellular and protein products that cannot be obtained from other sources. Once a wound occurs, the blood starts to clot within a few minutes to stop bleeding. One of the key cells during these phases are platelets that have been shown to be important regulators of hemostasis through fibrin clot formation [1,2]. Platelets release cytokines and growth factors that further attract macrophages and neutrophils to the defect sites; thereafter debris, necrotic tissue, and bacteria from the wound may be removed. By day 3, the proliferative phase begins and the blood clot within the wound is further supplied with a provisional matrix for cell migration, while the clot within the vessel lumen contributes to hemostasis [2]. Fibroblasts begin to produce collagen in a random order, and thereafter angiogenesis occurs at the same time when the wound gradually begins to gain initial stability. During the final remodeling phase, collagen is replaced by organized collagen fibrils that provide enhanced strength to the injured site where tissue regeneration takes place (Figure 2.1) [3]).

Blood includes mainly four components: plasma, red blood cells, white blood cells, and platelets. Particularly, platelets are reported as the responsible component for the activation and release of crucial growth factors including platelet-derived growth factor (PDGF), coagulation factors, adhesion molecules, cytokines, and angiogenic factors, which enables the recruitment and activity of fibroblasts, leukocytes, macrophages, and mesenchymal stem cells (MSCs). Coagulation factors, growth factors, and cytokines released in the clot by activated platelets organize complex physiological events resulting in tissue repair, vascular remodeling, and tissue regeneration [2,4,5].

2.2 Cell components of PRF

Platelet concentrate therapy has been developed in order to naturally accelerate the regenerative potential of platelets contained in blood. PRF is formulated by separation of blood after centrifugation into various components including red blood cells, plasma, white blood cells, and platelets. The final naturally derived PRF is a concentrate of white blood cells, platelets, and fibrin. It has been shown that the initially developed PRF (also termed L-PRF) concentrates contain 97% platelets and more than 50% leukocytes within a high-density fibrin network when compared to whole blood [6]. PRF variants are mostly solid or dense gels and cannot be injected although recently the development of an injectable liquid-PRF is formulated utilizing lower centrifugation forces for shorter time periods later discussed in this chapter. Furthermore, low centrifugation forces utilizing the "low-speed centrifugation concept" have demonstrated that newer preparations of PRF (now termed advanced-PRF or A-PRF) can additionally provide an increase in platelets and neutrophilic granulocytes within the PRF clot and prolong the release of certain growth factors [7].

Leukocytes are the other major cell type found in PRF playing a prominent role in wound healing. Interestingly, studies from basic sciences have revealed the potent and large impact of leukocytes during tissue regeneration [8–10]. PRF contains a higher number of leukocytes when compared to the first-generation platelet concentrates, PRP, and PRGF. The amount of white blood cells in PRF has been determined at around 50% (with variability depending on the human

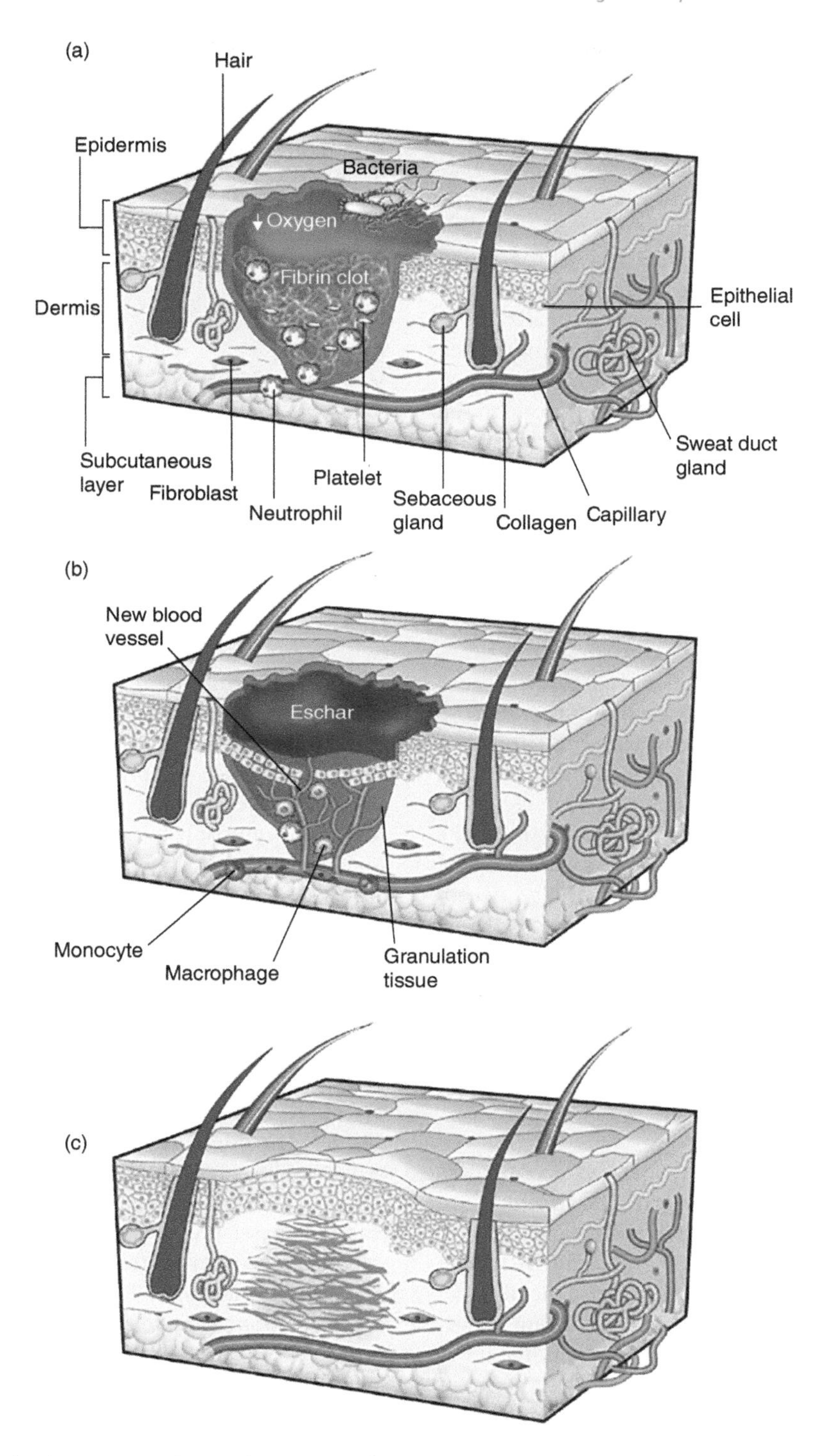

Figure 2.1 The three stages of wound repair: (a) Inflammatory (b) Proliferative, and (c) Remodeling phase. Source: Gurtner *et al.* 2008 [3]. Reproduced with permission of Nature Publishing Group.

donor) and newer formulations have further shown enhancements in total leukocyte numbers. Leucocytes are cells that play a key role in wound healing due to their anti-infectious action as well as immune regulation via the secretion of key immune cytokines such as interleukin (IL)-1β, IL-6, IL-4, and tumor necrosis factor alpha (TNF-α) [2,4,5]. While their role in immune defense is well characterized, they also serve the function as regulators controlling the ability for biomaterials to adapt to new host environments. In a previous study, one of the interesting findings when quantifying cells found in the PRF matrix histologically was the observation that the majority of leukocytes were found near the bottom of the fibrin clot [7]. Based on this finding, it became clear that centrifugation speeds (g-forces) were evidently too high pushing leukocytes down to the bottom of centrifugation tubes and away from the PRF matrix clot. In order to redistribute leukocyte cell numbers across the entire PRF matrix, lower centrifugation speeds were investigated as later described in detail in Chapter 3. Since macrophages supply a continuing source of chemotactic agents necessary to stimulate fibrosis and angiogenesis, fibroblasts construct new ECM necessary to support cell ingrowth, newer formulations of PRF (A-PRF, i-PRF) are therefore increasingly more bioactive.

2.3 Advantages of a three-dimensional fibrin network

Fibrin is the activated form of a plasmatic molecule called fibrinogen. The combination of properties including cells, and growth factors in a three-dimensional fibrin matrix as found in PRF acts to synergistically lead to a fast and potent increase in tissue regeneration. This soluble fibrillary molecule is massively present both in plasma and in the α-granules that are the most abundant platelet granule. Fibrin plays a determining role in platelet aggregation during hemostasis. It has been reported that fibrin alone

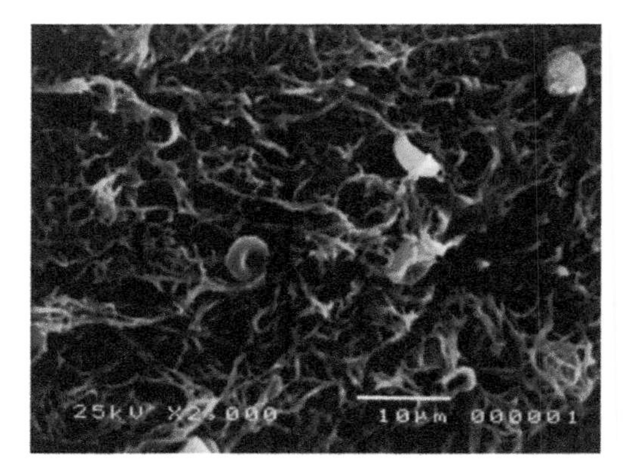

Figure 2.2 SEM examination of the fibrin clot revealed a dense and mature fibrin matrix with a very low quantity of identifiable bodies (RBCs, leukocytes, or platelet aggregates) trapped inside (original magnification x2,000). Source: Dohan Ehrenfest DM. *et al.* 2010 [6]. Reproduced with permission of the American Academy of Periodontology.

(without growth factors or living cells) is able to act as a provisional matrix allowing cell invasion and tissue regeneration [11–13]. PRF therefore has numerous additional advantages since it consists of an intimate assembly of cytokines, glycanic chains, and structural glycoproteins enmeshed within a slowly polymerized fibrin network (Figure 2.2). The trapped growth factors influence ECM, which allows migration, division, and phenotypic change of endothelial cells, thus leading to angiogenesis [14–16].

The PRF scaffold itself has further been identified as a biological three-dimensional network. Micropores composed of thin fibrin fibers form within clots and can function as scaffolds for cell migration, proliferation, and differentiation as well as for delivery of growth factors. Platelets are theoretically trapped massively within the fibrin network and keep growth factors contained within this three-dimensional PRF mesh followed by the slow and gradual release of growth factors over time [17]. The clot also provides a matrix scaffold for the recruitment of tissue cells to the injured site. Specifically, fibrin in conjunction with fibronectin acts as a provisional matrix for the influx of monocytes, fibroblasts, and endothelial cells. In summary, the initial limitations of PRP have led to the emergence of a second generation platelet concentrate, which takes advantage of the fact that without anti-coagulants, a fibrin matrix that incorporates the full set of growth factors trapped within its matrix are slowly released over time in a natural manner [8–10].

More recently, reports have revealed that stem cells existing naturally in blood vessels (mesenchymal stem cells (MSCs)) contribute to promote wound healing directly [18,19]. Although found in extremely low levels, MSCs have the potential to differentiate themselves into adipocytes, osteoblasts, and chondrocytes. MSCs also express several growth factors, including fibroblast growth factor 2 (FGF-2) and vascular endothelial growth factor (VEGF), which promote the proliferation of vascular endothelial cells, vascular stability, and the development of a long-lasting functional vascular network [20]. Future research investigating the impact of MSCs in blood are necessary. While PRF does not contain MSCs in high quantity, it may represent a potential future strategies to isolate MSCs relatively easily at low cost.

2.4 Growth factors in blood

It is also important to understand that inflammation and wound healing are controlled under high regulation by an array of growth factors. Growth factors can either stimulate or inhibit cellular migration, adhesion, proliferation, and differentiation. While growth factors exist in all tissues, it is important to note that blood serves as the main reservoir of numerous growth factors and cytokines promoting angiogenesis and tissue regeneration for wound healing. Growth factors usually exist as inactive or partially active precursors that require proteolytic activation, and may further require binding to matrix molecules for activity or stabilization. Growth factors also typically have short biological half-lives. For example, platelet-derived growth factor (PDGF) has a half-life of less than 2 minutes when injected intravenously [21]. Namely, as many cellular processes involved in morphogenesis require a complex network of several signaling pathways and usually more than one growth factor, recent research efforts have focused on schemes for sequential delivery of multiple growth factors [22]. Unlike recombinant growth factors, platelet concentrates create the opportunity to deliver many autologous growth factors simultaneously. Platelets and macrophages release an abundance of factors including transforming growth factor beta-1 (TGF-β1), PDGF, vascular endothelial growth factor (VEGF), epidermal growth factor (EGF), and insulin- like growth factor (IGF) [23,24]. Below their individual roles are briefly described.

TGF-β1: Transforming growth factor β (TGF-β) is a superfamily of more than 30 members described in the literature as fibrosis agents [25,26]. Platelets are known to be a major source of TGF-β production. The role of TGF-β mediates tissue repair, immune modulation, and extracellular matrix synthesis. Bone morphogenetic proteins (BMPs) are also part of the TGF subfamily. TGF-β1, the predominant isoform, is important in wound healing, with roles in inflammation, angiogenesis, re-epithelialization, and connective tissue regeneration [21]. This growth factor is crucial during bone formation contributing to osteoblast precursors in chemotaxis and mitogenesis, and stimulates osteoblast deposition of mineralized tissue on the bone collagen matrix. It is also reported that TGF-β1 can upregulate VEGF, thereby favoring angiogenesis and recruitment of inflammatory cells. Although its effects in terms of proliferation are highly variable, for the great majority of cell types, it constitutes the most powerful fibrosis agent among all cytokines and the growth factor commonly released from autogenous bone during tissue repair and remodeling [21].

PDGF: Platelet-derived growth factors (PDGFs) are essential regulators for the migration, proliferation, and survival of mesenchymal cell lineages and promotes collagen production for remodeling of ECM during wound healing [27–32]. Platelets are the major source of PDGF with various groups divided into homo- (PDGF-AA, PDGF-BB, PDGF-CC, and PDGF-DD) and hetero-dimeric (PDGF-AB) polypeptide dimers linked by disulfide bonds. They are present in large amounts in platelet α-granules. Interestingly, PDGF is accumulated in high quantities in the PRF matrix and are considered one of the important released molecules over time from PRF. It is important to note that since PDGF has an extremely short half-life, the PRF matrix acts to support its slow and gradual release over time. PDGF is also a major mitogen for osteoblasts and undifferentiated osteoprogenitor cells, fibroblasts, smooth muscle cells, and glial cells. Since it plays such a critical role in the mechanisms of physiologic healing, a commercially available recombinant source (rhPDGF-BB) was made available having received FDA approval for the regeneration of various defects in medicine and dentistry.

VEGF: Vascular endothelial growth factor (VEGF) is secreted by activated thrombocytes and macrophages to damaged sites to promote angiogenesis. The VEGF family is related to PDGF, and includes VEGF-A, -B, -C, -D, and -E. VEGF has previously been isolated and described as the most potent growth factor leading to angiogenesis of tissues, stimulating new blood vessel formation and, therefore, for bringing nutrients and increased blood flow to the site of injury [20,33]. It has potent effects on tissue remodeling and the incorporation of recombinant human VEGF into various bone biomaterials has been demonstrated to increase new bone formation, thereby pointing to the fast and potent effects of VEGF [34].

EGF: The EGF family stimulates chemotaxis and angiogenesis of endothelial cells and mitosis of mesenchymal cells. It further enhances epithelization and markedly shortens the overall healing process when administered. EGF is upregulated after acute injury and acts to significantly increase the tensile strength of wounds. EGF receptor is expressed on most human cell types including those that play a critical role during wound repair such as fibroblasts, endothelial cells, and keratinocytes [35].

IGF: Insulin-like growth factors (IGFs) are positive regulators of proliferation and differentiation of most cell types, which act as cell-protective agents [36]. This growth factor is released from platelets during their activation and degranulation and stimulates differentiation and mitogenesis of mesenchymal cells. Although IGFs are cell proliferative mediators, they also constitute the major axis of programmed cell apoptosis regulation, by inducing survival signals protecting cells from many apoptotic stimuli [36].

2.5 PRP versus PRF for growth factor release

The release profile of growth factors has been an important and highly debated research topic over the past years. These differ significantly between PRP and PRF. Development of PRF enabled to control and enrich growth factors from platelet concentrates by allowing a slower and gradual release of growth factors over time. The fact that this second generation of platelet concentrate contains leukocytes within the fibrin matrix also allowed for an enhanced secretion of growth from these cells involved in tissue regeneration [37]. Growth factor release from three different platelet concentrates including PRP, L-PRF, A-PRF were reported by Kobayashi *et al.* (Figures 2.3 and 2.4) [14]. PRF (L-PRF and A-PRF) released a higher total amount of growth factors when compared to PRP over a 10-day period.

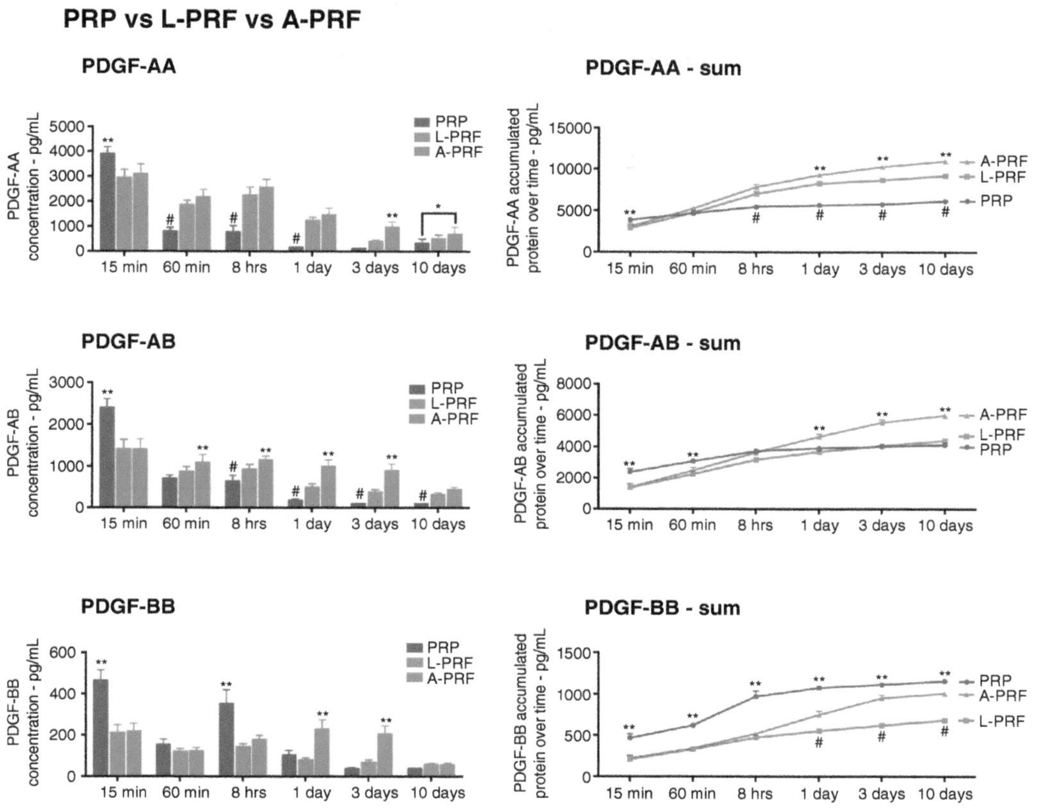

Figure 2.3 Growth factor release from PRP and PRF at each time point of PDGF-AA, -AB, and -BB over a 10-day period. Notice that while PRP has significantly higher growth factors released at early time points, over a 10-day period, significantly higher levels are most commonly found with A-PRF due to the slow and gradual release of growth factors utilizing slower centrifugation speeds. Source: Kobayashi *et al.* 2016 [14]. Reproduced with permission of Springer.

In order to characterize precisely growth factor release over an extended period of time, analysis by our research team investigated common blood proteins including PDGF-AA, -AB, and -BB at each of the following early and late time periods including 15 mins, 60 mins, 8 hours, 24 hours, 3 days, and 10 days (Figure 2.3). Interestingly, at an early time point (15 minutes), significantly higher levels of PDGF-AA is released from PRP when compared to L-PRF or A-PRF, while significantly lower levels were observed at 60 minutes demonstrating that PRP rapidly releases PDGF-AA between 0 and 15 minutes and thereafter significantly less release is observed compared to PRF up to 10 days (Figure 2.3). While no significant differences at early time points was detected between A-PRF and L-PRF (up to 1 day), by 3 days A-PRF showed significantly higher growth factor release of PDGF-AA when compared to either PRP and L-PRF (Figure 2.3). Furthermore, the total PDGF-AA accumulated proteins over time demonstrated that while PRP showed significantly lowest levels from 8 hours until 10 days, whereas in contrast, significantly higher levels were detected for A-PRF from 1 to 10 days when compared to PRP and PRF (Figure 2.3). Moreover, PDGF-AA was found released from all platelet concentrations at 6- to 10-fold higher concentrations when compared to PDGF-AB and PDGF-BB. Similar trends were also observed for PDGF-AB and PDGF-BB.

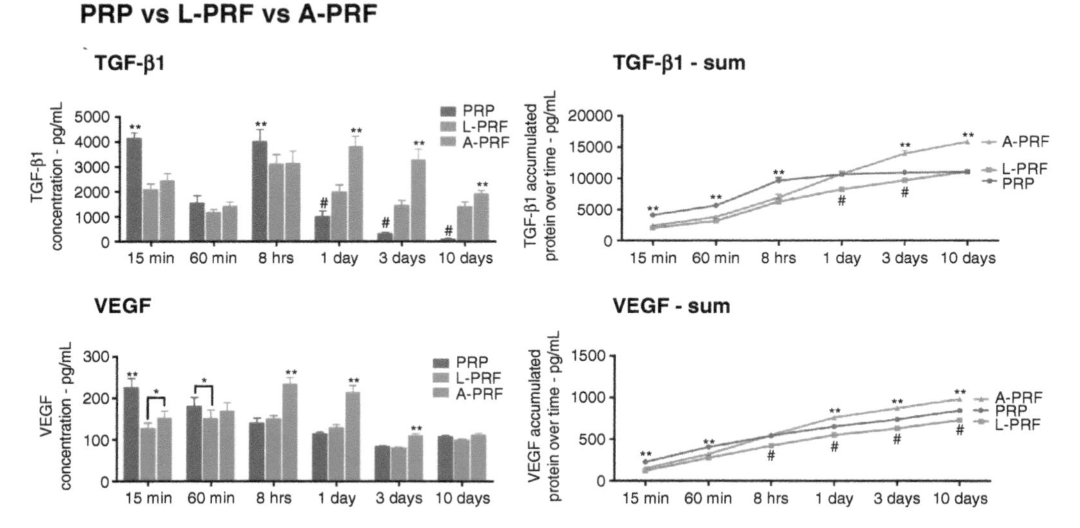

Figure 2.4 Growth factor release from PRP and PRF at each time point of TGF-β1 and VEGF over a 10-day period. Once again it was found that PRP released higher growth factors at early time points; however, A-PRF demonstrated significantly highest release at later time points. Overall, more growth factor release from A-PRF was observed when compared to the other modalities. Source: Kobayashi *et al.* 2016 [14]. Reproduced with permission of Springer.

The release of TGF-β1 and VEGF were also calculated and a similar trend was observed whereby PRP promoted the early release of growth factors at 15 minutes and 8 hours when compared to PRF (L-PRF or A-PRF) (Figure 2.4). Thereafter, PRP levels dropped considerably and both standard L-PRF and A-PRF showed significant elevated levels of both TGF-β1 and VEGF concentrations. Parallel to the results obtained with PDGF, total protein release was significantly highest for A-PRF at 3 and 10 days for TGF-β1, and 1, 3, and 10 days for VEGF when compared to PRP and L-PRF.

In general, the release of EGF and IGF were lower in quantity when compared to PDGF, TGF-β1, and VEGF concentrations. Different trends were observed between the release profiles of EGF and IGF [14]. Total protein accumulation demonstrated highest total EGF for A-PRF with lowest being PRP. Moreover, significantly higher levels of IGF were observed for PRP at 15 minutes, 60 minutes, and 8 hours compared to PRF. Overall, PRP can be recommended for fast delivery of growth factors, whereas A-PRF is better-suited for long-term delivery up to a 10-day period.

2.6 L-PRF versus A-PRF vs A-PRF+—new findings with the low-speed centrifugation concept and low-time induces even higher growth factor release

The gradual release of growth factors to their surrounding tissues are more commonly known as suitable factors for tissue engineering. Something worth noting is that the development of the low-speed centrifugation concept later described in detail in Chapter 3, standard L-PRF has been further improved to support more growth factor release in A-PRF and A-PRF+ [24]. It was reported by Ghanaati *et al.* in 2014 that cells within the original PRF matrix were surprisingly found gathered at the bottom of the PRF matrix [7]. In principle, less centrifugation time would reduce cell pull-down by centrifugation g-forces, which increases the total number of cells left contained within the top layer of PRF enabling a higher number of leukocytes "trapped" within the fibrin matrix.

In a second study by our group, the newer formulation of A-PRF (A-PRF+, which is not only lower centrifugation speed but also time—1300 rpm for 8 min) has been shown to increase growth factor release of TGF-beta1, PDGF-AA, PDGF-AB, PDGF-BB, VEGF, IGF, and EGF (Figures 2.5 and 2.6) [24]. The release of growth factors including PDGF-AA, -AB, and -BB are shown in Figure 2.5. While the trends are slightly different between all investigated growth factors, A-PRF+ demonstrated a significant increase in growth factor release at either 1, 3, or 10 days when compared to all other groups. L-PRF demonstrated significantly lower values when compared A-PRF and A-PRF+ (Figure 2.5). Therefore, in conclusion it was found that the total growth factor release could be enhanced by reducing both centrifugation speed and time in A-PRF+.

The release of TGF-β1 also demonstrated a similar trend whereby A-PRF+ demonstrated significantly highest values at 1, 3, and 10 days and the total release of growth factors after a 10-day period was nearly 3 times significantly higher when compared to L-PRF (Figure 2.6). Interestingly, A-PRF+ demonstrated a higher release of VEGF at an early time point of 1 day; however, little change was observed in the total release at 10 days (Figure 2.6). EGF and IGF-1 further confirmed that

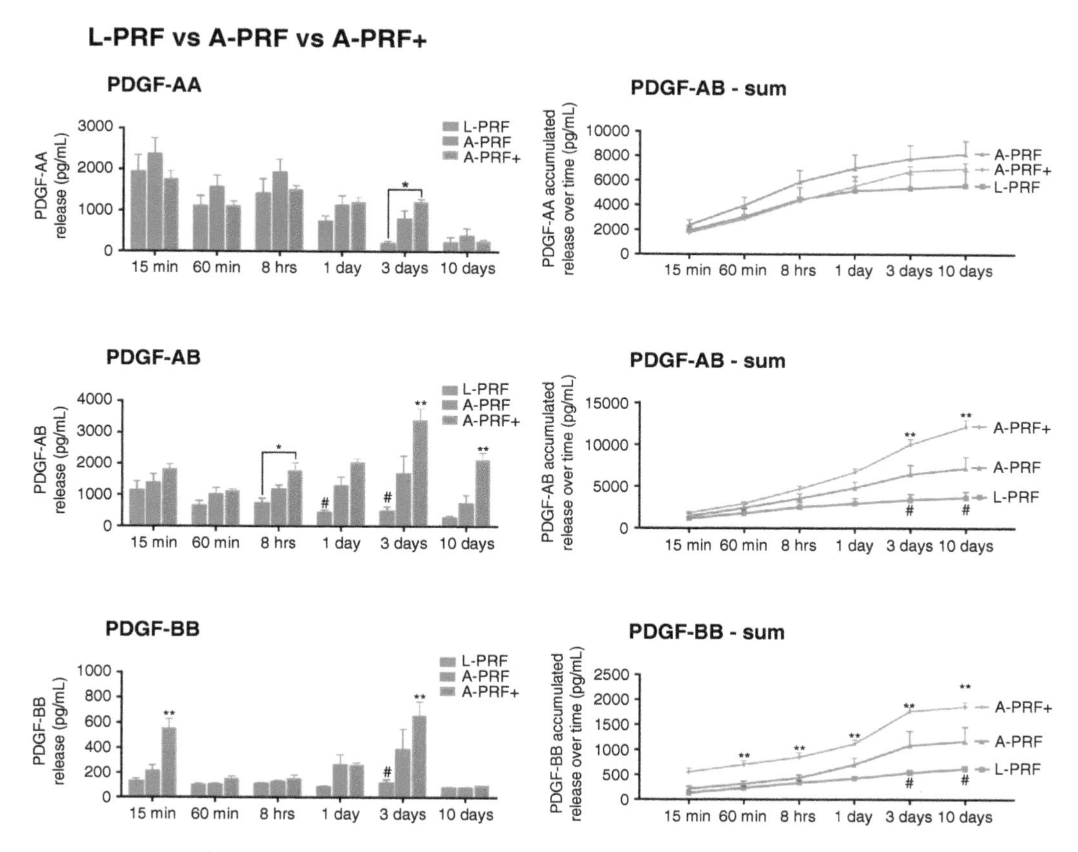

Figure 2.5 Growth factor release resulting from the slow speed centrifugation concept at each time point of PDGF-AA, -AB, and -BB over a 10-day period. In general, it was found that A-PRF+ demonstrated significantly highest growth factor release when compared to all other modalities after a 10-day period. Source: Fujioka-Kobayashi *et al.* 2017 [24]. Reproduced with permission of the American Academy of Periodontology.

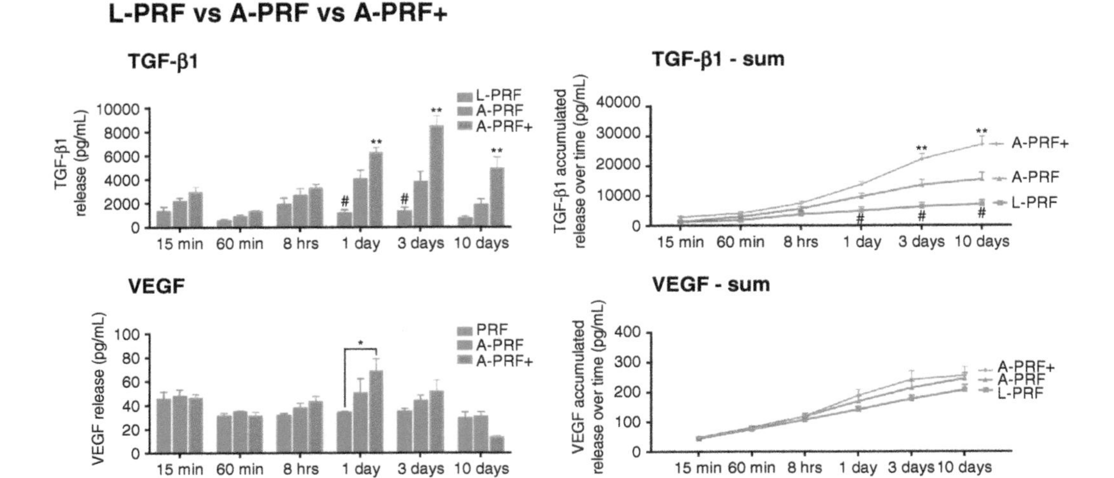

Figure 2.6 Growth factor release from slow speed concept at each time point of TGF-β1, VEGF over a 10-day period. Source: Fujioka-Kobayashi *et al.* 2017 [24]. Reproduced with permission of the American Academy of Periodontology.

the low speed centrifugation concept favored the release of both growth factors from A-PRF+ when compared to A-PRF and L-PRF [24]. Overall, lower centrifugation speeds and times (A-PRF, A-PRF+) demonstrated a significant increase in growth factor release of PDGF, TGF- β1, EGF, and IGF with A-PRF+ being highest of all groups.

2.7 i-PRF versus PRP—growth factor release

Since PRP is liquid in nature, it was originally proposed that PRP be combined with various bone biomaterials, most notably bone-grafting materials. Very recent data from our laboratories has reported that growth factor release with PRP is released very early in the delivery phase, whereas a preference would be to deliver growth factors over an extended period of time during the entire regenerative phase [14,38,39]. Moreover, the technique for PRP preparation requires the additional use of bovine thrombin or $CaCl_2$ in addition to coagulation factors, which leads to a decrease in the healing potential. In some cases, the entire protocol to prepare PRP needs several separation phases lasting upward of 1 hour making it inefficient for everyday medical purposes. For these reasons, i-PRF has been developed as an injectable-PRF in liquid formulation by drawing blood rapidly in a specific centrifugation tube at a very low speed of 700 rpm (60 g) for an even shorter centrifugation time (3 minutes) with one centrifugation cycle. The i-PRF must be utilized within 15 minutes of collection due to the fact it does not contain anti-coagulants and is therefore able to coagulate within a short period of time. This new formulation can be utilized for a variety of procedures including mixing with bone grafts to form a stable fibrin bone graft for improved handling to improve graft stability. The principle for i-PRF remains the same—it contains a larger proportion of leukocytes and blood plasma proteins due to lower centrifugation speeds and time.

The release of growth factors from PRP and i-PRF were compared in a third study by our group as depicted in Figure 2.7. While all growth factors investigated demonstrated a significantly higher early (15 minutes) release from PRP when compared to i-PRF, the total release of growth factors showed

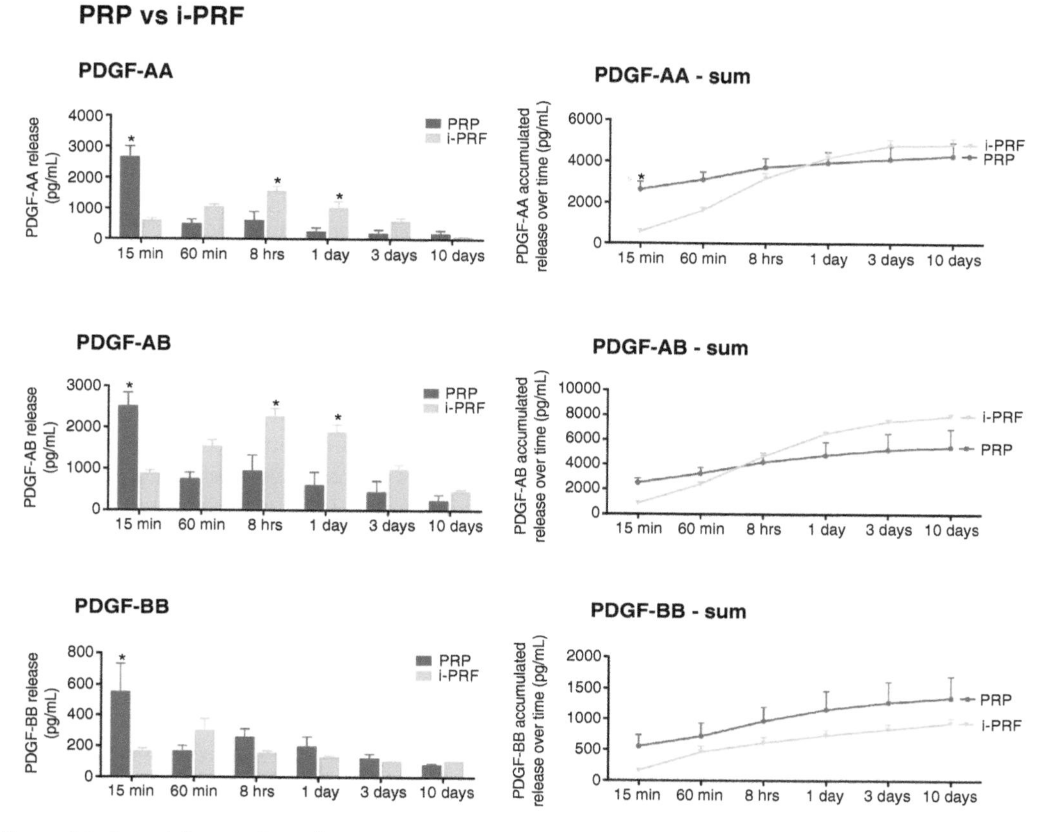

Figure 2.7 Growth factor release from i-PRF compared with PRP at each time point for growth factors PDGF-AA, -AB, and -BB over a 10-day period. Reprinted with permission from Miron *et al.* 2017.

that PDGF-AA, PDGF-AB, EGF, and IGF-1 all demonstrated higher released levels from i-PRF when compared to PRP (Figure 2.7, data not shown). Interestingly, however, total growth factor release of PDGF-BB, VEGF, and TGF-β1 were significantly higher in PRP when compared to i-PRF. Methods to further understand these variations are continuously being investigated in our laboratory as well as others. It may be hypothesized that the differences in spin protocols are suggested to have collected slightly different cell populations and/or total growth factors responsible for the variations in release over time. The advantages of i-PRF are that it remains a 100% autologous product with the benefit of forming a fibrin clot while maintaining comparable growth factor release to PRP.

2.8 Cell behavior in response to L-PRF, A-PRF, and A-PRF+

Our group was then interested to investigate the various PRF formulations (L-PRF, A-PRF, A-PRF+) on cell behavior. All PRF formulations utilizing the low-speed concept showed excellent biocompatibility and cellular activity in vitro [24]. Both A-PRF and A-PRF+ demonstrated significantly higher levels of human gingival fibroblast migration and proliferation when compared to

L-PRF (Figure 2.8A). Furthermore, gingival fibroblasts cultured with A-PRF+ demonstrated significantly higher mRNA levels of TGF-β, PDGF, and collagen1 at either 3 or 7 days (Figure 2.8B). It was also shown that A-PRF and A-PRF+ samples were able to locally demonstrate up to a 300% significant increase in collagen1 synthesis (Figure 2.8C). Not surprisingly, collagen remains one of the key factors during tissue wound healing and remodeling [40–42]. Therefore, the three-fold increase in collagen type 1 synthesis when cells were exposed to A-PRF and A-PRF+ further demonstrates the regenerative potential of the newer PRF formulations centrifuged at lower g-forces and lower centrifugation times.

2.9 Cell behavior in response to PRP, i-PRF

Thereafter, our group was interested to determine cellular differences between PRP and i-PRF. Both formulations, PRP and i-PRF, exhibited high biocompatibility of human gingival fibroblasts as well as significantly induced higher cell migration when compared to control tissue-culture plastic in vitro (Figure 2.9) [43]. It was found that i-PRF induced significantly higher migration, whereas PRP demonstrated significantly highest cellular proliferation (Figure 2.9A). Furthermore, i-PRF showed significantly highest mRNA levels of TGF-β at 7 days, PDGF at 3 days, and collagen1 expression at both 3 and 7 days when compared to PRP (Figure 2.9B). Both PRP and i-PRF demonstrated significantly higher collagen synthesis compared to control tissue culture plastic (Figure 2.9C). It is interesting to point out that although both PRP and i-PRF induced significantly higher cell activity when compared to controls, slight differences where observed between the groups and this may be due to the slight differences in released growth factors. Further investigation is therefore needed to fully characterize the regenerative potential of PRP versus i-PRF.

2.10 Future prospective

The trend in dentistry has gradually shifted toward more bioactive materials including cell-based therapies. Autologous PRF has therefore been introduced and utilized as an extremely physiological, safe, and reliable biomaterial for wound healing in the body since it is derived from 100% natural human blood. This chapter illustrates the various components of PRF including the function of acting as a 1) growth factor reserve and delivery system, 2) biocompatible scaffold, and 3) reservoir for living autologous cells capable of contributing to wound healing. Major advances have been recognized over recent years in the architectures of PRF growth factor-delivery systems that allow the controlled release of growth factors in a well-ordered manner. However, there remains several challenges that linger as potential future research. These include the optimal growth factor concentrations of PRF to allow more favorable release in various tissue defects. Another interesting hurdle currently being studied is the effect of patient variability and hematocrit differences on final PRF scaffolds. It has been suggested that the relative content of each factor and the kinetics of growth factor release from PRF scaffolds to their microenvironment may vary depending on donor characteristics, production methods, and platelet count enrichment. Furthermore, this chapter focused primarily on soft-tissue wound healing using PRF; however, the regeneration of the oral cavity requires the regeneration of many cell types including both hard and soft tissues collectively. Future research is therefore presently ongoing. Nevertheless, PRF serves as an ideal scaffold for tissue regeneration fulfilling the three main criteria of tissue engineering including: scaffold, cells, and growth factors. It has further been validated that the low-speed centrifugation concept releases higher growth factors as well as presents higher cellular bioactivity from A-PRF+ when compared to L-PRF.

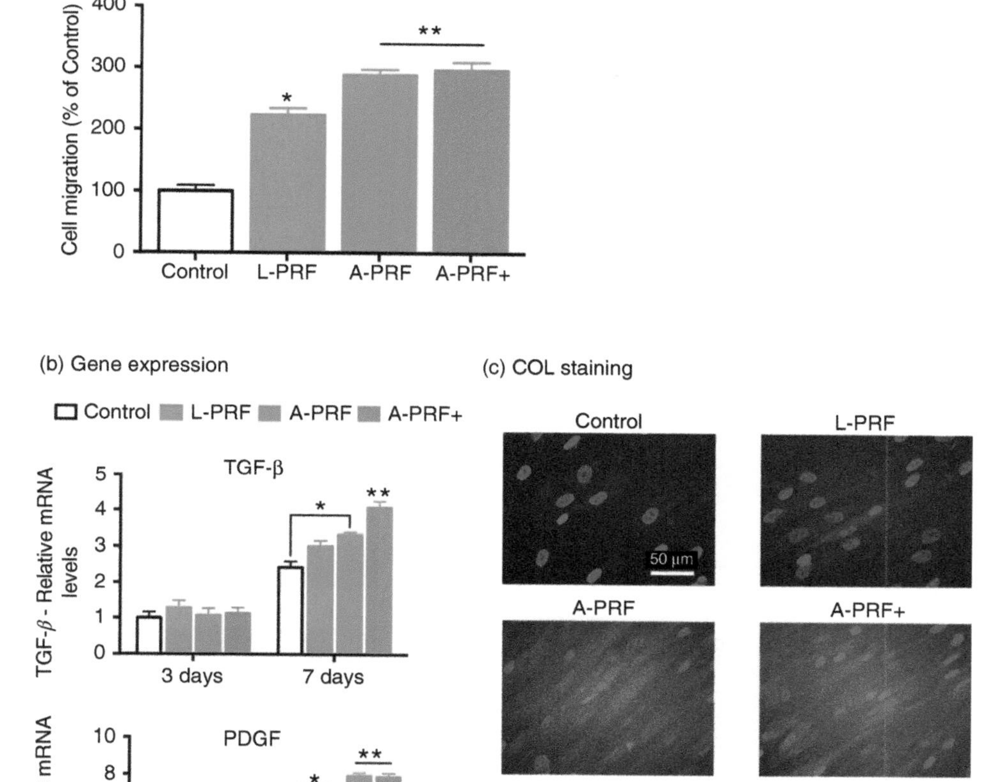

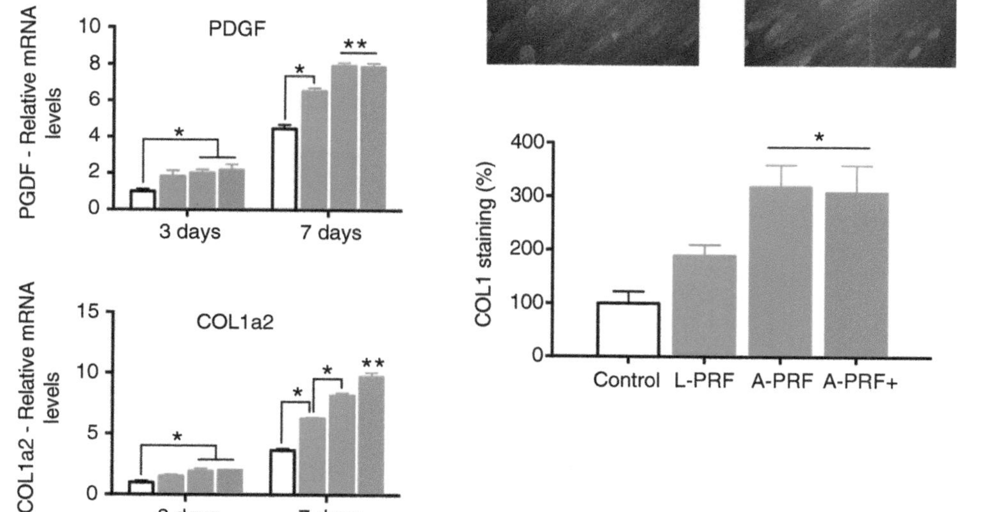

Figure 2.8 Human gingival fibroblast behavior exposed to L-PRF, A-PRF, and A-PRF+. (A) Cell migration, (B) gene expression, and (C) collagen synthesis on human gingival fibroblasts. Source: Fujioka-Kobayashi *et al.* 2017 [24]. Reproduced with permission of the American Academy of Periodontology.

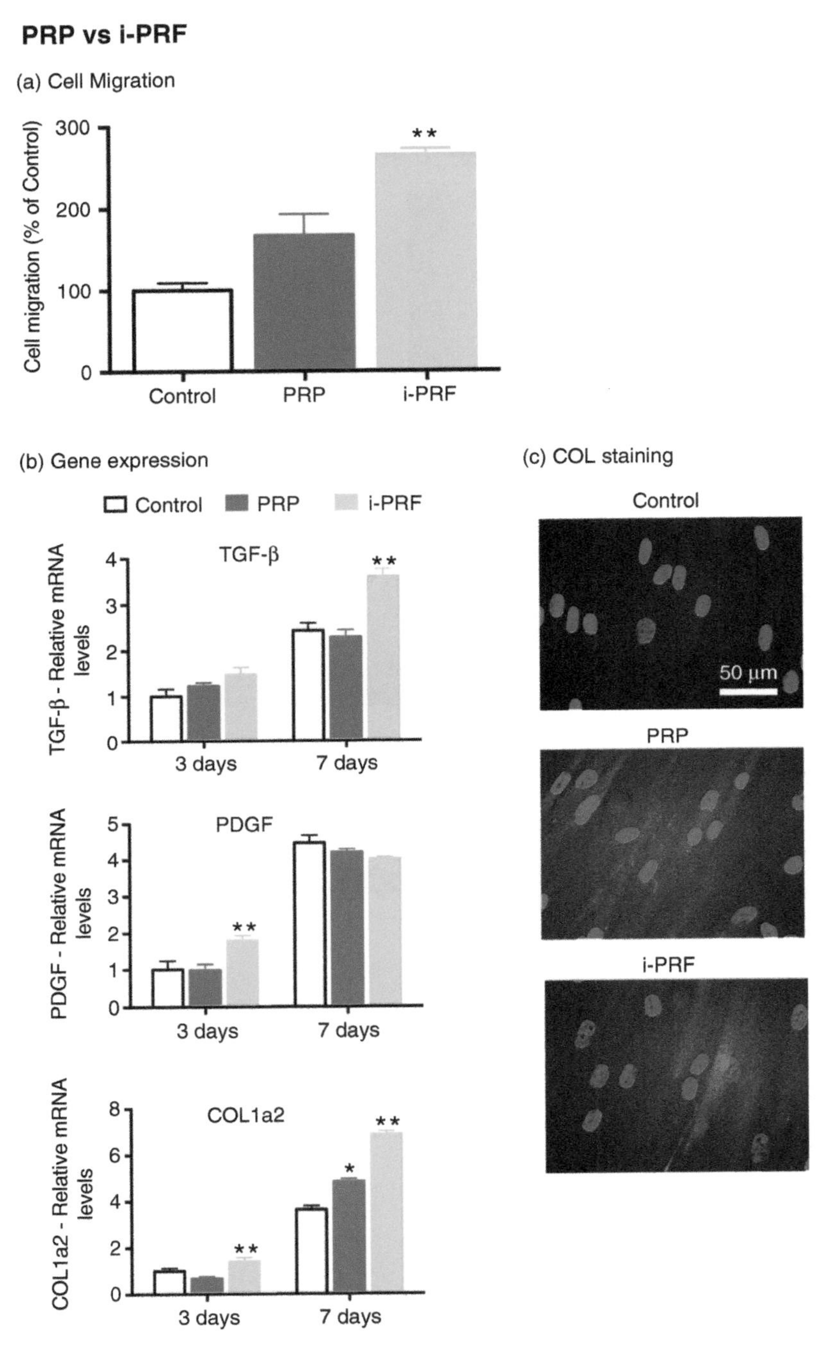

Figure 2.9 Human gingival fibroblast behavior exposed to i-PRF versus PRP. (A) Cell migration, (B) gene expression, and (C) collagen synthesis. Reprinted with permission from Miron *et al.* 2017.

References

1 Guo S, Dipietro LA. Factors affecting wound healing. J Dent Res. 2010;89(3): 219–29.
2 Tonnesen MG, Feng X, Clark RA, editors. Angiogenesis in wound healing. Journal of Investigative Dermatology Symposium Proceedings; 2000: Nature Publishing Group.
3 Gurtner GC, Werner S, Barrandon Y, Longaker MT. Wound repair and regeneration. Nature. 2008;453(7193): 314–21.
4 Gosain A, DiPietro LA. Aging and wound healing. World journal of surgery. 2004; 28(3):321–6.
5 Eming SA, Brachvogel B, Odorisio T, Koch M. Regulation of angiogenesis: wound healing as a model. Progress in histochemistry and cytochemistry. 2007; 42(3):115–70.
6 Dohan Ehrenfest DM, Del Corso M, Diss A, Mouhyi J, Charrier JB. Three-dimensional architecture and cell composition of a Choukroun's platelet-rich fibrin clot and membrane. J Periodontol. 2010;81(4):546–55.
7 Ghanaati S, Booms P, Orlowska A, Kubesch A, Lorenz J, Rutkowski J, et al. Advanced platelet-rich fibrin: a new concept for cell-based tissue engineering by means of inflammatory cells. The Journal of oral implantology. 2014;40(6):679–89.
8 Kawazoe T, Kim HH. Tissue augmentation by white blood cell-containing platelet-rich plasma. Cell transplantation. 2012; 21(2-3):601–7.
9 Perut F, Filardo G, Mariani E, Cenacchi A, Pratelli L, Devescovi V, et al. Preparation method and growth factor content of platelet concentrate influence the osteogenic differentiation of bone marrow stromal cells. Cytotherapy. 2013;15(7): 830–9.
10 Pirraco RP, Reis RL, Marques AP. Effect of monocytes/macrophages on the early osteogenic differentiation of hBMSCs. Journal of tissue engineering and regenerative medicine. 2013;7(5):392–400.
11 Chase AJ, Newby AC. Regulation of matrix metalloproteinase (matrixin) genes in blood vessels: a multi-step recruitment model for pathological remodelling. Journal of vascular research. 2003; 40(4):329–43.
12 Mazzucco L, Borzini P, Gope R. Platelet-derived factors involved in tissue repair-from signal to function. Transfusion medicine reviews. 2010;24(3):218–34.
13 Nguyen LH, Annabi N, Nikkhah M, Bae H, Binan L, Park S, et al. Vascularized bone tissue engineering: approaches for potential improvement. Tissue engineering Part B, Reviews. 2012;18(5):363–82.
14 Kobayashi E, Fluckiger L, Fujioka-Kobayashi M, Sawada K, Sculean A, Schaller B, et al. Comparative release of growth factors from PRP, PRF, and advanced-PRF. Clinical oral investigations. 2016.
15 Burnouf T, Goubran HA, Chen T-M, Ou K-L, El-Ekiaby M, Radosevic M. Blood-derived biomaterials and platelet growth factors in regenerative medicine. Blood reviews. 2013;27(2):77–89.
16 Reed GL, editor Platelet secretory mechanisms. Seminars in thrombosis and hemostasis; 2004: Copyright© 2004 by Thieme Medical Publishers, Inc., 333 Seventh Avenue, New York, NY 10001, USA.
17 Dohan DM, Choukroun J, Diss A, Dohan SL, Dohan AJ, Mouhyi J, et al. Platelet-rich fibrin (PRF): a second-generation platelet concentrate. Part II: platelet-related biologic features. Oral surgery, oral medicine, oral pathology, oral radiology, and endodontics. 2006;101(3): e45–50.
18 Gruber R, Kandler B, Holzmann P, Vogele-Kadletz M, Losert U, Fischer MB, et al. Bone marrow stromal cells can provide a local environment that favors migration and formation of tubular structures of endothelial cells. Tissue engineering. 2005;11(5-6):896–903.

19 Au P, Tam J, Fukumura D, Jain RK. Bone marrow-derived mesenchymal stem cells facilitate engineering of long-lasting functional vasculature. Blood. 2008; 111(9):4551–8.
20 Lozito TP, Taboas JM, Kuo CK, Tuan RS. Mesenchymal stem cell modification of endothelial matrix regulates their vascular differentiation. Journal of cellular biochemistry. 2009;107(4):706–13.
21 Clark RA. Fibrin and wound healing. Annals of the New York Academy of Sciences. 2001;936(1):355–67.
22 Shaikh FM, Callanan A, Kavanagh EG, Burke PE, Grace PA, McGloughlin TM. Fibrin: a natural biodegradable scaffold in vascular tissue engineering. Cells, tissues, organs. 2008;188(4):333–46.
23 Nurden AT. Platelets, inflammation and tissue regeneration. Thrombosis and haemostasis. 2011;105 Suppl 1:S13–33.
24 Fujioka-Kobayashi M, Miron RJ, Hernandez M, Kandalam U, Zhang Y, Choukroun J. Optimized Platelet Rich Fibrin With the Low Speed Concept: Growth Factor Release, Biocompatibility and Cellular Response. J Periodontol. 2017;88(1):112–121. Epub 2016 Sep 2.
25 Border WA, Noble NA. Transforming growth factor beta in tissue fibrosis. The New England journal of medicine. 1994;331(19):1286–92.
26 Bowen T, Jenkins RH, Fraser DJ. MicroRNAs, transforming growth factor beta-1, and tissue fibrosis. The Journal of pathology. 2013;229(2):274–85.
27 Martin P, Leibovich SJ. Inflammatory cells during wound repair: the good, the bad and the ugly. Trends in cell biology. 2005; 15(11):599–607.
28 Tsirogianni AK, Moutsopoulos NM, Moutsopoulos HM. Wound healing: immunological aspects. Injury. 2006;37 Suppl 1:S5–12.
29 Adamson R. Role of macrophages in normal wound healing: an overview. Journal of wound care. 2009;18(8):349–51.
30 Davis VL, Abukabda AB, Radio NM, Witt-Enderby PA, Clafshenkel WP, Cairone JV, et al. Platelet-rich preparations to improve healing. Part I: workable options for every size practice. The Journal of oral implantology. 2014;40(4):500–10.
31 Davis VL, Abukabda AB, Radio NM, Witt-Enderby PA, Clafshenkel WP, Cairone JV, et al. Platelet-rich preparations to improve healing. Part II: platelet activation and enrichment, leukocyte inclusion, and other selection criteria. The Journal of oral implantology. 2014;40(4):511–21.
32 Ghasemzadeh M, Hosseini E. Intravascular leukocyte migration through platelet thrombi: directing leukocytes to sites of vascular injury. Thrombosis and haemostasis. 2015;113(6):1224–35.
33 Kato J, Tsuruda T, Kita T, Kitamura K, Eto T. Adrenomedullin: a protective factor for blood vessels. Arteriosclerosis, thrombosis, and vascular biology. 2005;25(12):2480–7.
34 Shamloo A, Xu H, Heilshorn S. Mechanisms of vascular endothelial growth factor-induced pathfinding by endothelial sprouts in biomaterials. Tissue engineering Part A. 2012;18(3-4):320–30.
35 Babensee JE, McIntire LV, Mikos AG. Growth factor delivery for tissue engineering. Pharmaceutical research. 2000;17(5):497–504.
36 Giannobile WV, Hernandez RA, Finkelman RD, Ryan S, Kiritsy CP, D'Andrea M, et al. Comparative effects of platelet-derived growth factor-BB and insulin-like growth factor-I, individually and in combination, on periodontal regeneration in Macaca fascicularis. Journal of periodontal research. 1996;31(5):301–12.
37 Eren G, Gurkan A, Atmaca H, Donmez A, Atilla G. Effect of centrifugation time on growth factor and MMP release of an experimental platelet-rich fibrin-type product. Platelets. 2016;27(5):427–32.
38 Lucarelli E, Beretta R, Dozza B, Tazzari PL, O'Connel SM, Ricci F, et al. A recently developed bifacial platelet-rich fibrin matrix. European cells & materials. 2010;20:13–23.
39 Saluja H, Dehane V, Mahindra U. Platelet-Rich fibrin: A second generation

platelet concentrate and a new friend of oral and maxillofacial surgeons. Annals of maxillofacial surgery. 2011;1(1):53–7.

40 Chu GH, Ogawa Y, McPherson JM, Ksander G, Pratt B, Hendricks D, et al. Collagen wound healing matrices and process for their production. Google Patents; 1991.

41 Clark R. The molecular and cellular biology of wound repair: Springer Science & Business Media; 2013.

42 Chattopadhyay S, Raines RT. Review collagen-based biomaterials for wound healing. Biopolymers. 2014;101(8): 821–33.

43 Miron RJ, Fujioka-Kobayashi M, Hernandez M, Kandalam U, Zhang Y, Ghanaati S, Choukroun J. Injectable platelet rich fibrin (i-PRF): opportunities in regenerative dentistry? Clin Oral Investig. 2017 Feb 2. doi: 10.1007/ s00784-017-2063-9. [Epub ahead of print].

3

Introducing the Low-Speed Centrifugation Concept

Joseph Choukroun and Shahram Ghanaati

Abstract

This chapter describes the development of platelet rich fibrin (PRF) as a fully autologous blood concentrate system. The low-speed centrifugation concept (LSCC) indicates that reducing the relevant centrifugation force (RCF) advances PRF matrices with an enhanced number of inflammatory cells and platelets. This effect was shown in Advanced PRF (A-PRF) and Advanced PRF plus (A-PRF+) as solid PRF-based matrices. In this context, A-PRF+ prepared according to the LSCC, compared to PRF, exhibited an enhanced number of platelets and leukocytes and showed significantly higher growth factor release concentrations over 10 days. Moreover, further RCF reduction based on the LSCC allowed for the development of an injectable PRF (i-PRF) without the use of anticoagulants. I-PRF, prepared with the lowest RCF, includes the highest number of leukocytes and platelets, illustrating the effect of the LSCC on this blood concentrate system. Leukocytes are the main protagonists in wound healing and the regeneration process. Their presence in advanced PRF-based matrices and i-PRF highlights their enhanced regeneration capacity. This chapter highlights PRF-based matrices and their use for a wide range of clinical applications in dentistry, maxillofacial surgery, and other medical fields, due to their simplified preparation process and the effectiveness of this system as a minimally invasive approach.

Highlights

- Development of solid PRF (A-PRF, A-PRF+)
- Development of injectable PRF (i-PRF)
- Role of platelets and leukocytes
- Clinical insights into the future use of A-PRF and i-PRF

3.1 Introduction

In the last decades, different concepts have been introduced for clinically relevant tissue regeneration in impaired regions. In this context, the application of pure biomaterials in terms of guided bone regeneration (GBR) [1] and guided tissue regeneration (GTR) [2–4] are well-accepted models as minimally invasive approaches in regenerative medicine. Furthermore, to enhance the regenerative capacity of biomaterials, concepts such as cell-based tissue engineering have shown promising results in many preclinical studies. The combination of biomaterials with several primary mesenchymal or endothelial cells leads to rapid anastomosis formation and enhanced vascularization after in vivo implantation in small animal models [5,6]. However, cell isolation and pre-cultivation need strict sterile settings and elaborate conditions. Therefore, the limited applicability of these methods simultaneously with the surgical intervention in addition to the time

Platelet Rich Fibrin in Regenerative Dentistry: Biological Background and Clinical Indications, First Edition.
Edited by Richard J. Miron and Joseph Choukroun.

required are the main drawbacks for clinical translation.

The need for new strategies to modify these issues with less-complex methods led to the introduction of an autologous blood concentrate system termed platelet rich plasma (PRP). In this system, the patient's own blood is first treated with anticoagulants and bovine serum and is then centrifuged in two centrifugation steps. Through these manufacturing processes, the gained blood concentrate is based on platelets, while leukocytes, which physiologically exist within the peripheral blood, are minimized and excluded [7]. The application of PRP has been widely studied and has shown positive outcomes in tissue regeneration [8]. In addition, plasma rich in growth factors (PRGFs) has been introduced as a blood-derived concentrate, focusing on the advantages of growth factors [9]. Similar to PRP, this blood concentrate requires external additives for processing [9]. However, the use of anticoagulants as external components and the preparation processes of these systems still provide limitations in clinical applications. Thus, the necessity for alternative strategies and feasible clinical applications is raised.

Aiming to develop an improved and facilitated preparation concept, a new blood concentrate system, platelet rich fibrin (PRF), was introduced as the first total autologous concept without additional anticoagulants [10]. In this concept, the need for anticoagulants was excluded, which significantly reduced the risk of trans-contamination. Moreover, the elimination of anticoagulants allowed the physiological cell functions to take place after centrifugation without inhibition or manipulation. The main goal was to simplify the preparation process and to minimize the required preparation steps and time in order for this method to be more suitable for clinical applications, as time is one of the most precious factors in the clinic. In this system, peripheral blood is collected from the patient in specific tubes and immediately processed by one-step centrifugation. This process activates the coagulation cascade and leads to three-dimensional fibrin clot formation. After centrifugation, the blood is separated into a red cell fraction and the PRF clot, which has to be gently isolated. The resulting clot consists of an upper buffy coat part, which is adjacent to the eliminated red blood phase. The clot body as a fibrin network is enriched with platelets and concentrated with a variety of leukocytes, which physiologically exist within the peripheral blood. Furthermore, after clotting, the growth factor release in the PRF has been described as slow and continuous, lasting up to 10 days [11].

3.2 Development of advanced solid PRF matrices following the low speed centrifugation concept (LSCC)

For the preparation of solid PRF according to Choukroun's established protocol [10], glass tubes were used to collect blood. The specific glass surface allows for the activation of the coagulation cascade during the centrifugation process to generate a solid fibrin clot. Moreover, the application of a high relative centrifugation force (RCF); that is, 708 g, is required [10]. In this RCF range, the fibrin network exhibits a dense structure with minimal interfibrous space [12]. The fibrin scaffold includes, apart from the platelets, different inflammatory cells, such as leukocytes and their subfamilies, lymphocytes, macrophages, and stem cells. Moreover, the cellular distribution pattern is mostly accumulated within the proximal part close to the buffy coat, whereas the platelet density is decreased toward the distal part (Figure 3.1).

Modification of the preparation protocol by reducing the applied RCF resulted in an improved preparation protocol for advanced solid PRF (A-PRF) using 208 g[12] (Figure 3.1). The advanced fibrin clot showed a more porous structure with a larger interfibrous space compared to that of PRF [12]. Furthermore, cells, especially platelets, were observed in even distributions throughout

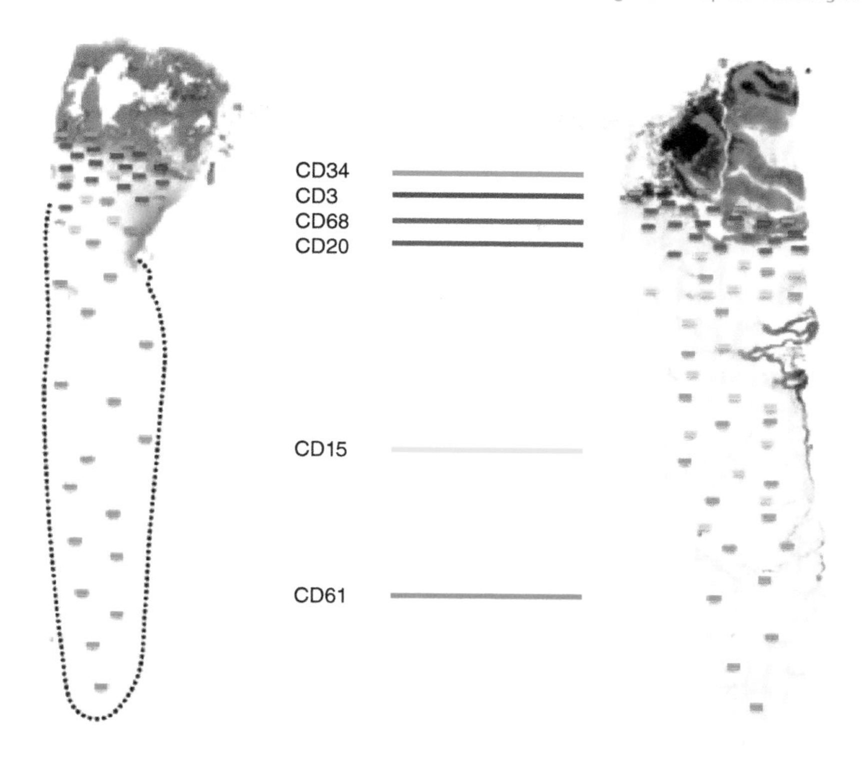

Figure 3.1 Total scan of PRF (left) with Hemp;E staining. Total scan of A-PRF (right) with Masson-Goldner staining. Immunohistochemistry markers: CD3 = T-lymphocytes; CD 15 = neutrophilic granulocytes; CD 20 = B-lymphocytes; CD34 = stem cells; CD61 = platelets; and CD68 = monocytes. Different colors illustrate the distribution pattern of the particular cell types.

the entire clot (Figure 3.1). The reduction of the RCF used led not only to a more even cellular distribution but also to an enhanced number of the included inflammatory cells and platelets. Thereby, histological analysis of A-PRF showed a significantly higher number of neutrophilic granulocytes, a leukocyte subfamily, compared to that in PRF [12]. In addition, different inflammatory cells were also observed in the middle and distal parts of the A-PRF clot, illustrating the influence of the applied RCF on the particular cell types (Figure 3.1). Furthermore, in vivo pre-clinical investigations showed the role of the clot structure in the vascularization and regeneration processes. Comparative histological analysis demonstrated that, due to its porous structure, A-PRF significantly facilitated the cellular penetration into the fibrin scaffold, showing a significantly improved vascularization pattern 10 days after subcutaneous implantation in mice compared to PRF (Figure 3.2) [13].

PRF is a complex system consisting of numerous biologically active cells and signaling molecules. To understand the role of these components, further studies were necessary. Various in vitro investigations showed a correlation between reducing the RCF in terms of the low-speed centrifugation concept (LSCC) and enhancing the growth factor release. Over 10 days, PRF matrices showed a slow and continuous accumulated growth factor release, such as platelet-derived growth factor (PDGF), transforming growth factors (TGF), and vascular endothelial growth factor (VEGF). However, other blood concentrates, such as PRP, showed

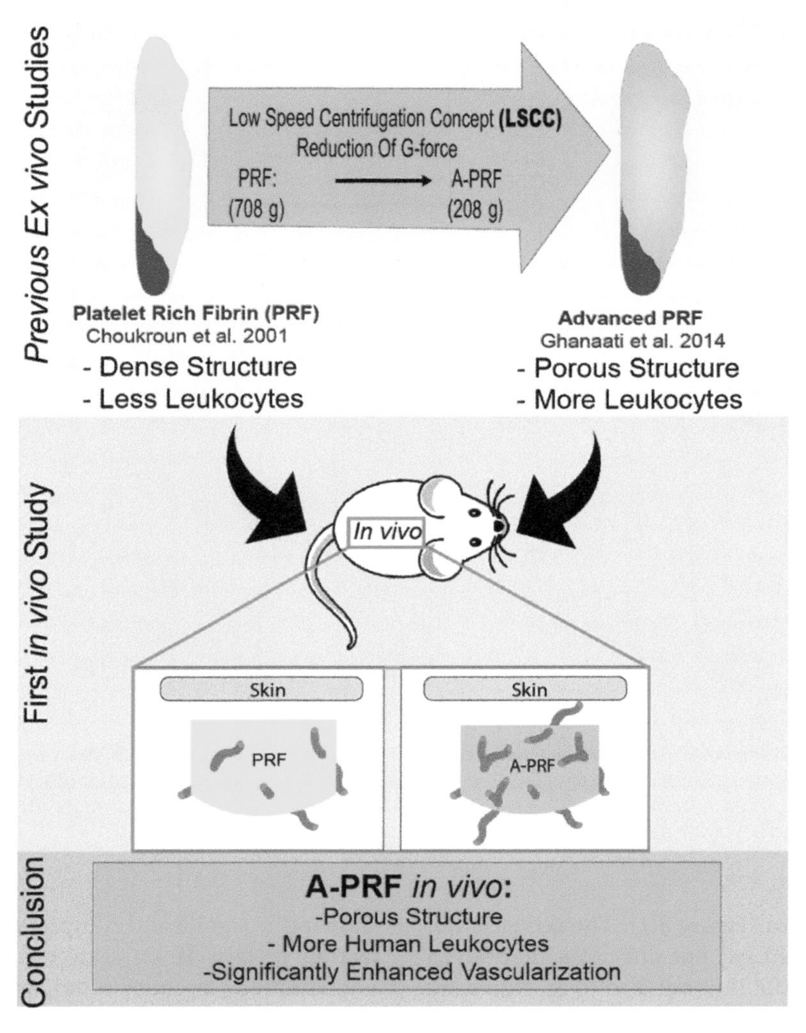

Figure 3.2 Comparative illustration of PRF and A-PRF. In vivo results highlight the enhanced regeneration capacity of A-PRF based on the LSCC.

enhanced accumulated growth factor release activity at early time points, that is, up to 8 hours, which was then significantly lower compared to that in PRF matrices close to day 10 [11]. One explanation for this observation is the solid PRF structure, which functions as a reservoir of growth factors and leads to gradual and sustained growth factor release. However, specific growth factors, for example, VEGF, showed no significant difference between PRF and A-PRF when comparing the accumulated release over 10 days [14]. This observation called for further modification of A-PRF to optimize the growth factor release.

In the course of developing A-PRF, the essential impact of the applied centrifugation force on the clot quality and composition became obvious. Thus, special emphasis was placed on the functional integrity and clot formation in terms of structure and consistency to be suitable for clinical handling. Therefore, it was established that preparation protocols other than A-PRF led to either a comparable dense structure as PRF or no clot formation. Therefore,

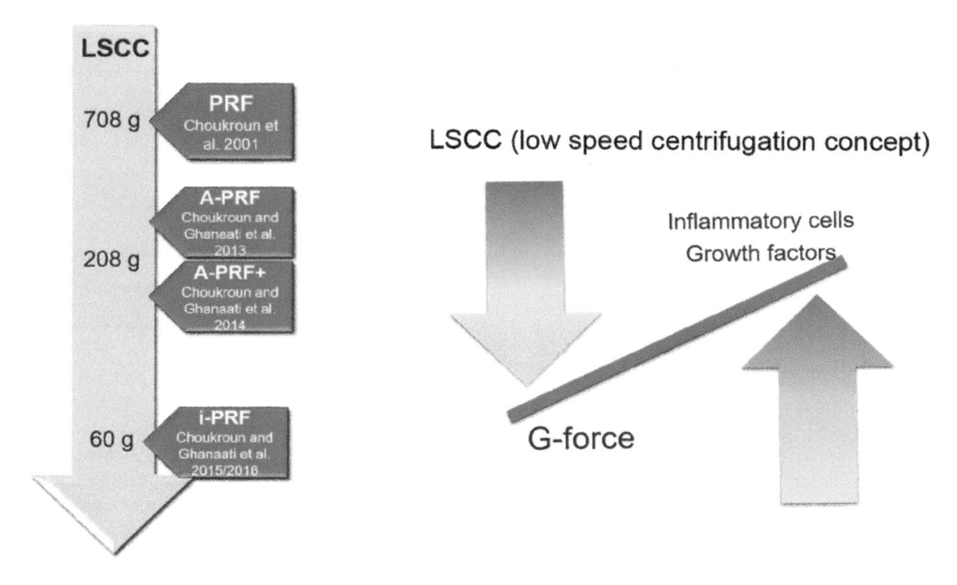

Figure 3.3 Development of solid and injectable PRFs following the low-speed centrifugation concept (LSCC).

attention was directed to the centrifugation time to improve the growth factor release along with maintaining the porous and stable A-PRF structure. A slight decrease in the centrifugation period by maintaining the RCF range within 208 g resulted in an improved clot termed Advanced PRF plus (A-PRF+), indicating its supplemented characteristics (Figure 3.3). Moreover, clinical handling was simplified in this protocol, as A-PRF+ barely needs to be processed in order to separate the clot from the red cell fraction. After centrifugation, the clot is most likely directly detached from the adjacent red cell phase and can be immediately transferred to the application region. In terms of structural integrity, A-PRF+ showed similar porosity to A-PRF when examining the fibrin network [14]. Additionally, the cellular distribution pattern showed evenly dispersed platelets over the entire clot [14]. In contrast to A-PRF, A-PRF+ had an improved growth factor release pattern. In this context, a comparative in vitro study over 10 days showed that A-PRF+ has the potential to release significantly enhanced accumulated growth factors, especially VEGF, compared to PRF and A-PRF [14]. These findings could be related to the binding affinity of the various growth factors to fibrin and fibrinogen and to the impact of the centrifugation time on the activated cells within the A-PRF+ clot. Moreover, the interaction between A-PRF+ and possible host cells was studied in an in vitro cell cultivation model using gingival fibroblasts. It was obvious that the cellular migration and proliferation rate in A-PRF and A-PRF+ were significantly higher than those in PRF. When interacting with A-PRF and A-PRF+, these cells showed enhanced growth factor release and increased mRNA levels of type 1 collagen [15]. These observations underline that, by means of the LSCC, advanced PRF matrices exhibit an improved regeneration capacity with direct impact on cellular function and growth factor release.

The LSCC indicates that, by reducing the relevant centrifugation force (RCF), the regeneration capacity of PRF matrices can be improved [16]. The total number of platelets and leukocytes within the PRF, A-PRF, and A-PRF+ matrices as a stepwise RCF reduction was analyzed using flow cytometry. Interestingly, the total platelet number significantly increased from PRF to A-PRF and A-PRF+. However, the total leukocyte number was only significantly higher when comparing A-PRF+ to PRF, whereas no statistically

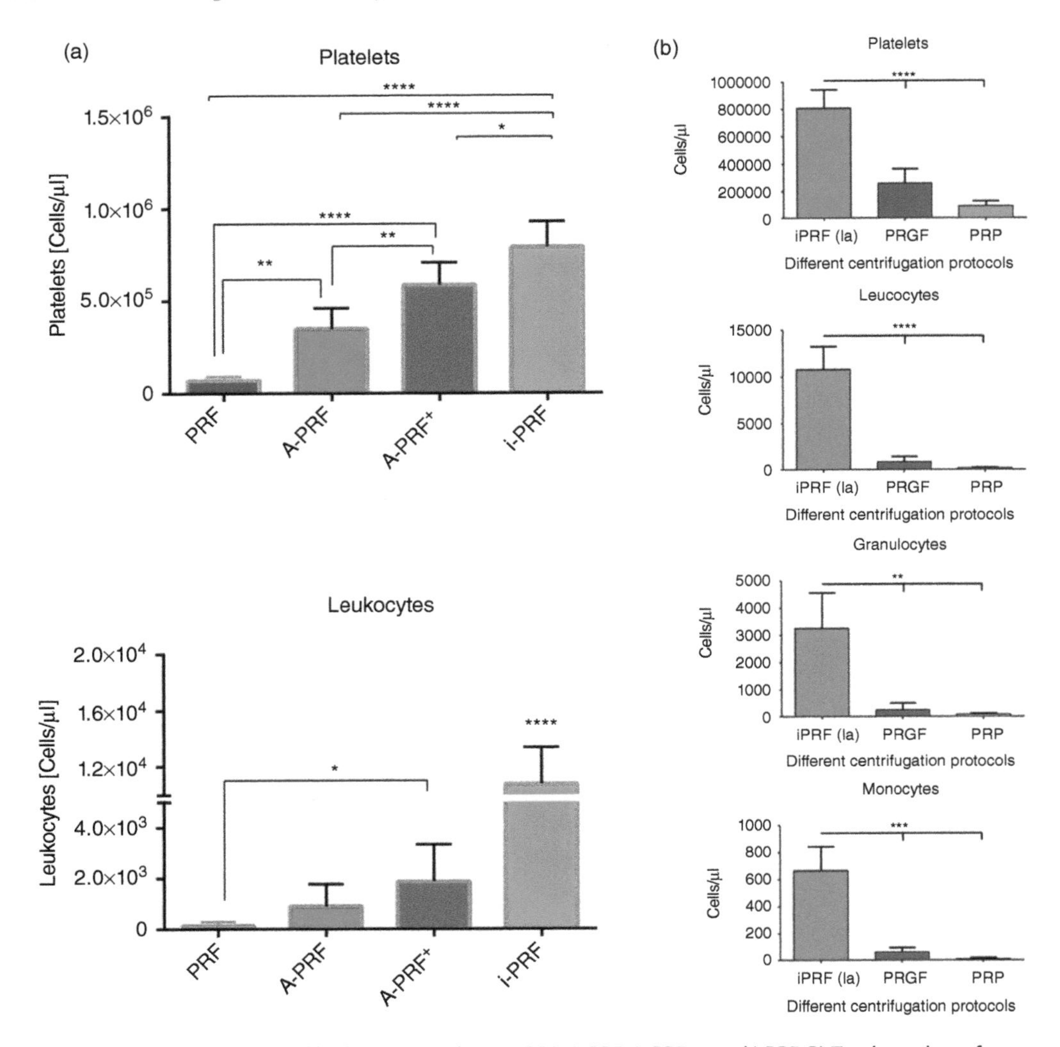

Figure 3.4 A) Total platelet and leukocyte numbers in PRF, A-PRF, A-PRF+, and i-PRF. B) Total number of platelets, leukocytes, granulocytes, and monocytes in i-PRF compared to PRP and PRGF. (*P<0.5), (**P<0.1), (***P<0.01), (****P<0,001).

significant difference was observed in the case of A-PRF compared to PRF (Figure 3.4). The correlation between the included leukocytes number and the enhanced growth factor release in A-PRF+ suggested that leukocytes could be one factor to improve growth factor release in PRF matrices. These findings again emphasize the impact of the preparation setting and the applied RCF on the composition and regenerative capacity of PRF matrices to highlight the optimized A-PRF+ regenerative potential.

3.3 Development of an injectable PRF (i-PRF) following the low speed centrifugation concept (LSCC)

Several indication fields were successfully established for the use of solid PRF-based matrices alone or in combination with biomaterials. However, in clinical settings, there is still an existing necessity for a fluid biological system. Accordingly, great interest was directed to the question of whether further reduction of RCF and fine tuning of the centrifugation setting, that is, revolution per minute (rpm) and centrifugation time, would enable the manufacturing of a fluid PRF matrix. To remove the need for external anticoagulants in order to generate an effective total autologous and fluid blood concentrate system, specific plastic tubes were developed to collect blood. In contrast to the glass tubes used in solid PRF matrices, the characteristics of the plastic surface do not activate the coagulation cascade during centrifugation. Thereby, according to the low speed centrifugation concept (LSCC) [16], further reduction of the RCF to 60 g and the use of plastic tubes allowed for the introduction of an injectable PRF matrix (i-PRF) without using anticoagulants (Figure 3.3). After centrifugation, the blood is separated into a yellow orange upper phase (i-PRF) and a red lower phase (red cell fraction). I-PRF is collected using a syringe by controlled aspiration of the upper fluid phase (Figure 3.5A). The collected i-PRF maintains its fluid phase for up to 10 to 15 minutes after centrifugation. Remarkably, the reduction of the RCF led to an enrichment of i-PRF with platelets and leukocytes. Consequently, flow cytometry showed that i-PRF includes the highest number of platelets and leukocytes among all the solid PRF-based matrices (Figure 3.4). Moreover, a comparative analysis of the total cells number in i-PRF and further liquid blood concentrates systems such as PRGF and PRP showed a significantly higher number of platelets, leukocytes, monocytes and granulocytes in i-PRF than in PRP and PRGF. However, no statistically significant difference was observed between PRP and PRGF (Figure 3.4). These observations highlight that by using the LSCC, solid PRF-based matrices could be improved into highly cell-rich injectable PRF with enhanced regenerative potential [16].

The introduction of i-PRF has since broadened the fields of PRF application in various medical and surgical indications, especially in combination with biomaterial-based regenerative medicine. Consequently, i-PRF made scientific promises in terms of clinically applicable cell-based tissue engineering. Biomaterials such as bone substitute materials can be easily combined with fluid i-PRF. Furthermore, standard GTR techniques using collagen-based biomaterials can be improved by loading with a dose of autologous cell-rich fluid fibrin matrix (i-PRF). The conditioning of biomaterials using i-PRF in terms of biomaterial functionalization and biologization, regardless of their origin, provide the patient's own concentrated regenerative components to accelerate the regeneration process (Figure 3.5C,D,E).

3.4 Platelets and leukocytes are key elements in the regeneration process

To understand the role of PRF-based matrices, such as A-PRF+ and i-PRF, in the generation process, it is essential to understand the physiological function of its components. Wound healing as a common event after every surgical intervention illustrates the crucial role of platelets and leukocytes in tissue regeneration. This process undergoes three overlapping phases, including inflammation, proliferation and new tissue formation [17]. Immediately after an injury, platelets form a plug for initial hemostasis, which is then replaced by a fibrin clot. Once activated, these cells release various signaling molecules such as platelet-derived growth factors (PDGFs), which are responsible for the regeneration process, vascular endothelial growth factor (VEGF) and transforming growth factor beta (TGF β) [18]. While the fibrin scaffold provides a framework for infiltrating and migrating inflammatory cells, leukocytes are common players for regeneration in various tissue types. The recruitment of these cells is accompanied by increased angiogenesis and lymphangiogenesis, which are of great importance for wound healing [19]. In addition, leukocytes are involved in the cellular

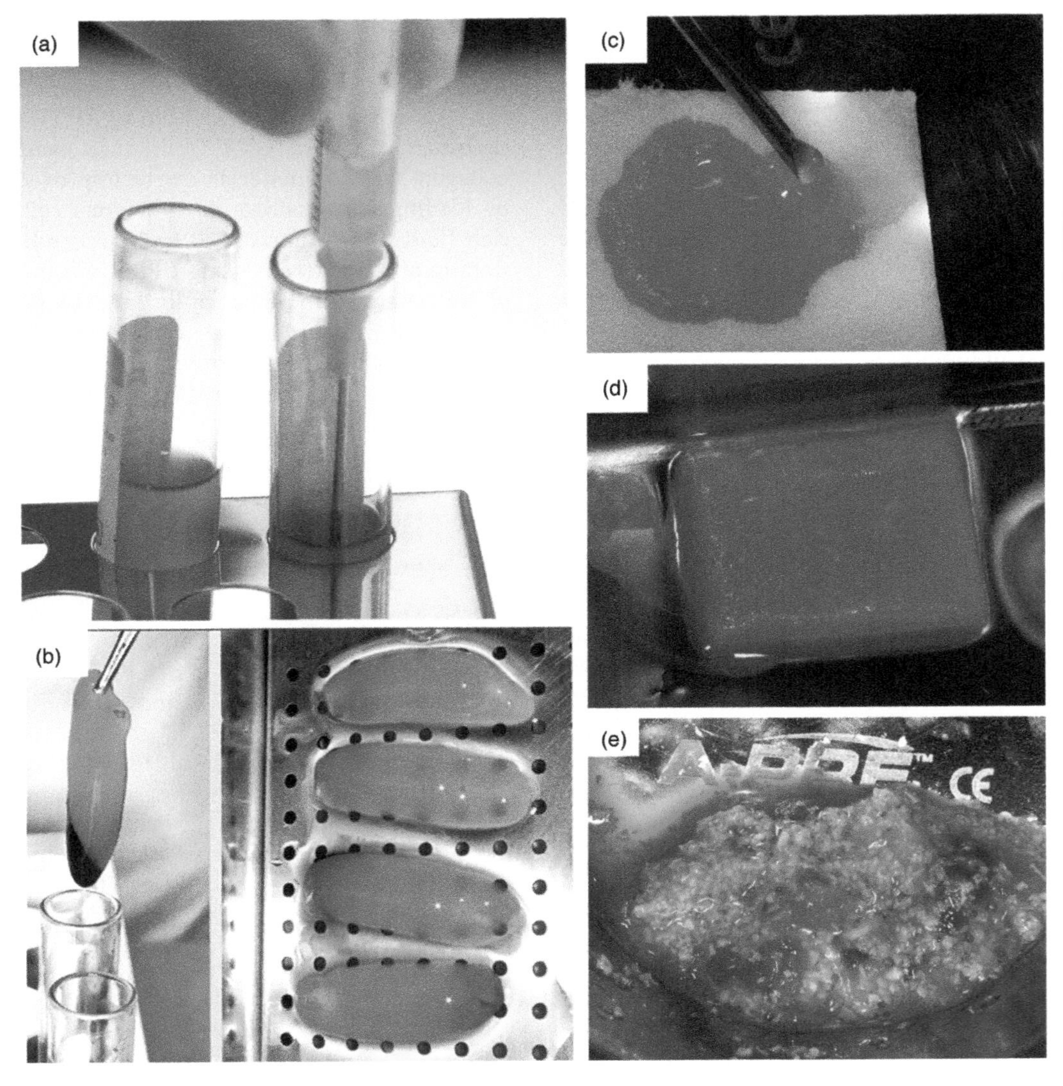

Figure 3.5 A) Injectable PRF (i-PRF) collection. B) A-PRF+ clots after centrifugation. C) The application of i-PRF on a collagen-based biomaterial. D) Collagen-based biomaterial loaded with i-PRF. E) Combination of A-RPF+, i-PRF, and a bone substitute material.

cross talk between several cells during bone regeneration [20]. Neutrophilic granulocytes present within the initial reaction as the first recruited cells after an injury. These cells are important for the early inflammation stage in wound healing. Their phagocytotic potential and neutrophilic extracellular traps eliminate pathogens and thus reduces the risk of wound infections [21,22]. Moreover, recent studies have reported on the regenerative potential of neutrophilic granulocytes by supporting lymphangiogenesis and secreting VEGF-D in a murine model [23]. The role of neutrophils is not limited to soft-tissue regeneration, but neutrophils are also involved in new bone formation. In the early phase up to 48 h, isolated human fracture hematoma includes neutrophil granulocytes, which have been shown to synthetize extracellular matrix in order to support new bone formation [24]. Furthermore, neutrophils contribute to the recruitment of monocytes to the inflammation site, which have been reported to be involved in the regeneration and vascularization of the wounded area [25,26]. After their recruitment to the injured region, monocytes differentiate into macrophages [27]. In addition to their phagocytic activity, macrophages release several immunomodulatory factors and cytokines to support collagen production and wound repair [28,29]. Monocytes have been shown to express osteogenic molecules including bone morphogenetic protein 2 (BMP-2) [20,30,31]. Different studies have shown that new bone formation was effectively promoted in critically sized bone defects in animals that were treated with a BMP-2 carrying biomaterials compared to a control group [32,33]. Interestingly, these cells were previously shown to be involved in the mononuclear-based integration process of collagenous biomaterials [2,34]. Monocytes and macrophages are also of prime importance in the biomaterial-based tissue regeneration process. After biomaterial implantation, adequate vascularization is needed to supply oxygen and nutrients and to enhance the biomaterial regenerative capacity. An in vivo study in a subcutaneous implantation model demonstrated that compared to the implantation of pure bone substitute material, the implantation of monocytes isolated from the peripheral blood combined with a synthetic bone substitute material contribute to a significantly enhanced vascularization pattern. These findings highlight the role of these cells in the fields of guided bone regeneration (GBR) [35]. Thus, i-PRF-matrix with enhanced monocyte concentrations could serve as an autologous source of regenerative cells to support guided bone and tissue regeneration. Moreover, lymphocytes are integral components of the immune system that participate in the process of wound healing. Lymphocyte sublines, such as T-lymphocytes, were shown to have an influence on the osteogenic differentiation of human mesenchymal stromal cells in vitro [36]. Additionally, T-lymphocytes and B-lymphocytes are involved in bone fracture healing; thus, the loss of B-cells was clinically associated with impaired human fracture healing [37–39]. Improved PRF-based matrices offer an easy and accessible autologous system including all the aforementioned cells embedded in a fibrin network. Thus, the application of A-PRF+ and i-PRF as a "biocatalyst" within the impaired region could accelerate the wound healing by providing the needed cells immediately after injury so that less cell recruitment is required. The combination with biomaterials is a promising approach in guided bone and tissue regeneration to enhance the capacity of the applied biomaterials and to enhance their bioactivity.

3.5 Clinical insights

After the introduction of PRF in 2001 and its modification (A-PRF+ and i-PRF), the clinical application of PRF penetrated many surgical fields. Due to the easy accessibility, minimal invasivity and time saving preparation, the role of PRF-based matrices gained in importance. Especially in oral and maxillofacial surgery, the application of PRF matrices meets various indications. Jaw atrophy after tooth loss, trauma, or diseases is a major limiting factor for dental implantation. Therefore, different approaches, such as guided bone regeneration, have been established for bone augmentation and regeneration. Consequently, A-PRF+ and i-PRF are widely used either as a prophylactic measure in terms of socket preservation[40] after tooth extraction to prevent jaw atrophy and support the wound healing or in combination with bone substitute materials[41] to accelerate and enhance the regeneration process in the bone augmentation bed and to provide enhanced bone formation. Moreover, soft-tissue regeneration in periodontology is a further representative field for the application of PRF-based matrices; specifically, the introduction of i-PRF facilitated its application in this field. In this context, PRF-based matrices are disseminated in the treatment of chronic periodontitis[42] and the regeneration of gingival recession [43]. Furthermore, necrosis, such as bisphosphonate-associated osteonecrosis of the jaw, suffers from limited vascularization and impaired wound healing [44]. Conventional treatment of this pathology indicates the excision of the affected region as an elective surgical treatment [44]. However, with the introduction of PRF, further minimal invasive possibilities became available for clinical application. Consequently, the use of PRF as a membrane or i-PRF injections showed promising clinical outcomes [45]. Generally, chronic wounds such as those observed in diabetic feet or in patients with impaired regeneration potential lack different growth factors [46]. PRF-based matrices, especially those prepared according to the LSCC (low-speed centrifugation concept), provide a reservoir of autologous inflammatory cells and continuous growth factor release [15]. Thereby, the application of PRF-based matrices as wound dressings is widespread in various medical fields. These clinical observations demonstrated an improved and accelerated wound healing in chronic wounds treated with PRF matrices.

The development of i-PRF further provides new insights and extended the application possibilities to orthopedic surgery [47], arthritic joint therapy and sports medicine [48]. Temporomandibular joint (TMJ) dysfunction is accompanied by chronic pain. The injection of i-PRF within the TMJ showed reduced pain and improves clinical outcomes. Thus, the application of i-PRF in fields of pain management could reduce the need for painkillers and their side effects, especially in chronic pain patients. Moreover, i-PRF is also used in aesthetic medicine for skin rejuvenation as an autologous material to reduce the risk of contamination and infection related to external materials. Thereby, PRF-based matrices as a complex system of different autologous components showed numerous application areas reflecting its effectiveness and practical implementation. However, ongoing research and clinical studies will further evaluate the role of the improved PRF-based matrices and the effect of the LSCC on the clinical outcomes and patient benefits.

3.6 Conclusion

Platelet rich fibrin (PRF) is a totally autologous blood concentrate system that does not require the use of external anticoagulants. This system is characterized by a simplified and appropriate preparation process to be suitable for everyday clinical application. By means of the low speed centrifugation concept (LSCC), the modification of the preparation protocol, that is, the reduction of the applied relevant centrifugation force, resulted in advanced PRF (A-PRF, A-PRF+) and fluid injectable PRF (i-PRF). Compared to PRF, these novel PRF matrices are significantly enriched with various inflammatory cells such as leukocytes and platelets. Moreover, the LSCC led to the development of a more porous clot structure in order to serve as a scaffold and growth factor reservoir, facilitating the regeneration process.

References

1 Schlee M, Rothamel D. Ridge augmentation using customized allogenic bone blocks: proof of concept and histological findings., Implant Dent. 2013;222:12–8. doi:10.1097/ID.0b013e3182885fa1.
2 Ghanaati S, Schlee M, Webber MJ, Willershausen I, Barbeck M, Balic E,

Görlach C, Stupp SI, Sader RA, Kirkpatrick CJ, Ghanaati S. Evaluation of the tissue reaction to a new bilayered collagen matrix in vivo and its translation to the clinic, Biomed. Mater. 2011;6:15010–12. doi:10.1088/1748-6041/6/1/015010.
3 Ghanaati S, Kovács A, Barbeck M, Lorenz J, Teiler A, Sadeghi N, Kirkpatrick CJ, Sader R. Bilayered, non-cross-linked collagen matrix for regeneration of facial defects after skin cancer removal: a new perspective for biomaterial-based tissue reconstruction., J. Cell Commun. Signal. 2016;10:3–15. doi:10.1007/s12079-015-0313-7.
4 Lorenz J, Blume M, Barbeck M, Teiler A, Kirkpatrick CJ, Sader RA, Ghanaati S. Expansion of the peri-implant attached gingiva with a three-dimensional collagen matrix in head and neck cancer patients-results from a prospective clinical and histological study., Clin. Oral Investig. 2016. doi:10.1007/s00784-016-1868-2.
5 Ghanaati S, Unger RE, Webber MJ, Barbeck M, Orth C, Kirkpatrick JA, Booms P, Motta A, Migliaresi C, Sader RA, Kirkpatrick CJ. Scaffold vascularization in vivo driven by primary human osteoblasts in concert with host inflammatory cells, Biomaterials. 2011;32:8150–60. doi:10.1016/j.biomaterials.2011.07.041.
6 Unger RE, Ghanaati S, Orth C, Sartoris A, Barbeck M, Halstenberg S, Motta A, Migliaresi C, Kirkpatrick CJ. The rapid anastomosis between prevascularized networks on silk fibroin scaffolds generated in vitro with cocultures of human microvascular endothelial and osteoblast cells and the host vasculature, Biomaterials. 2010;31:6959–67. doi:10.1016/j.biomaterials.2010.05.057.
7 Anitua E, Sánchez M, Orive G, Andía I. The potential impact of the preparation rich in growth factors (PRGF) in different medical fields, Biomaterials. 2007;28:4551–60. doi:10.1016/j.biomaterials.2007.06.037.
8 Albanese A, Licata ME, Polizzi B, Campisi G. Platelet-rich plasma (PRP) in dental and oral surgery: from the wound healing to bone regeneration., Immun. Ageing. 2013;10:23. doi:10.1186/1742-4933-10-23.
9 Anitua E, Andia I, Sanchez M. PRGF plasma rich growth factors, Dent. Dialogue. 2004:1–9.
10 Choukroun J, Adda F, Schoeffler C, Vervelle A. Une opportunité en paro-implantologie: le PRF, Implantodontie. 2001;42:55–62.
11 Kobayashi E, Flückiger L, Fujioka-Kobayashi M, Sawada K, Sculean A, Schaller B, Miron RJ. Comparative release of growth factors from PRP, PRF, and advanced-PRF, Clin. Oral Investig. 2016:1–8. doi:10.1007/s00784-016-1719-1.
12 Ghanaati S, Booms P, Orlowska A, Kubesch A, Lorenz J, Rutkowski J, Landes C, Sader R, Kirkpatrick C, Choukroun J. Advanced Platelet-Rich Fibrin: A New Concept for Cell-Based Tissue Engineering by Means of Inflammatory Cells, J. Oral Implantol. 2014;40:679–89. doi:10.1563/aaid-joi-D-14-00138.
13 Kubesch A, Barbeck M, Orlowska A, Booms P, Al-Maawi S, Sader RA, Kirkpatrick CJ, Choukroun J, Ghanaati S. Pre-clinical in vivo evaluation of Platelet-rich fibrin (PRF) scaffolds: G-force reduction in advanced platelet-rich fibrin (A-PRF) scaffolds increases scaffold integration and vascularization: First pre-clinical in vivo evaluation, (n.d.) JMSM, submitted.
14 El Bagdadi K, Yu X, Al-Maawi S, Dias A, Dohle E, Kubesch A, Booms P, Sader R, Kirkpatrick J, Choukroun J, Ghanaati S. Reduction of relative centrifugal forces influences the growth factor release within the solid PRF-based matrices: A proof of concept of LSCC (Low Speed Centrifugation Concept), ETOJ. in revision, (2016).
15 Fujioka-Kobayashi M, Miron RJ, Hernandez M, Kandalam U, Zhang Y, Choukroun J. Optimized Platelet Rich Fibrin With the Low Speed Concept: Growth Factor Release, Biocompatibility and Cellular Response., J. Periodontol. 2016:1–17. doi:10.1902/jop.2016.160443.

16 Choukroun J, Ghanaati G. Reduction of relative centrifugation force within PRF-(Platelet-Rich-Fibrin) concentrates advances patients' own inflammatory cells and platelets: First introduction of the Low Speed Centrifugation Concept, ETOJ, in revision (2016).
17 Nurden AT. Platelets, inflammation and tissue regeneration., Thromb. Haemost. 2011:S13–33. doi:10.1160/THS10-11-0720.
18 Jenne CN, Urrutia R, Kubes P. Platelets: bridging hemostasis, inflammation, and immunity., Int. J. Lab. Hematol. 2013;35:254–61. doi:10.1111/ijlh.12084.
19 Soloviev DA, Hazen SL, Szpak D, Bledzka KM, Ballantyne CM, Plow EF, Pluskota E. Dual Role of the Leukocyte Integrin M 2 in Angiogenesis, J. Immunol. 2014; 193:4712–21. doi:10.4049/jimmunol.1400202.
20 Ekström K, Omar O, Granéli C, Wang X, Vazirisani F, Thomsen P. Monocyte exosomes stimulate the osteogenic gene expression of mesenchymal stem cells., PLoS One. 2013;8:e75227. doi:10.1371/journal.pone.0075227.
21 Brinkmann V, Reichard U, Goosmann C, Fauler B, Uhlemann Y, Weiss DS, Weinrauch Y, Zychlinsky A. Neutrophil extracellular traps kill bacteria., Science. 2004;303:1532–5. doi:10.1126/science.1092385.
22 Mócsai A. Diverse novel functions of neutrophils in immunity, inflammation, and beyond., J. Exp. Med. 2013;210: 1283–99. doi:10.1084/jem.20122220.
23 Tan KW, Chong SZ, Wong FHS, Evrard M, Tan SM-L, Keeble J, Kemeny DM, Ng LG, Abastado J-P, Angeli V. Neutrophils contribute to inflammatory lymphangiogenesis by increasing VEGF-A bioavailability and secreting VEGF-D., Blood. 2013;122:3666–77. doi:10.1182/blood-2012-11-466532.
24 Bastian OW, Koenderman L, Alblas J, Leenen LPH, Blokhuis TJ. Neutrophils contribute to fracture healing by synthesizing fibronectin+ extracellular matrix rapidly after injury., Clin. Immunol. 2016;164:78–84. doi:10.1016/j.clim.2016.02.001.
25 Gurtner G, Werner S, Barrandon Y, Longaker M. Wound repair and regeneration, Nature. 2008;453:314–21. doi:10.1038/nature07039.
26 Krieger JR, Ogle ME, McFaline-Figueroa J, Segar CE, Temenoff JS, Botchwey EA. Spatially localized recruitment of anti-inflammatory monocytes by SDF-1α-releasing hydrogels enhances microvascular network remodeling., Biomaterials. 2016;77:280–90. doi:10.1016/j.biomaterials.2015.10.045.
27 Gurtner GC, Werner S, Barrandon Y, Longaker MT. Wound repair and regeneration., Nature. 2008;453:314–21. doi:10.1038/nature07039.
28 Leoni G, Neumann P-A, Sumagin R, Denning TL, Nusrat A. Wound repair: role of immune-epithelial interactions., Mucosal Immunol. 2015;8:959–68. doi:10.1038/mi.2015.63.
29 Murray PJ, Wynn TA. Protective and pathogenic functions of macrophage subsets., Nat. Rev. Immunol. 2017;11:723–37. doi:10.1038/nri3073.
30 Pirraco RP, Reis RL, Marques AP. Effect of monocytes/macrophages on the early osteogenic differentiation of hBMSCs., J. Tissue Eng. Regen. Med. 2013;7:392–400. doi:10.1002/term.535.
31 Omar OM, Granéli C, Ekström K, Karlsson C, Johansson A, Lausmaa J, Wexell CL, Thomsen P. The stimulation of an osteogenic response by classical monocyte activation., Biomaterials. 2011;32:8190–204. doi:10.1016/j.biomaterials.2011.07.055.
32 Peng K-T, Hsieh M-Y, Lin CT, Chen C-F, Lee MS, Huang Y-Y, Chang P-J. Treatment of critically sized femoral defects with recombinant BMP-2 delivered by a modified mPEG-PLGA biodegradable thermosensitive hydrogel., BMC

Musculoskelet. Disord. 2016;17:286. doi:10.1186/s12891-016-1131-7.

33 Kolk A, Tischer T, Koch C, Vogt S, Haller B, Smeets R, Kreutzer K, Plank C, Bissinger O. A novel nonviral gene delivery tool of BMP-2 for the reconstitution of critical-size bone defects in rats., J. Biomed. Mater. Res. A. 2016;104:2441–55. doi:10.1002/jbm.a.35773.

34 Ghanaati S. Non-cross-linked porcine-based collagen I-III membranes do not require high vascularization rates for their integration within the implantation bed: A paradigm shift, Acta Biomater. 2012;8:3061–72. doi:10.1016/j.actbio.2012.04.041.

35 Barbeck M, Unger RE, Booms P, Dohle E, Sader RA, Kirkpatrick CJ, Ghanaati S. Monocyte preseeding leads to an increased implant bed vascularization of biphasic calcium phosphate bone substitutes via vessel maturation, J. Biomed. Mater. Res. - Part A. 2016:1–8. doi:10.1002/jbm.a.35834.

36 Grassi F, Cattini L, Gambari L, Manferdini C, Piacentini A, Gabusi E, Facchini A, Lisignoli G. T cell subsets differently regulate osteogenic differentiation of human mesenchymal stromal cells in vitro., J. Tissue Eng. Regen. Med. 2016;10:305–14. doi:10.1002/term.1727.

37 Ono T, Okamoto K, Nakashima T, Nitta T, Hori S, Iwakura Y, Takayanagi H. IL-17-producing γδ T cells enhance bone regeneration, Nat. Commun. 2016;7. doi:10.1038/ncomms10928.

38 Croes M, Cumhur Öner F, van Neerven D, Sabir E, Kruyt MC, Blokhuis TJ, Dhert WJ, Alblas J. Proinflammatory T cells and IL-17 stimulate osteoblast differentiation. 2016. doi:10.1016/j.bone.2016.01.010.

39 Yang S, Ding W, Feng D, Gong H, Zhu D, Chen B, Chen J. Loss of B cell regulatory function is associated with delayed healing in patients with tibia fracture., APMIS. 2015;123:975–85. doi:10.1111/apm.12439.

40 Yelamali T, Saikrishna D. Role of platelet rich fibrin and platelet rich plasma in wound healing of extracted third molar sockets: a comparative study., J. Maxillofac. Oral Surg. 2015;14:410–6. doi:10.1007/s12663-014-0638-4.

41 Zhang Y, Tangl S, Huber CD, Lin Y, Qiu L, Rausch-Fan X. Effects of Choukroun's platelet-rich fibrin on bone regeneration in combination with deproteinized bovine bone mineral in maxillary sinus augmentation: A histological and histomorphometric study, J. Cranio-Maxillofacial Surg. 2012;40:321–8. doi:10.1016/j.jcms.2011.04.020.

42 Sharma A, Pradeep aR. Treatment of 3-Wall Intrabony Defects in Patients With Chronic Periodontitis With Autologous Platelet-Rich Fibrin: A Randomized Controlled Clinical Trial, J. Periodontol. 2011;82:1705–12. doi:10.1902/jop.2011.110075.

43 Eren G, Atilla G. Platelet-rich fibrin in the treatment of localized gingival recessions: a split-mouth randomized clinical trial, Clin. Oral Investig. 2013;18:1941–8. doi:10.1007/s00784-013-1170-5.

44 Mücke T, Krestan C, Mitchell D, Kirschke J, Wutzl A. Bisphosphonate and Medication-Related Osteonecrosis of the Jaw: A Review, Semin. Musculoskelet. Radiol. 2016;20:305–14. doi:10.1055/s-0036-1592367.

45 Soydan SS, Uckan U. Management of bisphosphonate-related osteonecrosis of the jaw with a platelet-rich fibrin membrane: Technical report, J. Oral Maxillofac. Surg. 2014;72:322–6. doi:10.1016/j.joms.2013.07.027.

46 Knighton DR, Ciresi KF, Fiegel VD, Austin LL, Butler EL. Classification and treatment of chronic nonhealing wounds. Successful treatment with autologous platelet-derived wound healing factors (PDWHF)., Ann. Surg. 204 (1986) 322–30. http://www.ncbi.nlm.nih.gov/pubmed/3753059 (accessed October 2, 2016).

47 Nacopoulos C, Dontas I, Lelovas P, Galanos A, Vesalas AM, Raptou P, Mastoris M, Chronopoulos E, Papaioannou N. Enhancement of bone regeneration with

the combination of platelet-rich fibrin and synthetic graft., J. Craniofac. Surg. 2014; 25:2164–8. doi:10.1097/SCS.0000000000001172.

48 Weber SC, Kauffman JI, Parise C, Weber SJ, Katz SD. Platelet-rich fibrin matrix in the management of arthroscopic repair of the rotator cuff: a prospective, randomized, double-blinded study., Am. J. Sports Med. 2013;41:263–70. doi:10.1177/0363546512467621.

4

Uses of Platelet Rich Fibrin in Regenerative Dentistry: An Overview

Richard J. Miron, Giovanni Zucchelli, and Joseph Choukroun

Abstract

It becomes very interesting to point out how rapidly platelet rich fibrin (PRF) has exponentially developed over the past half-decade. Despite its first publication in 2001, many clinicians (even those working within universities) had not yet discovered PRF until the years 2012-2014. It therefore took many clinicians by surprise that this relatively "new" regenerative modality could be utilized predictably for various clinical procedures in dentistry. Nowadays, over 500 scientific articles evaluating its use in vitro, in vivo, and clinically have documented its regenerative potential for the repair of either soft or hard tissues in the oral cavity. Some biomaterials have essentially been replaced by this completely natural modality to regenerate tissues at relatively no cost. Despite this, we continue to learn how PRF has a more pronounced effect on soft-tissue regeneration when compared to hard tissue formation. New surgical protocols have since been established and modified as we learn more regarding the biological potential of PRF. This chapter highlights the evolving discipline of platelet concentrates in regenerative dentistry and introduces its various clinical indications in an evidence-based manner.

Highlights

- PRF as a barrier membrane
- PRF as a plug during extraction socket healing
- PRF for soft-tissue root coverage
- PRF as a sole material in sinus elevation procedures
- PRF as a material for Schneiderian membrane repair
- PRF for periodontal regeneration

4.1 Introduction

Regenerative therapy in dentistry has been defined as the replacement and/or regeneration of oral tissues lost as a result of disease or injury. In dentistry, this endeavor is greatly complicated due to the nature of oral tissues being derived from both mesodermal and ectodermal germ layers. The regeneration of periodontal defects, for example, includes both mineralized tissues (cementum and alveolar bone) as well as soft tissues (the periodontal ligament) as well as the overlaying epithelial/connective tissues. Each of these is derived from various tissue origins. These cell populations are further gathered in complex fashions residing in specialized extracellular matrices that significantly complicates the regeneration of their tissues [1,2].

In the late 1990s, a variety of regenerative strategies was conducted investigating the use of recombinant growth factors and bioactive modifiers. These included recombinant

Platelet Rich Fibrin in Regenerative Dentistry: Biological Background and Clinical Indications, First Edition.
Edited by Richard J. Miron and Joseph Choukroun.

bone morphogenetic proteins (BMPs) for bone regeneration, and platelet-derived growth factors (PDGF) or enamel matrix derivate (EMD) for periodontal regeneration. Furthermore, other attempts were being investigated including barrier membranes for guided tissue/bone regeneration to selectively allow repopulation of tissues by creating a barrier between soft and hard tissues. Regenerative modalities were also concurrently being investigated in the field of maxillofacial surgery exploring the effects of platelet rich plasma (PRP). Shortly thereafter, a second-generation platelet concentrate was introduced with the working name platelet rich fibrin (PRF) [3].

Unlike PRP, the use of PRF did not use additional anti-coagulants including bovine thrombin or calcium chloride during initial blood collection, and therefore did not interfere with the natural wound healing process. Fibrin is formed during the coagulation cascade and incorporates many cytokines found in blood as well as various cell types including platelets and leukocytes [4–6]. Despite the numerous reported cytokines, growth factors, and cell types found in PRF, many clinicians are most interested to study its potential for clinical applications. Therefore, the purpose of this chapter is to provide an overview of the current literature on PRF with respect to its use in various aspects of regenerative dentistry. Favoritism was granted to randomized clinical studies investigating the regenerative potential of PRF when compared to standardized controls or well-established standards in dentistry. Below is a list of clinical situations in which PRF has most often been utilized.

4.2 Extraction socket management with PRF

To date, the most common use of PRF has been for the management of extraction sockets (Figure 4.1) [7–10]. The main reported advantage is that since PRF is a natural fibrin matrix, it can be utilized alone thereby replacing either a bone grafting material and/or barrier membrane. It may also be utilized as a barrier membrane in guided tissue/bone regenerative procedures. Since it does not necessitate the use of other biomaterials to cover an exposed flap, it offers the added advantage of being capable of being left exposed to the oral cavity without risk of infection. Furthermore, since PRF is 100% autologous, it does not cause a foreign body reaction and thereby speeds the natural wound healing process without generating an immune response. PRF is typically stabilized by simply using an X suture within the socket (Figure 4.1). Primary closure is not a necessary requirement. It has been shown that within a 3-month healing period, the fibrin matrix is transformed into new tissue: bone in the socket with overlaying soft tissue [11]. Recently a randomized clinical trial demonstrated that PRF alone could minimize dimensional changes post-extraction, thereby improving new bone formation in extraction sockets prior to implant placement [11]. Furthermore, due to the presence of immune cells (leukocytes) contained within PRF, reports now indicate in a split-mouth design study that by placing PRF into third molar extraction sockets, a nearly 10-fold decrease in osteomyelitis infections can be expected when compared to controls (natural healing) [9]. Chapter 5 is dedicated to the current literature on this topic, and the role of PRF for the management of extraction socket healing.

4.3 Sinus elevations procedures with PRF

Parallel to its use in extraction socket management, PRF has also been used for sinus elevation procedures (Figures 4.2 and 4.3). In these indications, it may fulfill the task of being utilized as a sole grafting material, can be further used for the repair of the Schneiderian membrane, and has also been utilized

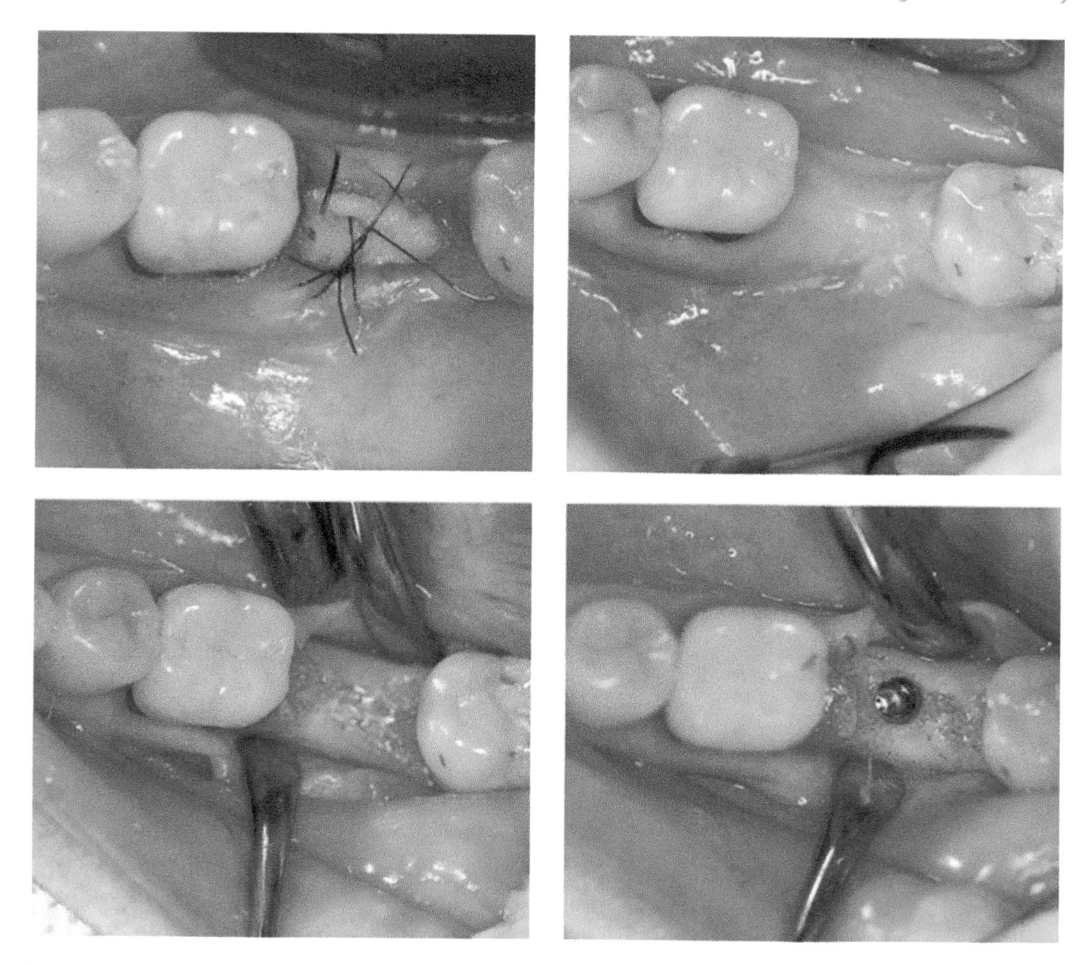

Figure 4.1 Extraction socket healing with PRF alone. PRF plugs were placed into an extraction site followed by a matrix suture. Following 3 months of healing, adequate new bone regeneration observed for the placement of a dental implant.

to close the window during the lateral sinus approach. While the success rate of the above mentioned procedures is reported very high [12–14], very few comparative studies have been reported. Others have shown additionally that PRF could be combined with a bone grafting material for sinus lift augmentation to decrease the overall healing time [15–18]. Chapter 6 and 7 focus on the complex anatomy of the sinus, and thereafter describes surgical protocols whereby PRF can be conservatively utilized successfully either alone or in combination with a bone grafting material.

4.4 Use of PRF for soft-tissue root coverage

One of the other most widespread uses for PRF in recent years has been for the management of root exposure (Figures 4.4–4.6). Since PRF has been shown to act more directly on soft-tissue regeneration, a variety of clinical studies have focused on the use of PRF during periodontal surgery of muco-gingival defects. Over a dozen randomized clinical studies have investigated the potential of PRF for soft-tissue management of Miller Class I and II defects [19–31]. It

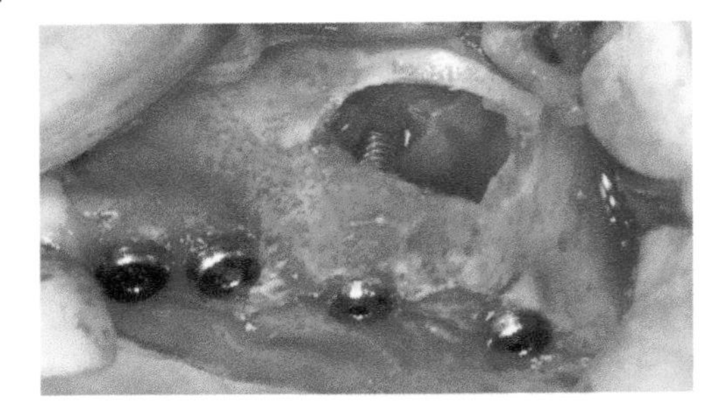

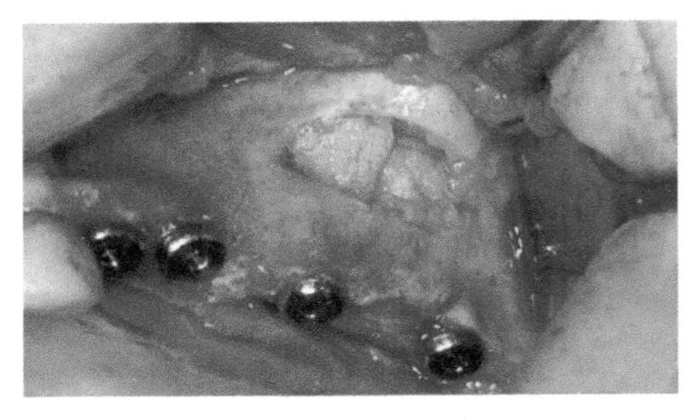

Figure 4.2 Sinus augmentation procedure performed with PRF utilized as a sole grafting material. Following implant placement, sinus cavity filled with PRF alone. Case performed by Dr. Alain Simonpieri.

is now known that PRF can be utilized in an evidence-based manner instead of connective tissue grafts in Miller Class I and 2 defects with a thick biotype where the use of PRF has been shown to improve vascularization, wound healing, and patient morbidity. Two reports have further demonstrated the advantages of PRF in pain management [25,26] with the potential to improve the epithelialization of palatal donor sites of CTGs [32]. Nevertheless, one of the limitations of PRF is the reported stability of the keratinized mucosa when compared to CTG over time [33]. Therefore, it remains a necessity to utilize CTG (either alone or in combination with PRF) for patients with thin tissue biotypes or in Miller Class III recessions where the recession extends past the mucogingival junction. Despite this, with proper patient selection, PRF has been shown equally as effective as CTG or utilizing a collagen-derived xenograft material for Miller Class I and II recession defects (Figures 4.7–4.9). It improves wound healing and speeds the re-vascularization of tissues with similar root coverage (%) without necessitating a second surgical site from the palate, or utilizing a foreign body collagen membrane. Chapter 8 highlights the randomized clinical trials and surgical techniques that have been modified to treat muco-gingival recessions.

4.5 Use of PRF for periodontal regeneration

Another area of research rapidly evolving is the use of PRF for periodontal regeneration of either intrabony or furcation defects. Since PRF can be utilized as a safe, natural method to repair tissues at low-cost, many investigators and clinicians in private office have attempted to use PRF for the regeneration of periodontal defects. Many randomized clinical trials are now available comparing PRF to open flap debridement alone or to other gold standards such as enamel matrix derivative (EMD) [34–44]. These reports have shown significant improvements in periodontal pocket depth reduction as well as clinical attachment level gains following regenerative periodontal therapy with PRF. Similar positive results have also been obtained for the treatment of furcation class II involvement [45–47]. The collected clinical trials now demonstrate that using PRF alone or combined with other biomaterials such as bone grafts leads to statistically superior results when compared to open flap debridement alone or bone grafting material alone. Chapter 9 highlights these findings and the essential need for further histological research to investigate periodontal regeneration in humans.

4.6 Use of PRF for the regeneration of soft tissues around implants

Similarly, an entire chapter is dedicated to the use of PRF around dental implants. A growing avenue of research has been the investigation and use of PRF for both

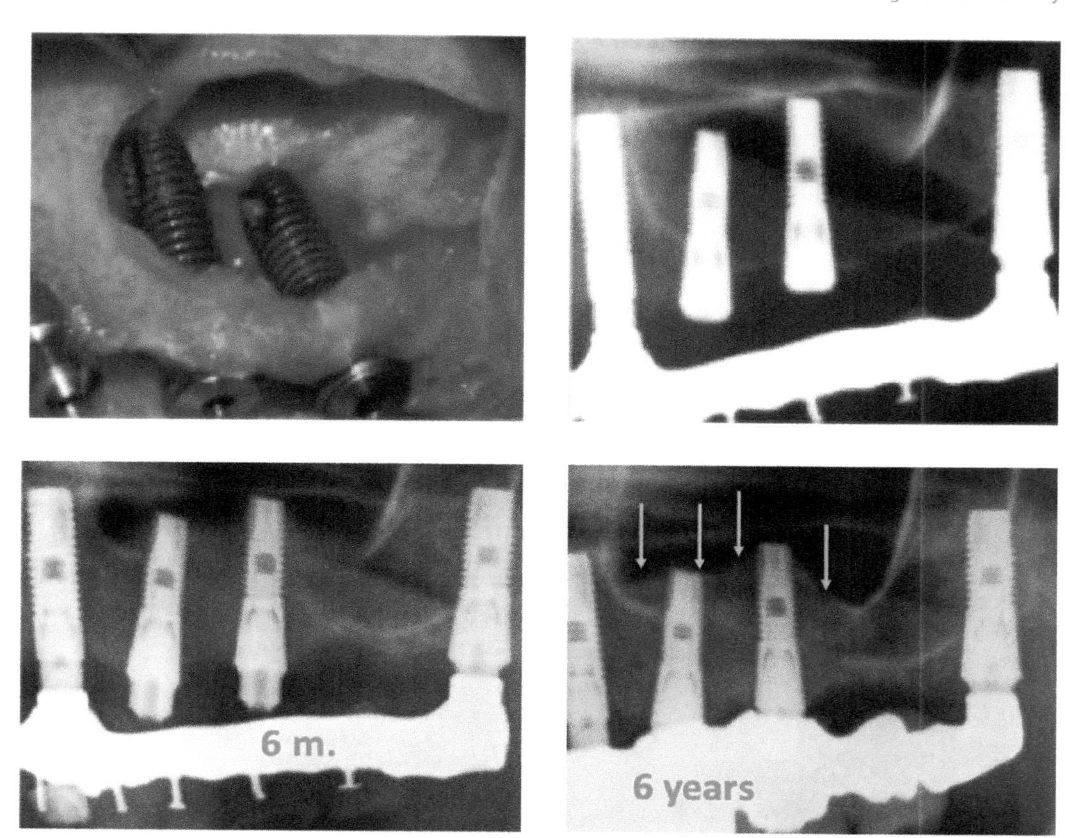

Figure 4.3 Sinus augmentation procedure performed with PRF utilized as a sole grafting material. Following implant placement, sinus cavity filled with PRF alone. X-rays taken at day 0, following 6 months, and following 6 years of healing. Notice the appreciable amount of new bone formation when PRF was utilized alone. Case performed by Dr. Alain Simonpieri.

improved osseointegration and soft-tissue healing around dental implants. In this context, PRF can be utilized quite conveniently as a low-cost biomaterial able to initiate the early healing of soft tissues around implants. While this area of clinical practice has become more common, limited to no available literature supporting its use exists, and the long-term evaluation of such protocols has seldom been investigated. Chapter 10 discusses this potential avenue of future research and the clinical concepts of utilizing PRF for dental implant osseointegration and/or soft-tissue augmentation around implants.

4.7 Use of PRF in guided bone regeneration

PRF has also frequently been utilized in combination with bone augmentation procedures. Reported advantages include an increased vascular supply as well as additional graft stability when PRF is utilized in combination with a bone grafting material. Despite this, very little research has addressed the true potential of PRF for bone regeneration procedures and much further research remains necessary. Chapter 11 provides an overview of the potential use of PRF during guided bone regeneration.

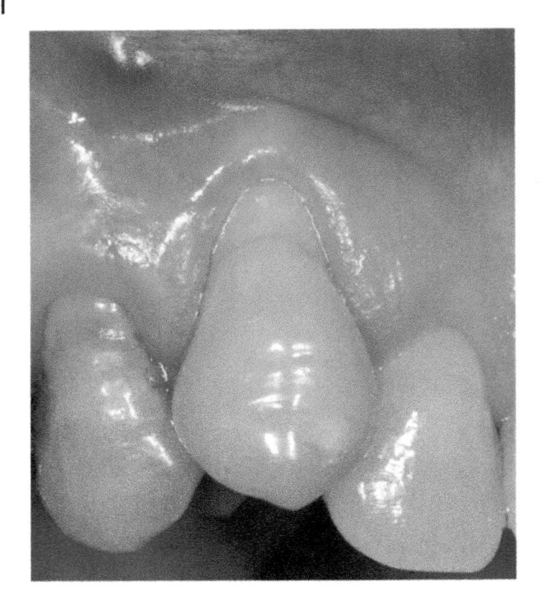
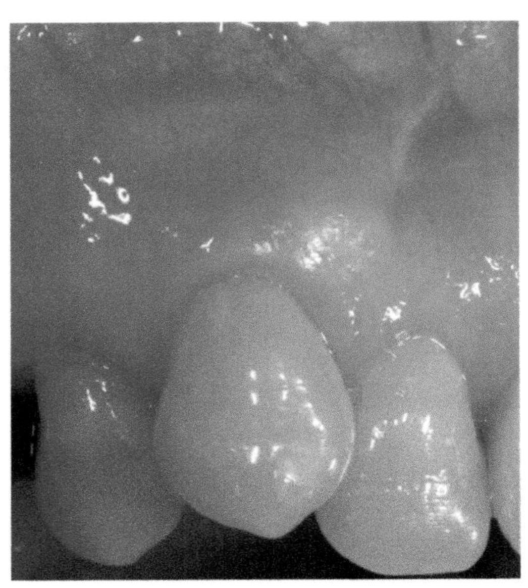

Figure 4.4 Gingival recession treated with PRF alone. Notice the final aesthetic outcomes as well as the increased vascularization when PRF is utilized. Case performed by Dr. Alexandre Aamir Aalam.

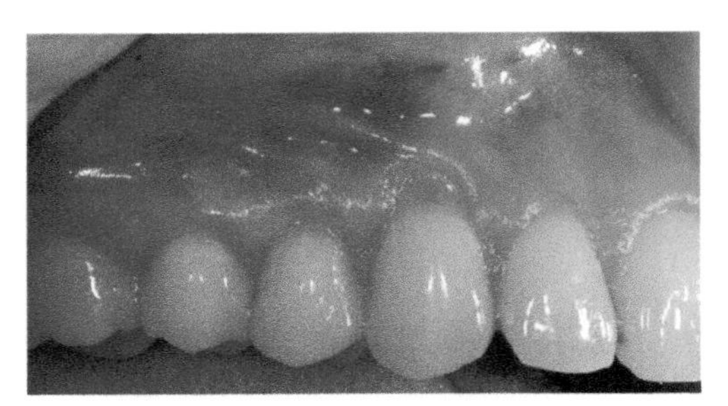
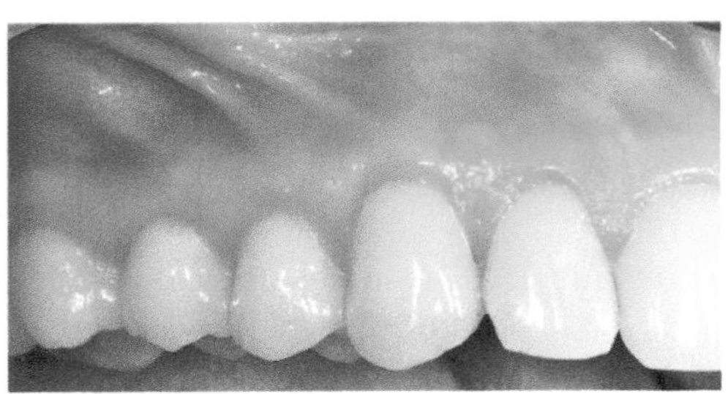

Figure 4.5 Multiple adjacent gingival recessions treated with PRF alone. Notice the final aesthetic outcomes with appreciable improvements in root coverage. Case performed by Dr. Alexandre Aamir Aalam.

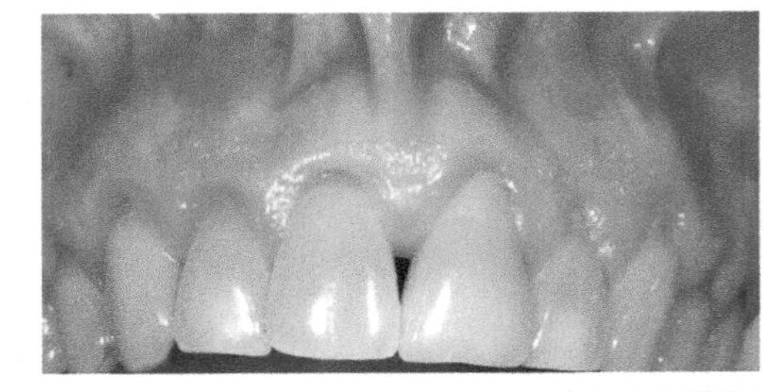
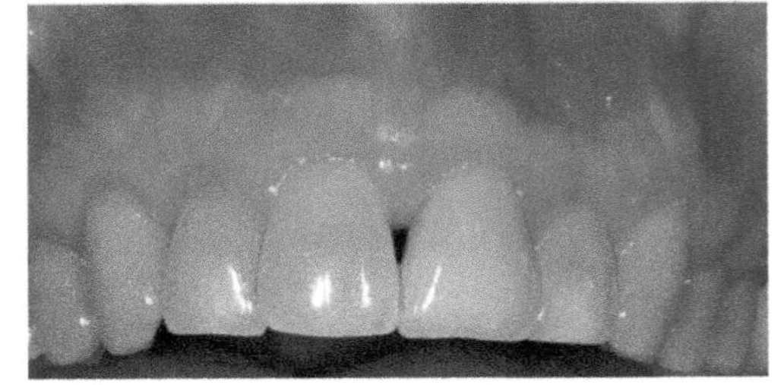

Figure 4.6 Multiple adjacent gingival recessions in the aesthetic zone treated with PRF alone. Notice the final aesthetic outcomes with appreciable improvements in root coverage. Case performed by Dr. Alexandre Aamir Aalam.

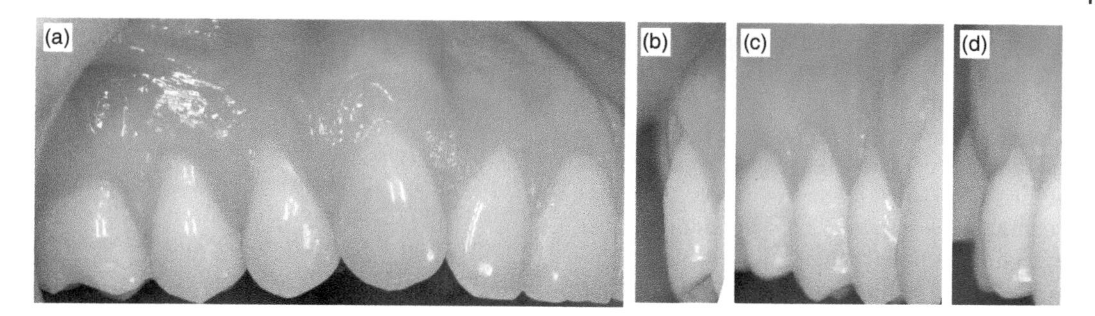

Figure 4.7 Multiple gingival recessions from canine to molar in the upper jaw. A) frontal view, B–D) lateral views (case performed by Dr. Giovanni Zucchelli)

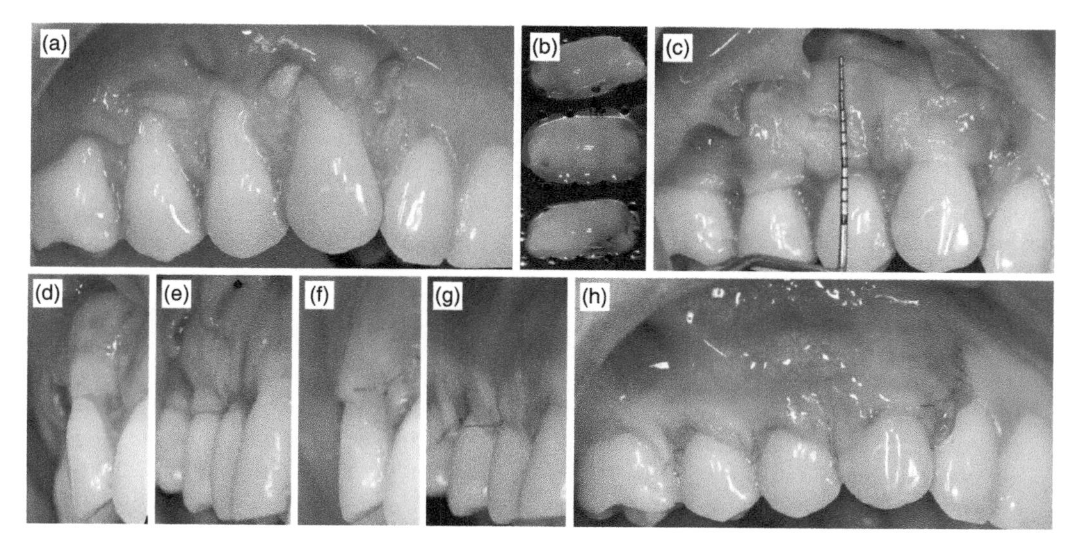

Figure 4.8 Surgical technique : A) A flap for multiple gingival recessions has been elevated with a split-full split thickness approach B) A-PRF prepared C) A-PRF has been applied to cover all teeth affected by gingival recessions. Multiple layers have been applied, D,E) lateral view showing the thickness of A-PRF material applied to the root exposures, F,G) lateral view showing the flap coronally advanced and covering completely the A-PRF material. H) frontal view showing the flap covering in excess all gingival recessions (case performed by Dr. Giovanni Zucchelli)

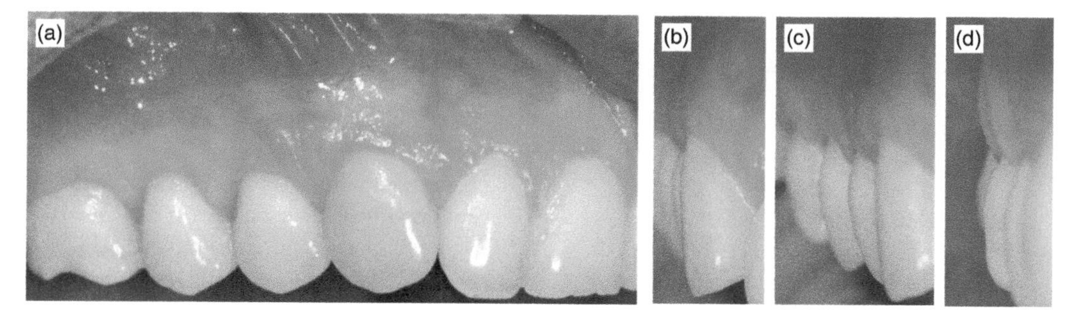

Figure 4.9 Six months follow-up. A) complete root coverage with increase in keratinized tissue height has been achieved in all treated gingival recessions B-D Lateral view showing the increase in gingival thickness at all teeth previously affected by gingival recessions (case performed by Dr. Giovanni Zucchelli)

4.8 Use of PRF in various other aspects of dentistry and medicine

The last chapters of this book are dedicated to the use of PRF in various other facets of dentistry and medicine where PRF has been seldom studied. This includes the use of an injectable PRF into osteoarthritic knees as a second-generation platelet concentrate without use of anti-coagulants. Furthermore, the development of injectable-PRF is also now utilized in the field of facial aesthetics in a similar manner to PRP (Chapter 13). Additionally, this technology is being studied in various other fields including temporomandibular joint disorders, pulp regeneration, treatment of osteonecrosis of the jaw, as well as in the field of orthopaedic medicine. These areas of research are briefly discussed in Chapters 14 and 15.

4.9 Conclusion

PRF has now been widely utilized in dentistry for a variety of procedures to help facilitate the repair and regeneration of oral tissues. In the early years, it was used as a scaffold matrix either alone or in combination with other biomaterials. Early attempts were made both successfully and unsuccessfully researching the benefits and limitations of this treatment modality in dentistry. Since then a great deal of information has been learned concerning the regenerative potential of PRF and its effect on various tissues in the oral cavity. The upcoming chapters will highlight the specific use of PRF across many procedures in clinical dentistry and more importantly discuss the evidence-based clinical trials leading to its recommended use.

References

1 Dangaria SJ, Ito Y, Walker C, Druzinsky R, Luan X, Diekwisch TG. Extracellular matrix-mediated differentiation of periodontal progenitor cells. Differentiation; research in biological diversity. 2009;78(2-3):79–90.
2 Hollander A, Macchiarini P, Gordijn B, Birchall M. The first stem cell-based tissue-engineered organ replacement: implications for regenerative medicine and society. Regenerative medicine. 2009; 4(2):147–8.
3 Choukroun J, Adda F, Schoeffler C, Vervelle A. Une opportunité en paro-implantologie: le PRF. Implantodontie. 2001;42(55):e62.
4 Kang YH, Jeon SH, Park JY, Chung JH, Choung YH, Choung HW, et al. Platelet-rich fibrin is a Bioscaffold and reservoir of growth factors for tissue regeneration. Tissue engineering Part A. 2011;17(3-4):349–59.
5 He L, Lin Y, Hu X, Zhang Y, Wu H. A comparative study of platelet-rich fibrin (PRF) and platelet-rich plasma (PRP) on the effect of proliferation and differentiation of rat osteoblasts in vitro. Oral surgery, oral medicine, oral pathology, oral radiology, and endodontics. 2009;108(5): 707–13.
6 Dohan Ehrenfest DM, Diss A, Odin G, Doglioli P, Hippolyte MP, Charrier JB. In vitro effects of Choukroun's PRF (platelet-rich fibrin) on human gingival fibroblasts, dermal prekeratinocytes, preadipocytes, and maxillofacial osteoblasts in primary cultures. Oral surgery, oral medicine, oral pathology, oral radiology, and endodontics. 2009;108(3): 341–52.
7 Girish Rao S, Bhat P, Nagesh KS, Rao GH, Mirle B, Kharbhari L, et al. Bone regeneration in extraction sockets with autologous platelet rich fibrin gel. Journal of maxillofacial and oral surgery. 2013; 12(1):11–6.
8 Suttapreyasri S, Leepong N. Influence of platelet-rich fibrin on alveolar ridge preservation. The Journal of craniofacial surgery. 2013;24(4):1088–94.

9 Hoaglin DR, Lines GK. Prevention of localized osteitis in mandibular third-molar sites using platelet-rich fibrin. International journal of dentistry. 2013;2013:875380.

10 Hauser F, Gaydarov N, Badoud I, Vazquez L, Bernard JP, Ammann P. Clinical and histological evaluation of postextraction platelet-rich fibrin socket filling: a prospective randomized controlled study. Implant dentistry. 2013;22(3): 295–303.

11 Temmerman A, Vandessel J, Castro A, Jacobs R, Teughels W, Pinto N, et al. The use of leucocyte and platelet-rich fibrin in socket management and ridge preservation: a split-mouth, randomized, controlled clinical trial. Journal of clinical periodontology. 2016.

12 Tajima N, Ohba S, Sawase T, Asahina I. Evaluation of sinus floor augmentation with simultaneous implant placement using platelet-rich fibrin as sole grafting material. The International journal of oral & maxillofacial implants. 2013;28(1): 77–83.

13 Mazor Z, Horowitz RA, Del Corso M, Prasad HS, Rohrer MD, Dohan Ehrenfest DM. Sinus floor augmentation with simultaneous implant placement using Choukroun's platelet-rich fibrin as the sole grafting material: a radiologic and histologic study at 6 months. J Periodontol. 2009;80(12):2056–64.

14 Simonpieri A, Choukroun J, Del Corso M, Sammartino G, Dohan Ehrenfest DM. Simultaneous sinus-lift and implantation using microthreaded implants and leukocyte- and platelet-rich fibrin as sole grafting material: a six-year experience. Implant dentistry. 2011;20(1): 2–12.

15 Inchingolo F, Tatullo M, Marrelli M, Inchingolo AM, Scacco S, Inchingolo AD, et al. Trial with Platelet-Rich Fibrin and Bio-Oss used as grafting materials in the treatment of the severe maxillar bone atrophy: clinical and radiological evaluations. European review for medical and pharmacological sciences. 2010; 14(12):1075–84.

16 Tatullo M, Marrelli M, Cassetta M, Pacifici A, Stefanelli LV, Scacco S, et al. Platelet Rich Fibrin (P.R.F.) in reconstructive surgery of atrophied maxillary bones: clinical and histological evaluations. International journal of medical sciences. 2012;9(10):872–80.

17 Zhang Y, Tangl S, Huber CD, Lin Y, Qiu L, Rausch-Fan X. Effects of Choukroun's platelet-rich fibrin on bone regeneration in combination with deproteinized bovine bone mineral in maxillary sinus augmentation: a histological and histomorphometric study. Journal of cranio-maxillo-facial surgery : official publication of the European Association for Cranio-Maxillo-Facial Surgery. 2012;40(4):321–8.

18 Choukroun J, Diss A, Simonpieri A, Girard MO, Schoeffler C, Dohan SL, et al. Platelet-rich fibrin (PRF): a second-generation platelet concentrate. Part V: histologic evaluations of PRF effects on bone allograft maturation in sinus lift. Oral surgery, oral medicine, oral pathology, oral radiology, and endodontics. 2006; 101(3):299–303.

19 Agarwal SK, Jhingran R, Bains VK, Srivastava R, Madan R, Rizvi I. Patient-centered evaluation of microsurgical management of gingival recession using coronally advanced flap with platelet-rich fibrin or amnion membrane: A comparative analysis. European journal of dentistry. 2016; 10(1):121–33.

20 Aleksic Z, Jankovic S, Dimitrijevic B, Divnic-Resnik T, Milinkovic I, Lekovic V. [The use of platelet-rich fibrin membrane in gingival recession treatment]. Srpski arhiv za celokupno lekarstvo. 2010;138(1-2):11–8.

21 Aroca S, Keglevich T, Barbieri B, Gera I, Etienne D. Clinical evaluation of a modified coronally advanced flap alone or in combination with a platelet-rich fibrin membrane for the treatment of adjacent

multiple gingival recessions: a 6-month study. Journal of periodontology. 2009;80(2):244–52.
22 Dogan SB, Dede FO, Balli U, Atalay EN, Durmuslar MC. Concentrated growth factor in the treatment of adjacent multiple gingival recessions: a split-mouth randomized clinical trial. Journal of clinical periodontology. 2015;42(9):868–75.
23 Eren G, Atilla G. Platelet-rich fibrin in the treatment of localized gingival recessions: a split-mouth randomized clinical trial. Clinical oral investigations. 2014;18(8): 1941–8.
24 Gupta S, Banthia R, Singh P, Banthia P, Raje S, Aggarwal N. Clinical evaluation and comparison of the efficacy of coronally advanced flap alone and in combination with platelet rich fibrin membrane in the treatment of Miller Class I and II gingival recessions. Contemporary clinical dentistry. 2015;6(2):153–60.
25 Jankovic S, Aleksic Z, Klokkevold P, Lekovic V, Dimitrijevic B, Kenney EB, et al. Use of platelet-rich fibrin membrane following treatment of gingival recession: a randomized clinical trial. The International journal of periodontics & restorative dentistry. 2012;32(2):e41–50.
26 Jankovic S, Aleksic Z, Milinkovic I, Dimitrijevic B. The coronally advanced flap in combination with platelet-rich fibrin (PRF) and enamel matrix derivative in the treatment of gingival recession: a comparative study. The European journal of esthetic dentistry : official journal of the European Academy of Esthetic Dentistry. 2010;5(3):260–73.
27 Keceli HG, Kamak G, Erdemir EO, Evginer MS, Dolgun A. The Adjunctive Effect of Platelet-Rich Fibrin to Connective Tissue Graft in the Treatment of Buccal Recession Defects: Results of a Randomized, Parallel-Group Controlled Trial. Journal of periodontology. 2015;86(11):1221–30.
28 Padma R, Shilpa A, Kumar PA, Nagasri M, Kumar C, Sreedhar A. A split mouth randomized controlled study to evaluate the adjunctive effect of platelet-rich fibrin to coronally advanced flap in Miller's class-I and II recession defects. Journal of Indian Society of Periodontology. 2013;17(5):631–6.
29 Rajaram V, Thyegarajan R, Balachandran A, Aari G, Kanakamedala A. Platelet Rich Fibrin in double lateral sliding bridge flap procedure for gingival recession coverage: An original study. Journal of Indian Society of Periodontology. 2015;19(6):665–70.
30 Thamaraiselvan M, Elavarasu S, Thangakumaran S, Gadagi JS, Arthie T. Comparative clinical evaluation of coronally advanced flap with or without platelet rich fibrin membrane in the treatment of isolated gingival recession. Journal of Indian Society of Periodontology. 2015;19(1):66–71.
31 Tunaliota M, Ozdemir H, Arabaciota T, Gurbuzer B, Pikdoken L, Firatli E. Clinical evaluation of autologous platelet-rich fibrin in the treatment of multiple adjacent gingival recession defects: a 12-month study. The International journal of periodontics & restorative dentistry. 2015;35(1):105–14.
32 Femminella B, Iaconi MC, Di Tullio M, Romano L, Sinjari B, D'Arcangelo C, et al. Clinical Comparison of Platelet-Rich Fibrin and a Gelatin Sponge in the Management of Palatal Wounds After Epithelialized Free Gingival Graft Harvest: A Randomized Clinical Trial. Journal of periodontology. 2016;87(2):103–13.
33 Moraschini V, Barboza Edos S. Use of Platelet-Rich Fibrin Membrane in the Treatment of Gingival Recession: A Systematic Review and Meta-Analysis. Journal of periodontology. 2016;87(3): 281–90.
34 Agarwal A, Gupta ND, Jain A. Platelet rich fibrin combined with decalcified freeze-dried bone allograft for the treatment of human intrabony periodontal defects: a randomized split mouth clinical trail. Acta odontologica Scandinavica. 2016;74(1):36–43.
35 Ajwani H, Shetty S, Gopalakrishnan D, Kathariya R, Kulloli A, Dolas RS, et al.

Comparative evaluation of platelet-rich fibrin biomaterial and open flap debridement in the treatment of two and three wall intrabony defects. Journal of international oral health : JIOH. 2015; 7(4):32–7.

36 Elgendy EA, Abo Shady TE. Clinical and radiographic evaluation of nanocrystalline hydroxyapatite with or without platelet-rich fibrin membrane in the treatment of periodontal intrabony defects. Journal of Indian Society of Periodontology. 2015;19(1):61–5.

37 Joseph VR, Sam G, Amol NV. Clinical evaluation of autologous platelet rich fibrin in horizontal alveolar bony defects. Journal of clinical and diagnostic research : JCDR. 2014;8(11):Zc43–7.

38 Panda S, Sankari M, Satpathy A, Jayakumar D, Mozzati M, Mortellaro C, et al. Adjunctive Effect of Autologus Platelet-Rich Fibrin to Barrier Membrane in the Treatment of Periodontal Intrabony Defects. The Journal of craniofacial surgery. 2016;27(3):691–6.

39 Pradeep AR, Nagpal K, Karvekar S, Patnaik K, Naik SB, Guruprasad CN. Platelet-rich fibrin with 1% metformin for the treatment of intrabony defects in chronic periodontitis: a randomized controlled clinical trial. Journal of periodontology. 2015;86(6):729–37.

40 Pradeep AR, Rao NS, Agarwal E, Bajaj P, Kumari M, Naik SB. Comparative evaluation of autologous platelet-rich fibrin and platelet-rich plasma in the treatment of 3-wall intrabony defects in chronic periodontitis: a randomized controlled clinical trial. J Periodontol. 2012;83(12): 1499–507.

41 Shah M, Patel J, Dave D, Shah S. Comparative evaluation of platelet-rich fibrin with demineralized freeze-dried bone allograft in periodontal infrabony defects: A randomized controlled clinical study. Journal of Indian Society of Periodontology. 2015;19(1):56–60.

42 Thorat M, Pradeep AR, Pallavi B. Clinical effect of autologous platelet-rich fibrin in the treatment of intra-bony defects: a controlled clinical trial. J Clin Periodontol. 2011;38(10):925–32.

43 Pradeep AR, Bajaj P, Rao NS, Agarwal E, Naik SB. Platelet-Rich Fibrin Combined With a Porous Hydroxyapatite Graft for the Treatment of Three-Wall Intrabony Defects in Chronic Periodontitis: A Randomized Controlled Clinical Trial. J Periodontol. 2012.

44 Sharma A, Pradeep AR. Treatment of 3-wall intrabony defects in patients with chronic periodontitis with autologous platelet-rich fibrin: a randomized controlled clinical trial. Journal of periodontology. 2011;82(12):1705–12.

45 Sharma A, Pradeep AR. Autologous platelet-rich fibrin in the treatment of mandibular degree II furcation defects: a randomized clinical trial. Journal of periodontology. 2011;82(10):1396–403.

46 Bajaj P, Pradeep AR, Agarwal E, Rao NS, Naik SB, Priyanka N, et al. Comparative evaluation of autologous platelet-rich fibrin and platelet-rich plasma in the treatment of mandibular degree II furcation defects: a randomized controlled clinical trial. Journal of periodontal research. 2013.

47 Pradeep AR, Karvekar S, Nagpal K, Patnaik K, Raju A, Singh P. Rosuvastatin 1.2 mg In Situ Gel Combined With 1:1 Mixture of Autologous Platelet-Rich Fibrin and Porous Hydroxyapatite Bone Graft in Surgical Treatment of Mandibular Class II Furcation Defects: A Randomized Clinical Control Trial. Journal of periodontology. 2016;87(1):5–13.

5

Use of Platelet Rich Fibrin for the Management of Extraction Sockets: Biological Basis and Clinical Relevance

Richard J. Miron and Jonathan Du Toit

Abstract

The use of platelet rich fibrin (PRF) has been most frequently utilized for the management of extraction sockets. Simply put, most clinician's first experience the wound healing properties and benefits of utilizing PRF during routine extraction socket healing. Interestingly, research over the past decade has shown that the main cause accelerating dimensional changes post-extraction is mainly due to the lack of blood supply resulting from tooth loss. In alveolar bone, the periodontal ligament contains the majority of blood supply and once removed, a rapid and drastic loss of bone around missing teeth is encountered, most notably on the thin facial and buccal bony walls. In this chapter, we outline the numerous currently available treatment options on the market and discuss their advantages and limitations. We then point to the prominent effects of utilizing PRF either as a sole grafting material or in combination with bone grafts to limit dimensional changes post-extraction. We provide evidence from randomized clinical trials and human histological samples describing the use of PRF for the management of extraction sockets.

Highlights

- Why does bone loss occur so rapidly following tooth extraction?
- How much dimensional change should we expect after tooth loss?
- What are the treatment options currently available on the market?
- How can we preserve alveolar bone following tooth loss?
- Clinical uses and indications of PRF for the management of extraction sockets—what are the advantages?
- What are the results from randomized clinical trials examining PRF as a sole biomaterial for the management of extraction sockets?
- Is there histological evidence supporting PRF as a sole biomaterial for extraction socket healing?

5.1 Introduction

It is well known that following tooth extraction, marked alterations in the bone-alveolar structure occurs [1,2]. In fact, one of the first publications on this topic dates back over 50 years published in the Australian Dental Journal [3]. It was found that specifically in the maxilla, natural healing following tooth extraction involved a great deal of bone loss and subsequent dimensional changes. With

Platelet Rich Fibrin in Regenerative Dentistry: Biological Background and Clinical Indications, First Edition.
Edited by Richard J. Miron and Joseph Choukroun.

the numerous advancements that have been made in implant dentistry over the past several decades, it becomes essential to better understand and characterize these changes with the aim of minimizing bone loss. As such, a great deal of research utilizing various bone grafts, barrier membranes, collagen sponges, and biological agents has been employed to overcome changes in bone morphology resulting from tooth loss.

Moreover, while we have learned that socket management can limit dimensional changes, to date no single therapy can predictably and systematically prevent change completely [4]. Furthermore, without a consistent and constant blood supply, bone cannot exist [5]. While bone-grafting materials are most commonly utilized and certainly limit dimensional changes post-extraction, a resulting 0.5–1 mm horizontal and vertical loss occurs mainly on the buccal surface [4]. This is primarily due to a drastic loss in blood supply resulting from extraction of the periodontal ligament, a tissue responsible for up to 90% of the blood supply found in alveolar bone [6].

Platelet concentrates have a complex history of development and reported research. As mentioned in Chapter 1, their first use dates back to the 1980s and 1990s where platelet rich plasma (PRP) was first utilized in regenerative dentistry specifically due to its ability to deliver supra-physiological doses of blood-derived growth factors capable of enhancing wound healing. They include, however, anti-coagulant additives; their main disadvantage. By preventing coagulation and fibrin clot formation, its use in secondary intention wound healing such as during extraction socket management was therefore considered limited.

More recently, a second-generation platelet concentrate has been investigated as a potential biomaterial capable of further minimizing dimensional changes [7]. PRF was developed with more ideal properties facilitating tissue regeneration and wound healing due to its ability to form a clot during extraction socket healing [7]. In fact, the great majority of clinicians first experience the use of PRF for extraction socket healing. This chapter aims to summarize the currently available literature describing the use of PRF for this topic. We first present the biological background of bone loss after extraction using studies characterizing dimensional changes that occur following tooth loss from both animal and human studies. Thereafter, we provide an overview of the currently available treatment options. To conclude, we summarize the clinical studies examining the use of PRF for the management of extraction sites.

5.2 Natural dimensional changes occurring post-extraction

Dimensional changes following tooth extraction remains inevitable. For these reasons, a variety of biomaterials have been developed and tested for their ability to minimize change that results following extraction. As mentioned in the introduction, over 50 years ago, Dr. Johnson began his studies to investigate the changes that were occurring in alveolar bone following tooth extraction [3]. While these preliminary findings were scarce, it fueled a great deal of research into this topic over the following decades to investigate more precisely the reasons and mechanisms for bone loss after tooth extraction.

Possibly the most-often cited pre-clinical study on alveolar bone remodeling was conducted by Auraujo and Lindhe in 2005. The greatest value to their research was the ability to investigate dimensional changes via histological assessment post-extraction in animals and not via manual probing or by measuring via ridge calipers [8]. Using a canine model, they showed convincingly that bone loss following tooth extraction occurred rapidly within an 8-week healing period (Figure 5.1). Within 2 weeks post-extraction, it was observed that a high number of bone-resorbing multi-nucleated osteoclasts were found on the buccal bone surface with lacunae (Figure 5.2) [8]. This was one of the first histological documentations

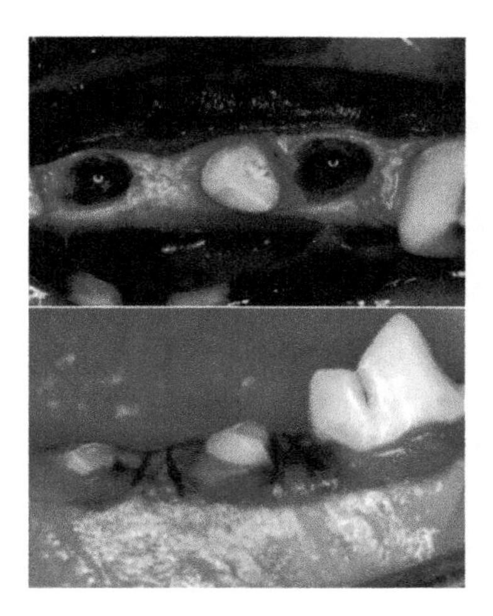

Aim of study: Characterize dimensional changes following tooth extraction after a 1, 2, 4 and 8 week healing period

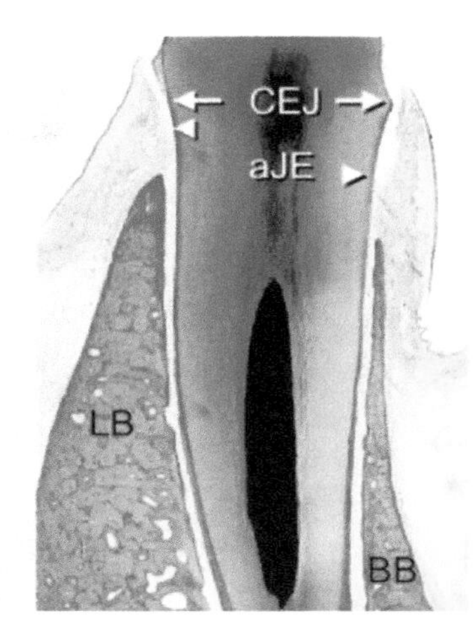

Figure 5.1 Clinical view of the experimental sites immediately after root extraction and placement of sutures (Upper left image). Clinical photograph illustrating the extraction sockets—distal roots—of the third and fourth mandibular pre-molars immediately after root extraction. Note that the buccal–lingual width of the extraction socket of the fourth pre-molar is wider than that of the third pre-molar (Bottom left Image). Histological assessment of a tooth prior to tooth extraction. Buccal–lingual section representing an involved tooth site. Note that the lingual bone crest is closer to the CEJ (arrows) at the lingual than at the buccal aspect of the tooth. The apical level (aJE) of the junctional epithelium (arrowheads). BB, buccal bone wall; LB, lingual bone wall; CEJ, cemento-enamel junction. Toluidine blue staining; original magnification × 16. Adapted from Araujo *et al.* 2005 [36]. Reproduced with permission of John Wiley & Sons.

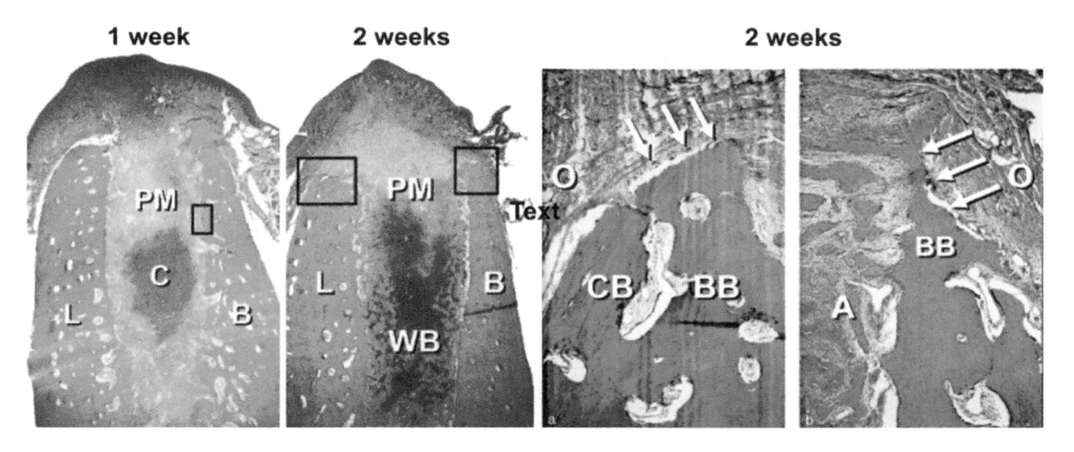

Figure 5.2 **A)** Overview of the extraction site after one and two weeks of healing. Note the large amounts of provisional matrix and, in the center of the socket, remaining blood clot. BC, blood clot, B, buccal; L, lingual; PM, provisional matrix. H&E staining; original magnification × 16. **B)** One week of healing. The crestal region of the lingual (a) and buccal (b) walls. The buccal bone crest is made exclusively of bundle bone while the lingual crest is comprised of a mixture of cortical bone and bundle bone. Note the presence of osteoclasts in the crestal regions of both walls (arrows). A, inner surface of the bone wall; BB, bundle bone; CB, cortical bone; O, outer surface of the bone wall; arrows, osteoclasts. H&E staining; original magnification × 50. Adapted from Araujo *et al.* 2005 [36]. Reproduced with permission of John Wiley & Sons.

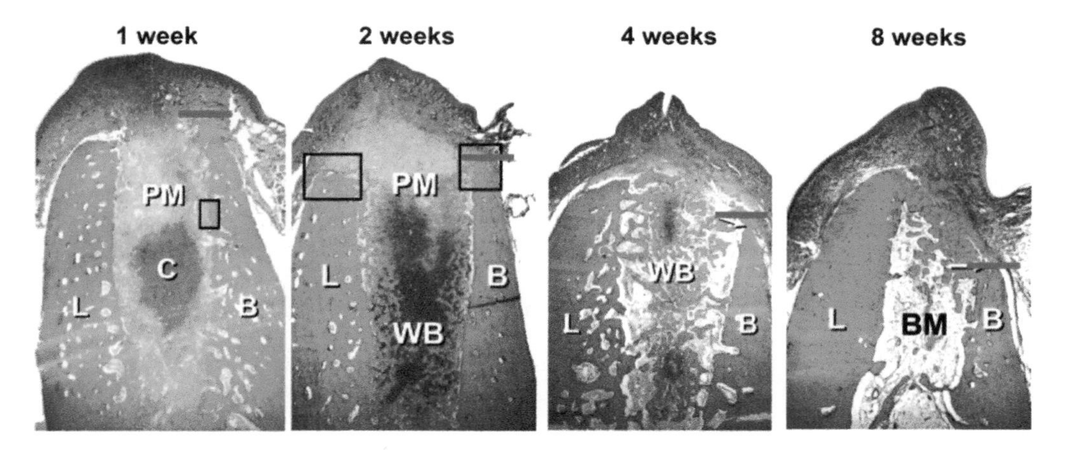

Figure 5.3 Overview of the extraction site after one, two, four, and eight weeks of healing. Note the large amount of provisional matrix and, in the center of the socket, remaining blood clot. BC, blood clot, B, buccal; L, lingual; PM, provisional matrix. H&E staining; original magnification × 16. Blue lines represent the vertical loss on the buccal surfaces. Adapted from Araujo *et al.* 2005 [36]. Reproduced with permission of John Wiley & Sons.

of the events following tooth loss in a controlled time-dependent manner. Such studies are not deemed possible in humans due to the inability to harvest tissue blocks from human patients. In conclusion, it was found that within 8 weeks post-extraction, a marked loss of bone was observed, most notably on the thin buccal surface (Figure 5.3) [8]. The authors state that the resorption of the buccal/lingual walls occurred in two overlapping phases including phase 1: "The bundle bone was resorbed and replaced with woven bone." And phase 2 "resorption that occurred from the outer surfaces of both bone walls." The hypothesized reason for fast bone resorption on the buccal bone wall was mainly due to the fact it is comprised solely of bundle bone and therefore modelling resulted in substantial vertical reduction of the buccal crest [8]. Scala and coworkers in 2014 carried out a similar study, looking at the socket healing patterns in monkeys [9]. The primate model may be more relevant since it bears more resemblance to humans. In that study, by day 30 half of the socket's bundle bone was lost and by day 90 greater than 90% was lost [9].

Interestingly, the advancements that have been made more recently in the field of cone-beam computed tomography (CBCT) have made possible the visualization of dimensional changes in humans by superimposing CBCT images from various healing periods (Figure 5.4). Utilizing this technology, Chappuis *et al.* investigated the dimensional changes occurring post-extraction following an 8-week healing period that corresponds with early implant placement [10]. The aims of this research were 1) to characterize the thickness and size of the buccal bone wall specifically in the aesthetic zone and 2) to evaluate both horizontal and vertical dimensional changes that were occurring following an 8-week healing period (Figure 5.5). It was found that 69% of human cases presented with a buccal wall surface thinner than 1 mm in thickness (Figure 5.5). Furthermore, it was observed that after an 8 week healing period, an average vertical bone loss of 5.2 mm was reported [10]. These changes were deemed to be 2.5 to 3 times more severe than those previously reported by Araujo and Lindhe and this was hypothesized to be caused by the animal's ability to regenerate at higher rates, as well as being utilized at surgery at a young age. Nevertheless, Figure 5.6 demonstrates the marked impact of tooth extraction on wound healing after only an 8-week period thereby requiring substantial new bone regeneration prior to implant placement in such cases.

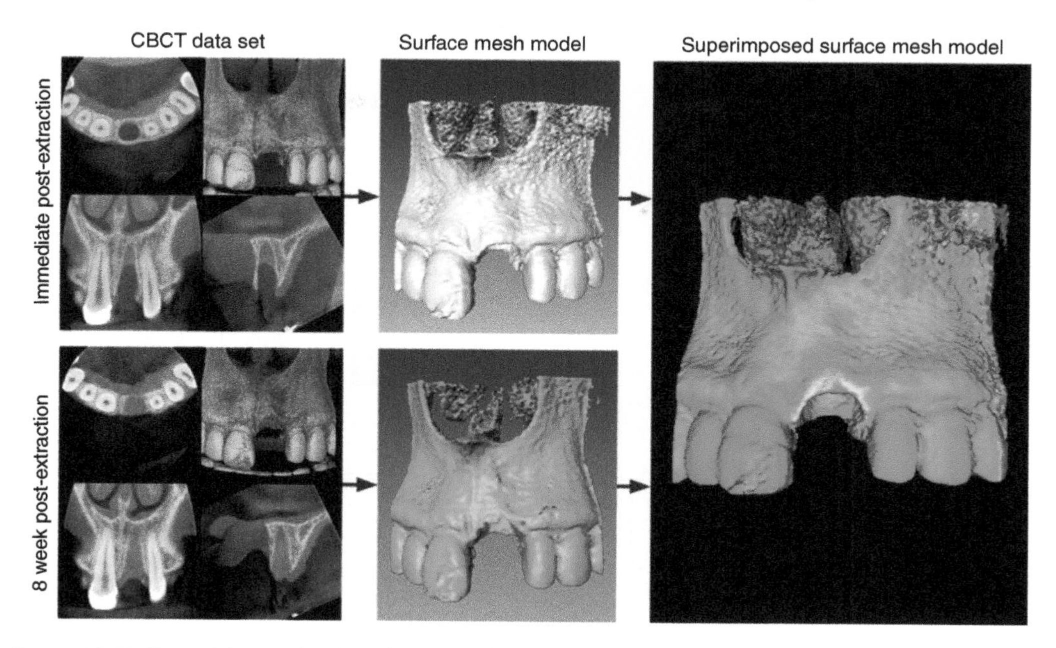

Figure 5.4 Radiographic examination. The DICOM files of the obtained CBCT datasets, immediately post-extraction and following eight weeks of healing, were converted into a surface mesh model with digital imaging software. The two-surface mesh models were superimposed and rigidly aligned with anatomical landmarks. The distance between the two- surface meshes was presented as color-coded figures to identify zones of facial bone resorption. Source: Chappuis *et al.* 2013 [10]. Reproduced with permission of SAGE Publications.

5.3 Conventional socket grafting and ridge preservation techniques

Over the past 10 years, much research has focused on minimizing the dimensional changes occurring post-extraction by utilizing a variety of bone biomaterials including but not limited to barrier membranes [11–14], bone grafting materials [12,14–16], and growth factor therapies [17–20]. The most commonly utilized materials are bone grafts classified into four categories including autogenous bone, allografts, xenografts, and various synthetically fabricated alloplasts (Figures 5.7 and 5.8). Furthermore, collagen barrier membranes have frequently been utilized to prevent soft-tissue infiltration favoring new bone formation (Figure 5.9) [21]. Despite these numerous attempts to prevent dimensional changes following extraction, no single therapy to date can predictably avoid at least some bone loss that occurs following tooth extraction [4,22–26]. Various systematic reviews have consistently shown that despite the technique utilized, dimensional changes in the 0.5 to 1 mm range are to be expected. Furthermore, over the past decade, research has also investigated the effect of raising a flap during tooth extraction. Since the periodontal ligament (the main source of blood supply) is removed following tooth loss, it has been the focus of much further research to evaluate the effect of raising a muco-periosteal flap (and thereby removing the blood supply from the periosteum) [27]. Today it is highly recommended that tooth extraction be performed as atraumatically as possible without the use of flap elevation. Various surgical techniques and instruments have been made available with this concept in mind.

Recently Morjaria *et al.* performed a systematic review of randomized controlled trials on bone healing after tooth extraction

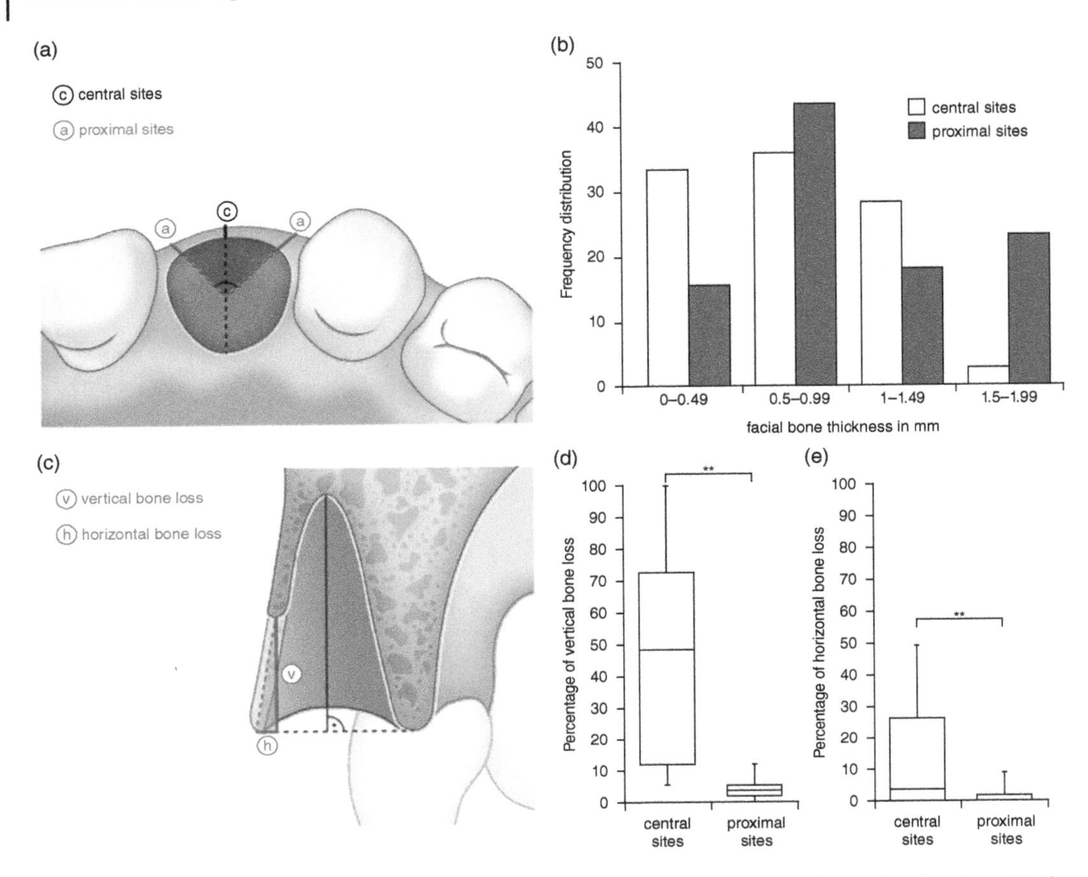

Figure 5.5 Baseline measurements and dimensional and vertical bone loss after eight weeks of healing. (A) The analysis was performed in central (c) and proximal sites (a) oriented at a 45° angle with the tooth axis as a reference. (B) Frequency distribution of facial bone wall thickness in central and proximal sites. (C) A horizontal reference line was traced connecting the facial and palatal bone wall for standardized measurements. The point-to-point distance between the two surfaces meshes with the respective angle to the reference line was obtained for each sample, and the vertical and horizontal bone losses were calculated accordingly. (D) Percentage of vertical bone loss in central and proximal sites. (E) Percentage of horizontal bone loss in central and proximal sites. $^{**}p < .0001$. Source: Chappuis *et al.* 2013 [10]. Reproduced with permission of SAGE Publications.

with or without an intervention [4]. Of the initial 2861 abstracts searched, 42 publications were kept and investigated for dimensional changes using control (no intervention), a graft and/or barrier membrane. In conclusion, it was found that limited data regarding the effectiveness of alveolar ridge preservation therapies were found when various modalities were compared, but all were superior to blank controls. The authors found that overall the socket intervention therapies did reduce alveolar ridge dimensional changes post-extraction, but were unable to prevent resorption [4]. In agreement with these findings, MacBeth *et al.* published a similar article in 2016 investigating two focused questions [28]. First, they studied the effect of alveolar ridge preservation on linear and volumetric alveolar site dimensions, keratinized measurements, histological characteristics, and patient-based outcomes when compared to unassisted socket healing. Secondly, they investigated the size effect of these outcomes in three different types of interventions including 1) guided bone regeneration, 2) socket grafting, and

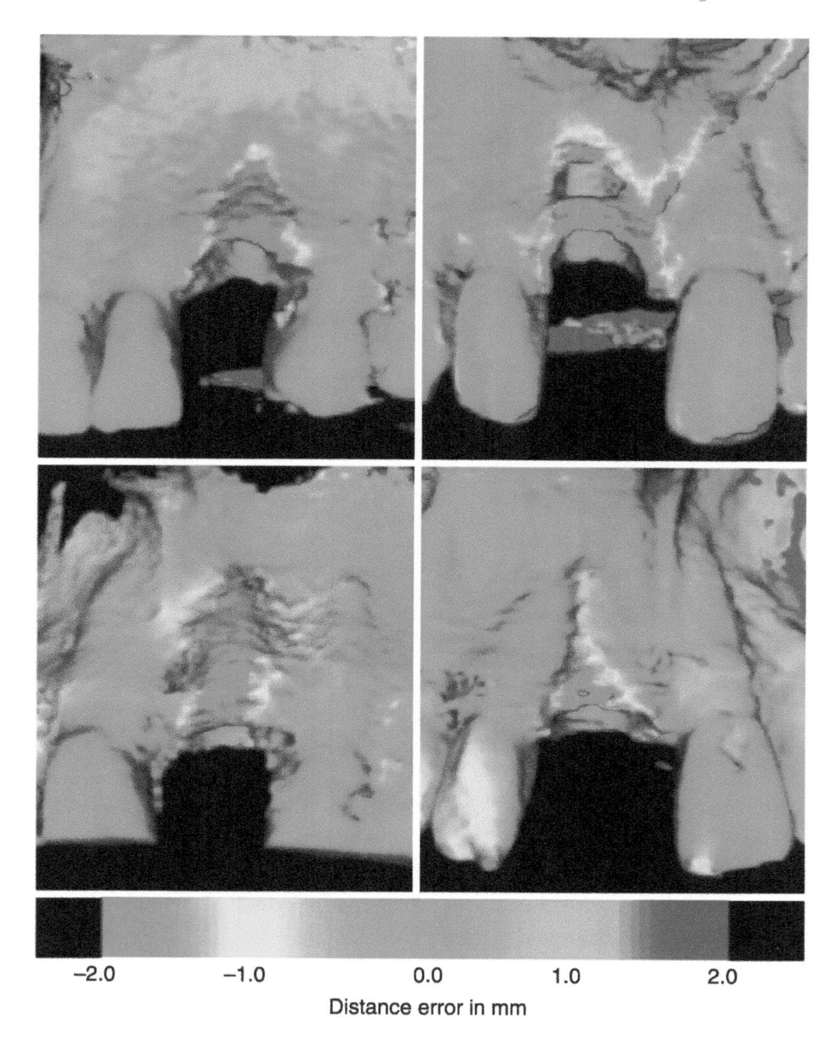

Figure 5.6 Characteristic bone resorption patterns. A thin-wall phenotype showed a facial bone wall thickness of ≤1 mm and revealed a progressive bone resorption pattern after eight weeks of healing. Source: Chappuis *et al.* 2013 [10]. Reproduced with permission of SAGE Publications.

3) socket seal [28]. Based on their findings, alveolar ridge preservation led to a significant reduction in the vertical bone dimensional change following tooth extraction when compared to unassisted socket healing. The reduction in horizontal alveolar bone dimensional change was found to be variable. No evidence was identified to clearly indicate the superior impact of a type of the various interventions (GBR, socket filler, and socket seal) on bone dimensional preservation, bone formation, keratinized tissue dimensions, and patient complications [28]. Therefore, and in summary, to date, two key findings have been revealed from the large number of studies investigating dimensional changes post-extraction:

1. To date, there are currently no available options to completely prevent dimensional changes following tooth extraction. Resorption of bundle bone will occur regardless of the alveolar ridge preservation technique utilized.

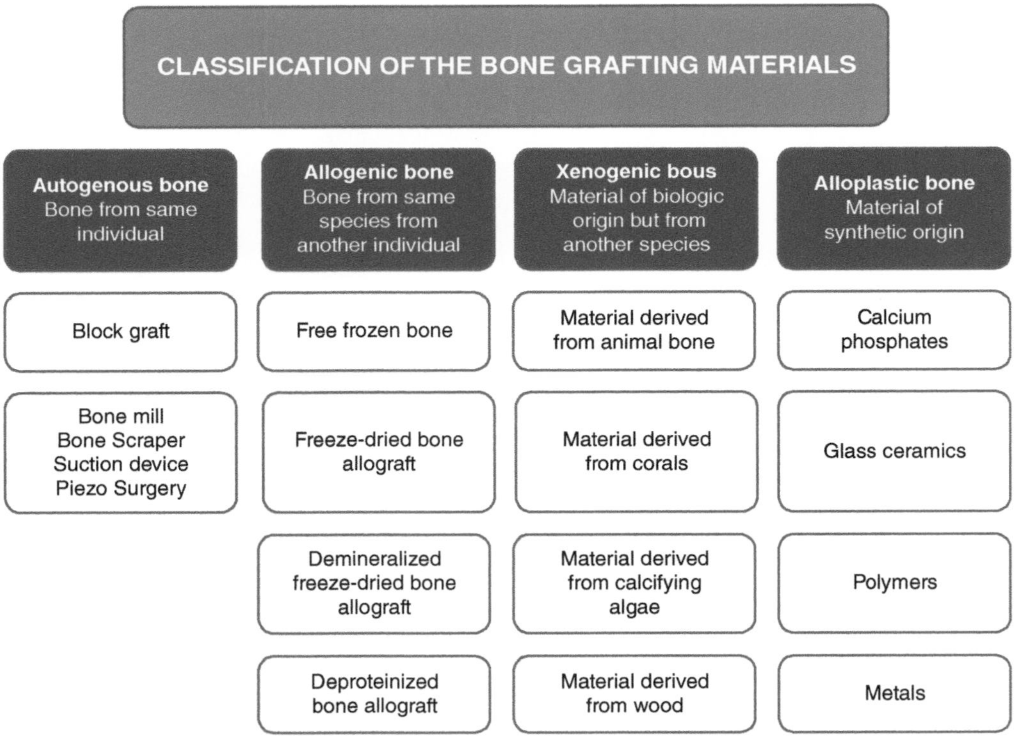

CLASSIFICATION OF THE BONE GRAFTING MATERIALS

Autogenous bone Bone from same individual	Allogenic bone Bone from same species from another individual	Xenogenic bous Material of biologic origin but from another species	Alloplastic bone Material of synthetic origin
Block graft	Free frozen bone	Material derived from animal bone	Calcium phosphates
Bone mill Bone Scraper Suction device Piezo Surgery	Freeze-dried bone allograft	Material derived from corals	Glass ceramics
	Demineralized freeze-dried bone allograft	Material derived from calcifying algae	Polymers
	Deproteinized bone allograft	Material derived from wood	Metals

Figure 5.7 Classification of bone grafting materials utilized in dentistry. Adapted from Dr. Simon Jensen. Osteology Meeting, Monaco, 2011.

2. There exists no ideal or favored method to preserve dimensional changes of the alveolar ridge including using GBR techniques, socket fillers, socket seals, or combinations of the above-mentioned techniques.

5.4 Immediate implant placement into fresh extraction sockets

One logical alternative strategy has been to place immediate implants into fresh extraction sockets prior to the resorption of bone. While hypothetically this seemed to logically favor the maintenance of bone around teeth, several reports have now shown that preventing buccal bone resorption by placing immediate implants has not been possible (Figure 5.10). In another classical study investigating immediate implant placement in beagle dogs, it was reported that horizontal resorption of the buccal bone dimension amounted to 56% loss [29]. Since then various attempts have been made to modify implant size and diameter as well as implant placement more lingually in order to prevent buccal bone loss. While implant survival rates remain high (in the 90%-95% range) [30–35], exposure of the mid-facial implant surface from mucosal recession has been a commonly reported problem as high as 40% [36–38]. Today, several criteria, including facial bone wall thickness, tissue biotype, implant type, size, and positioning within the extraction sockets, have all been factors affecting the final aesthetic outcomes [39,40]. Therefore, it is expected that changes in the vertical dimension most notably adjacent to the thinner buccal wall is common [1,2]. A recent systematic review showed that following immediate implant placement, an average

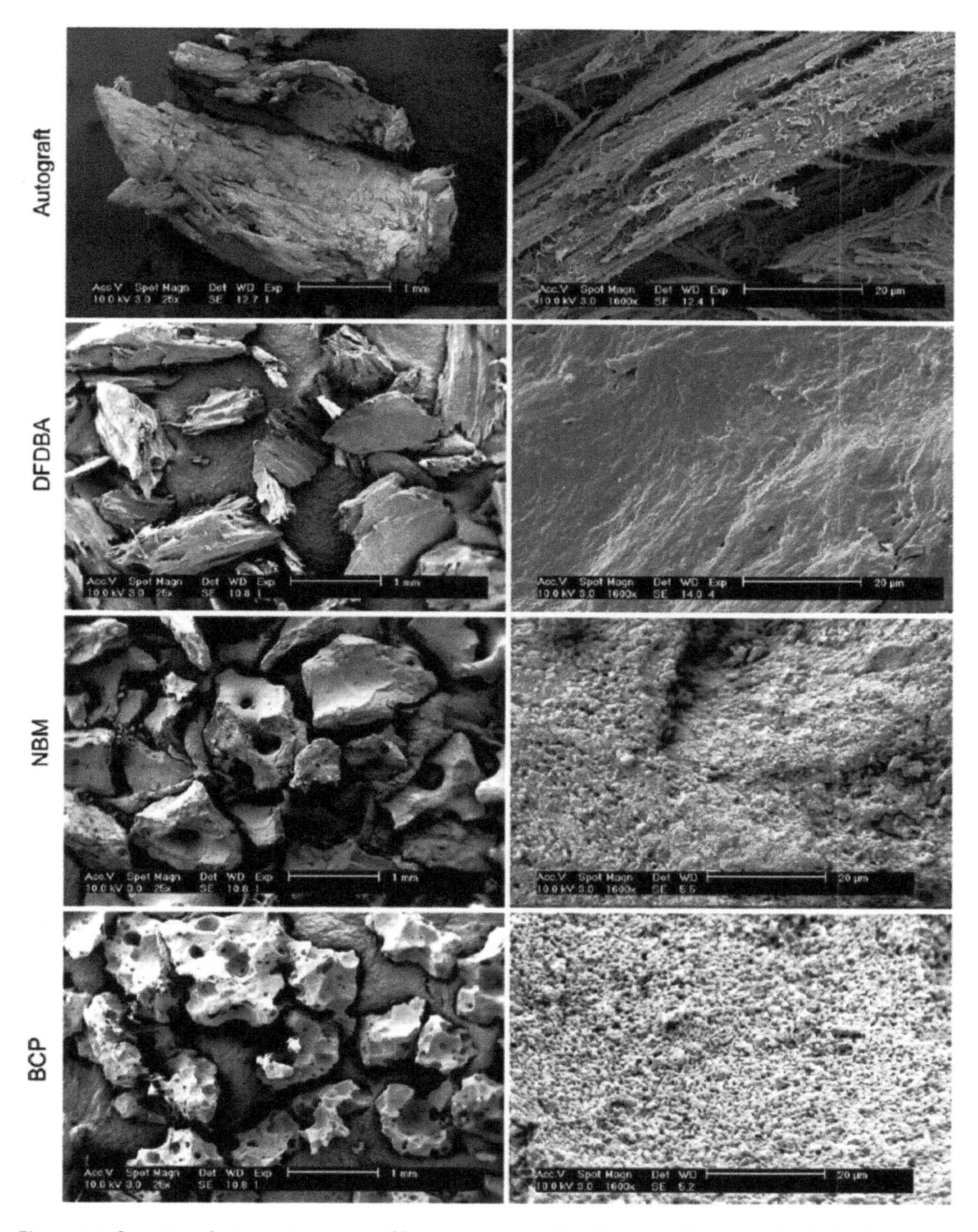

Figure 5.8 Scanning electron microscopy of four commonly utilized bone grafting materials in dentistry including autogenous bone harvested with a bone mill, a demineralized freeze-dried bone allograft (DFDBA), a commonly employed xenograft of bovine origin (natural bone mineral, NBM), and a synthetically fabricated biphasic calcium phosphate. Source: Miron *et al.* 2016 [54]. Reproduced with permission of Mary Ann Liebert, Inc.

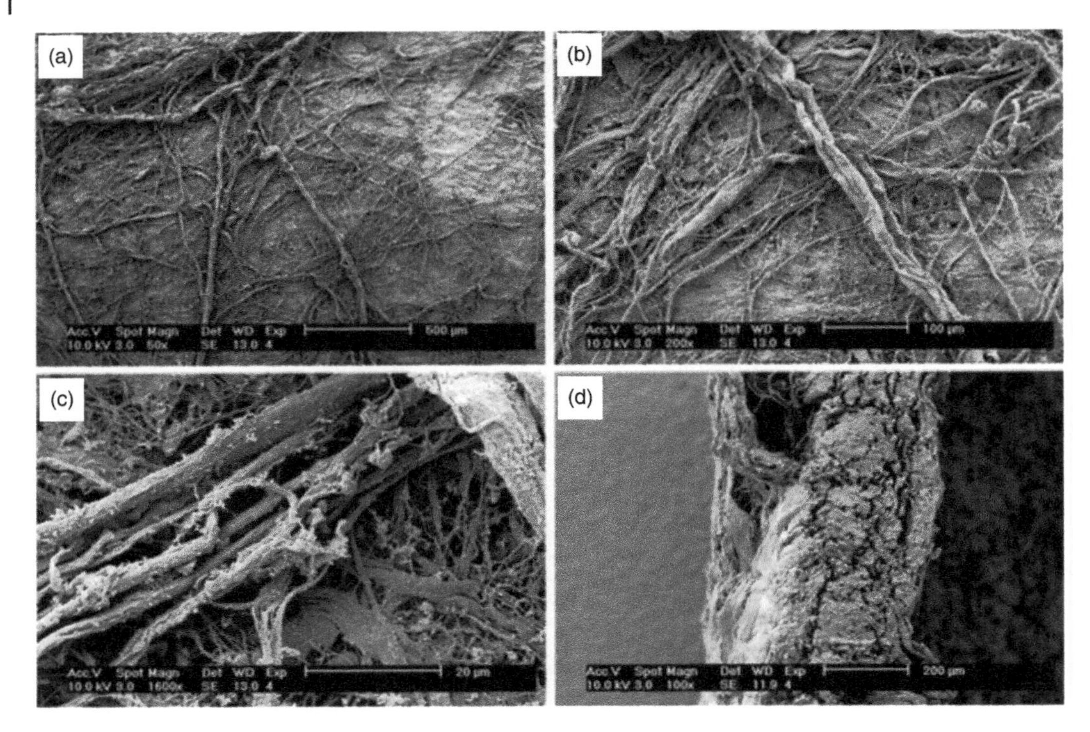

Figure 5.9 Scanning Electron Microscopy (SEM) analysis of collagen barrier membrane. a, b Membrane surface reveals many collagen fibrils that are intertwined with one another with various diameters and directions (magnification $A = \times 50$, $B = \times 200$). c High-resolution SEM demonstrates collagen fibrils ranging in diameter between 1 and 5 µm (magnification = ×1,600). d Cross-sectional view of collagen barrier membrane of approximately 300 µm (magnification = ×100). Source: Miron *et al.* 2013 [21]. Reproduced with permission of Springer-Verlag.

loss of 0.5-1 mm reduction in the vertical and horizontal aspects of the buccal bone was found between 4-12 months [41]. Importantly, however, and as previously discussed, the buccal bone surface in the aesthetic zone has been characterized as being 1 mm or less in 69% of cases [10], therefore, potentially creating mucosal recessions in the majority of these cases.

5.5 Overview of utilizing PRF in extraction sockets

5.5.1 Socket grafting and ridge preservation with PRF

As mentioned, alveolar bone is largely dependent on tooth structure/morphology and will rapidly undergo remodeling following extraction as a result of loss of the periodontal ligament's blood supply. Interestingly, PRF as a biomaterial for extraction socket management and healing has become a frequent topic of research in recent years. It has been hypothesized that ridge preservation may be achieved using PRF, where previously other bone products and biomaterials had been utilized. The rationale is to apply pro-angiogenic, positive inflammatory cytokines, and growth factors from PRF to stimulate healing in extraction sockets. The literature is abundant with reports advocating grafting of the socket immediately post-extraction, by xenografts, allografts, autografts, and alloplasts, as well as the sealing of the sockets by soft-tissue connective tissue grafts or barrier membranes. And whilst results have varied widely, there is strong evidence to graft the socket for ridge preservation. Systematic reviews of ridge preservation

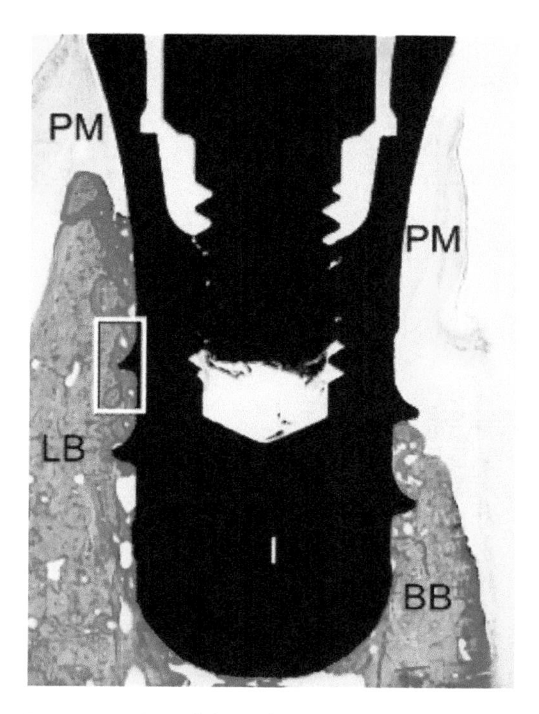

Figure 5.10 Buccal–lingual section representing one immediate implant site after three months of healing. Note the location of the bone crest at the buccal and lingual aspects of the implant. BB, buccal bone wall; I, implant; LB, lingual bone wall; PM, peri-implant mucosa. Toluidine blue staining; original magnification × 16. Source: Araujo *et al.* 2005 [36]. Reproduced with permission of John Wiley & Sons.

techniques report that regardless of the conventionally used materials or surgical technique, alveolar ridge preservation does reduce post-extraction bone loss [22,42]. The remaining question is whether PRF can achieve similar results for ridge preservation.

Table 5.1 presents the current studies evaluating dimensional changes post-extraction with PRF in comparison to control or to bone grafting material. Despite the wealth of reports and clinical experiences with clinicians that have utilized PRF for extraction socket healing from 2006 to present, few studies have in fact evaluated its performance in comparative human studies. Hauser and coworkers were one of the first to show that PRF was capable of inducing new bone formation in extraction sockets when compared to controls [43]. Analysis by micro-computed tomography showed better bone healing with improvements in the microarchitecture in the group treated with PRF. It was also shown that PRF had a significant effect on intrinsic bone tissue quality and preservation of the alveolar width. Interestingly, it was further determined that an invasive surgical procedure with a mucosal flap appeared to completely neutralize the advantages of PRF [43]. For these reasons, it is strongly recommended not to raise flaps during routine tooth extraction.

Girish Rao *et al.* evaluated a study sample consisting of 22 patients requiring bilateral transalveolar third molar extractions [44]. One side was randomly chosen as PRF and the other side was utilized as a blank control. Patients were called for a follow-up on the first day post-op, first week, 1 month, 3 months, and 6 months. Regeneration of bone was measured using serial radiographs (RVG) at day 0, as well as at 1, 3, and 6 months post-operation. The results demonstrated that a higher mean pixels was recorded in the PRF group when compared to controls at all time intervals, however, the reported difference was not deemed statistically significant likely as a result of patient size [44].

Another comparative study by Hoaglin and Lines investigating third molar socket fill was performed to determine the rate of alveolar infection (dry socket) with/without PRF [45]. This study demonstrated that PRF is capable of drastically decreasing the rate of post-op infections, which is later discussed in more detail in this chapter. A study by Suttapresyari and Leepong investigated the influence of PRF on early wound healing and preservation of the alveolar ridge shape following tooth extraction in 20 symmetrical premolar extraction sockets using a split-mouth design [46]. The evaluation of wound healing, alveolar ridge contour changes, and crestal bone resorption were performed in dental casts and periapical radiographs at 0, 1, 2, 4, 6, and 8 weeks post-extraction. PRF clinically showed earlier healing of soft-tissue coverage of socket orifices in the first 4 weeks, however, horizontal bone resorption

Table 5.1 Studies that have thus far utilized platelet rich fibrin (PRF) for extraction socket management.

Author	Defect	Number of Cases	Healing Period	Treatment	Dimensional Change of Bone	P value
Hauser (2013)	Premolar Extraction Sockets	23	8 weeks	control PRF PRF + MPF (flap)	−3.68 −0.48 −3.7	0.05
Girish Rao (2013)	3rd Molar Extraction Sockets	44	1, 3, 6 months	control PRF	979 units 1115 units	n.s.
Hoaglin (2013)	3rd Molar Osteomyelitis	200	7-10 days	control PRF	9.9 % infection 1% infection	0.05
Suttapreyasri (2013)	Premolar Extraction Sockets	20	0-8 weeks	blood clot PRF	1.33 mm 0.7 mm	n.s.
Das (2016)	Extraction sockets	30 cases	6 months	beta-TCP PRF	n.s. n.s.	no difference reported between groups
Temmerman (2016)	Single rooted maxillary and mandibular teeth	22	3 months	control PRF	−51.92% −22.84%	0.05

was not significantly different between control and tested groups. Radiographically, the overall resorption of marginal bone levels at the mesial and distal sites to the extraction socket were reported as 0.70 and 1.23 mm in the PRF group compared to 1.33 and 1.14 in the control group. The authors conclude that although PRF demonstrated faster bone healing compared to the control, no statistically significant difference was detected, potentially as a result of the limited sample size [46].

A clinical trial performed by Das and coworkers compared socket grafting of single-rooted teeth with beta-tri-calcium phosphate-collagen (β-TCP-Cl) versus PRF [47]. While both these materials have a rapid substitution rate, histologically β-TCP-Cl showed more mineral density and organizational maturation with less medullary spaces [47]. The study reported that PRF demonstrated equal ridge preservation and equal ability to minimize dimensional changes especially of the facial bone (PRF 1.5 mm loss; β-TCP-Cl 0.99mm).

Most recently, Andwandter investigated in a non-comparative human study healing of extraction sockets filled with PRF plugs in 18 patients [48]. Clinical bone sounding was performed using a customized acrylic stent and radiographic measurements were accomplished using CBCT, immediately after tooth extraction and after a 4-month healing period [48]. The authors report that the clinical observations demonstrated a mean horizontal resorption of 1.18±2.4 mm at the crest as well as a loss of 1.25±2.0 mm and 0.83±2.0 mm at 2 mm and 4 mm apical to the crest, respectively. The buccal plate demonstrated a mean vertical loss of 0.44±3.5mm. Moreover, the radiographic analysis demonstrated a mean vertical bone loss of 0.27±2.5 mm on the buccal and of 0.03±1.6 mm at the oral crest. The width of the alveolar ridge was reduced by 1.33mm±1.43 mm [48]. These reports are deemed comparable to the systematic reviews that have demonstrated an average mean loss of 0.5–1 mm of buccal bone resorption when a bone grafting material is utilized.

In a final randomized controlled clinical trial, Temmerman *et al.* investigated the influence of PRF as a socket filling material on ridge preservation [49]. Twenty-two patients in need of single bilateral and closely symmetrical teeth extractions in the maxilla or mandible were included and CBCT scans were obtained at day 0 and after a three-month healing period [49]. Mean ridge width differences between time points were measured at three levels below the crest on both the buccal and lingual sides (crest −1 mm (primary outcome variable), −3mm, and −5 mm) (Figure 5.11). It was found that mean vertical height changes at the buccal were −1.5 mm (±1.3) for control sites and 0.5 mm (±2.3) for test sites ($p < 0.005$). At the buccal side, control sites demonstrated mean losses of −2.1 (±2.5), −0.3 mm (±0.3), and −0.1 mm (±0.0), and test sites values were −0.6 mm (±2.2) ($p < 0.005$), −0.1 mm (±0.3), and 0.0 mm (±0.1) (Figure 5.12). Significant differences ($p < 0.005$) were found for total width reduction between test (−22.84%) and control sites (−51.92%) at 1 mm below crest levels. Significant differences were found for socket fill (visible mineralized bone) between test (94.7%) and control sites (63.3%) [49].

5.5.2 Preventing postoperative pain and infection

PRF has therapeutically been shown to reduce postoperative pain when placed in extraction sockets following third molar surgery [50]. Pain as a result of this procedure typically arises largely from soft-tissue incision, trauma, and stretching. Baseline variables were assessed preoperatively and included pain, the number of analgesics taken, as well as trismus, and swelling. These were assessed on short-term follow-up visits on days 1, 2, 3, and 7 [50]. The authors report a significant reduction in pain on days 1, 2, and 3, and in the number of analgesics taken on days 2 and 3 in the PRF groups. Therefore, the findings from this study

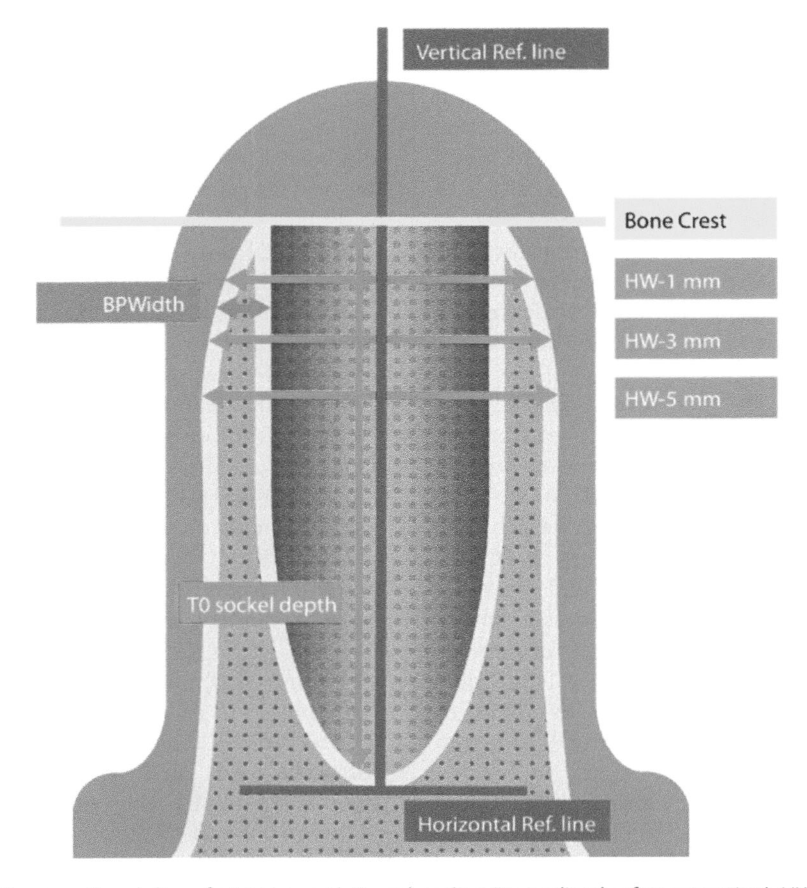

Figure 5.11 Cross-sectional slice of a test/control site at baseline (immediately after extraction). HW-1 mm, HW-3 mm, HW-5 mm are representing the measurements performed at three levels below the bone crest. The width of the buccal plate (BPwidth) was measured 1 mm below the crest. The depth of the socket was measured as the deepest point of the socket to the bone crest. Source: Temmerman *et al.* 2016 [49]. Reproduced with permissions of John Wiley & Sons.

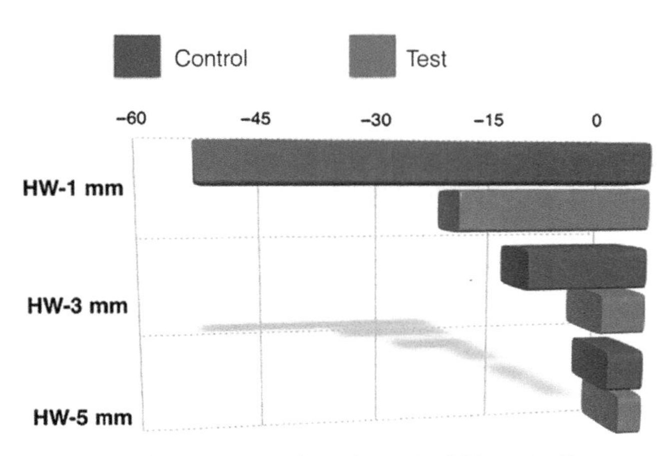

Figure 5.12 Changes in ridge height and width between control (unfilled sockets) and test (PRF) three months and baseline based on CBCT measurements expressed in %. Source: Temmerman *et al.* 2016 [49]. Reproduced with permissions of John Wiley & Sons.

indicated that 1) PRF was able to reduce postoperative pain largely due to the improvements in soft-tissue healing while reducing infections due to presence of microbial-fighting immune cells (leukocytes) and 2) this led to a reduction in the number of analgesics taken from these patients [50].

Interestingly, another study proposed using PRF to prevent postoperative infection in extraction sockets of mandibular third molars. The rationale is based on the local delivery of concentrated leukocytes, able to participate in an inflammatory response well understood to ward off infective pathogens. Data on PRF's performance in this regard are also few, though a retrospective report compared 200 mandibular third molar sites treated with/without PRF. The results showed only 2 cases of localized osteitis despite PRF treatment versus 19 cases in the control group (1 versus 9.5% respectively) [45]. Whilst the etiologies of localized osteitis are multiple and not well understood, the authors also point to the fact that the non-PRF treatment group (controls) required an additional 6.5 hours of clinical time to manage local infections necessitating extra surgical time and costs to resolve these problems. These authors demonstrate that preventative treatment of localized osteitis can be accomplished using a low-cost, autogenous, soluble, biologic material, and that PRF enhanced third-molar socket healing/clot retention and greatly decreased the clinical time required for postoperative management of infection [45].

In a final study carried out by a split-mouth randomized design, 78 mandibular third molar sockets treated with PRF were compared to 78 control sites [51]. Overall alveolar osteitis occurred more in their study but once again it was concluded that treating sockets with PRF reduced incidence of complication by about half (PRF 9% versus control 20.5%).

5.5.2.1 Histological evidence

Canine model: In 2014, Hatakeyama and coworkers created buccal dehiscences at four mandibular premolar sites following extraction in 12 beagle dogs [52]. Three different platelet concentrates including PRF were evaluated against a control. The authors evaluated several parameters including histology of block resections at the sockets. The reported results were information dense, although the following may be summarized:

- At an early healing period (4 weeks), there was varied new bone formation in the PRF group comparable to controls
- At a later healing period (8 weeks), bone formation had progressed in all groups although the bone formed in the PRF group had more mineralized tissue and a fine cortex when compared to the control group.

Based on these findings, it may therefore be concluded that a minimum of 8 weeks is necessary to improve new mineralized tissues when compared to controls. For these reasons, it is generally clinically recommended in humans that a 3- to 4-month waiting period is necessary prior to re-entry following socket grafting with PRF as described in Table 5.1.

Human study: Human histology from healed extraction sockets treated with PRF is quite scarce. Anwandter and coworkers presented a histological sample from their study yet data from all the samples was not reported. To date, only three known studies have harvested via trephined bone core biopsies to compare the histomorphometry in unfilled extraction sockets versus PRF. One of these studies reported on bone biopsy at a very late healing period after six months and thus will not be discussed [47]. In 2013, Hauser and coworkers retrieved trephined core biopsies during implant osteotomy preparation from extraction sockets that healed with PRF versus control unfilled sites. These were analyzed by microcomputed tomography, and higher bone density, trabecular number, and trabecular proximity was observed following healing with PRF.

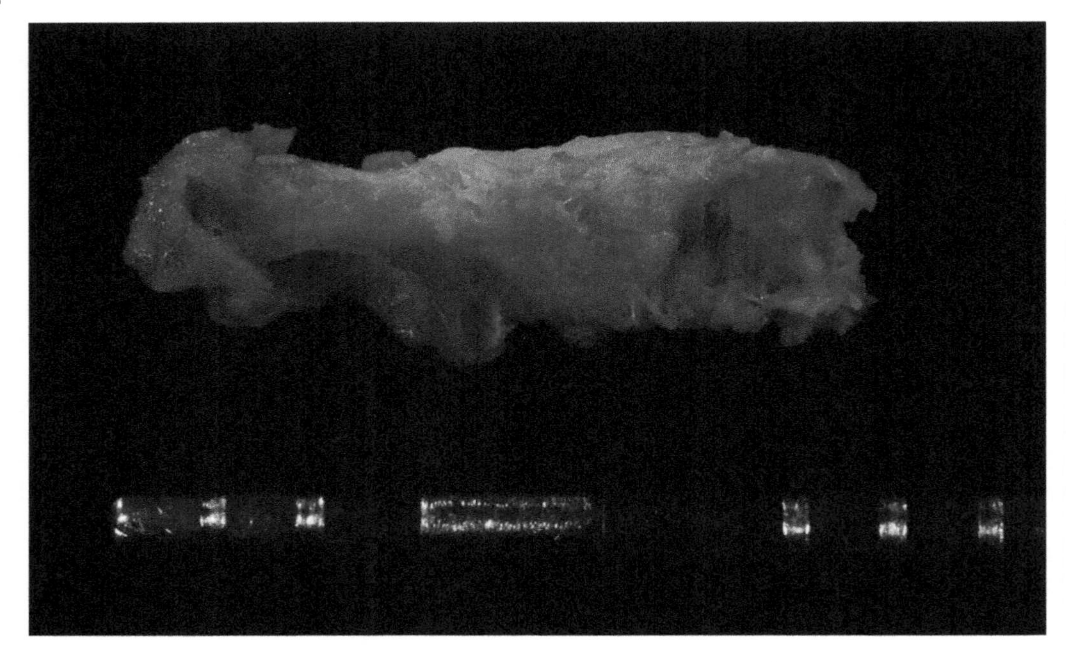

Figure 5.13 A 2 × 7 mm trephined bone biopsy from a human extraction socket filled with PRF plugs, retrieved after 90 days of healing. Source: Du Toit *et al.* 2016 [53]. Reproduced with permission of Quintessence Publishing Co., Inc.

The findings showed better bone healing with improvement of the microarchitecture and intrinsic bone tissue quality and preservation of the alveolar width in the group treated with PRF [43].

In 2016, Du Toit and coworkers designed a split-mouth randomized study with one site receiving PRF scaffolds when compared to unfilled controls in single rooted tooth extraction sockets in the maxilla. At implant placement, a trephined bone core biopsy was retrieved at each extraction socket after 90 days of healing (Figures 5.13 and 5.14) [53]. The undecalcified bone sections from these bone biopsies were photographed at ultra resolution and each tissue compartment was measured at high magnification using a software program (Figure 5.15). The program digitally calculated the surface areas for the total bone, newly formed osteoid, newly mineralized bone, and fibrovascular tissue (Figure 5.16). Eight human bone biopsies were successfully harvested from four patients. The findings resulted in a 9.9% ± 5.9% gain in newly formed osteoid in the PRF group versus 4% ± 2.1% for specimens derived from the control sites. Due to the low sample size, this was however not deemed significant ($P = .089$) (Figure 5.17) [53].

5.6 Discussion and future research

A wealth of literature has reported the regenerative potential of PRF in various clinical situation in dentistry over the past decade and research inquiries will continue. Despite this, to date, only few extraction socket studies have reported the effects of PRF in randomized clinical trials with little human histological data available. Therefore, much further investigation on tissue healing—both hard and soft tissue—requires greater exploration.

The effects of tooth loss on dimensional changes have now been extensively reported in the literature [4,8,10,22–26]. Due to considerable variations in humans, clinicians

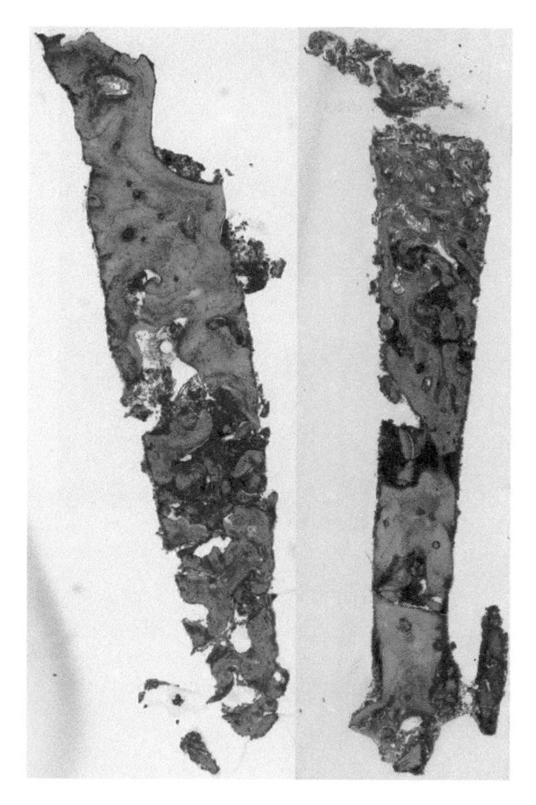

Figure 5.14 Two undecalcified sections of human bone derived from extraction sockets filled with PRF plugs, retrieved after 90 days of healing. Methylene blue-basic fuchsin, 10X magnification. Source: Du Toit *et al.* 2016 [53]. Reproduced with permission of Quintessence Publishing Co., Inc.

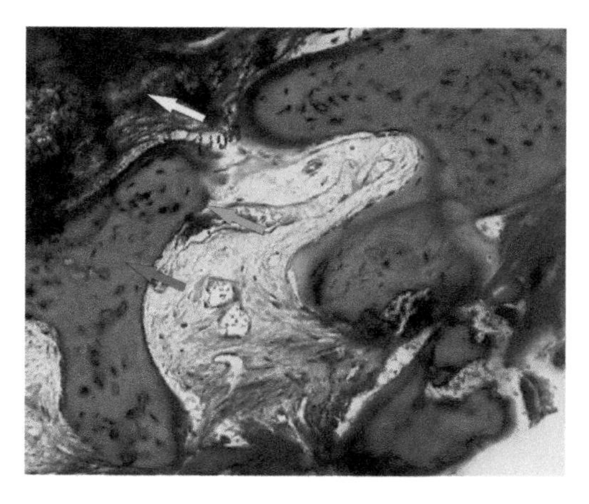

Figure 5.15 High magnification of a section of bone derived from PRF, at 90 days of healing, demonstrating new-mineralized bone (blue arrow), osteoid at the periphery (green arrow), and fibrovascular tissue (yellow arrow).

need to be aware that not all sockets resorb equally, not all patients are genetically predisposed to resorb equally, and that PRF may contribute to ridge preservation differently between sites and patients. For instance, Chappuis *et al.* showed convincingly that facial bone thickness in the aesthetic zone is a critical factor affecting potential facial bone resorption [10].

One potential benefit of socket grafting with PRF is the improvements in soft-tissue wound healing [54]. While no study to date has reported the soft-tissue wound healing quality specifically in extraction sockets, a plausible hypothesis may however be derived from the fact wound closure occurs more favorably following PRF use. From this point of view, patients that are currently taking high-dose bisphosphonates or having taken anti-resorptive medications for a number of years are at an increased risk of developing osteonecrosis of the jaw. It is therefore recommended that these patients are treated with PRF during routine extractions. PRF is an easy and simple technique, is derived from entirely autologous sources and is therefore entirely safe and biocompatible, does not provoke an immune response, and in various randomized clinical studies has been shown to preserve the dimensional changes occurring post-extraction in comparable fashion to bone grafts (at a fraction of the cost). Furthermore, analysis of pain and inflammation measures following socket grafting with PRF leads to a significant reduction in as early as two and three days post-surgery and the patients therefore take less medication as a result [50]. Additionally, the rate of infection post extraction, especially in mandibular third molars, has been decreased as much as 9.5-fold [45].

In summary, there is therefore benefit to utilize PRF for the preservation of the alveolar ridge, although its predictability and current indications for when to use the material alone versus when to perform ridge preservation in combination with a bone grafting material remains to be investigated. It must be noted that despite its use, changes

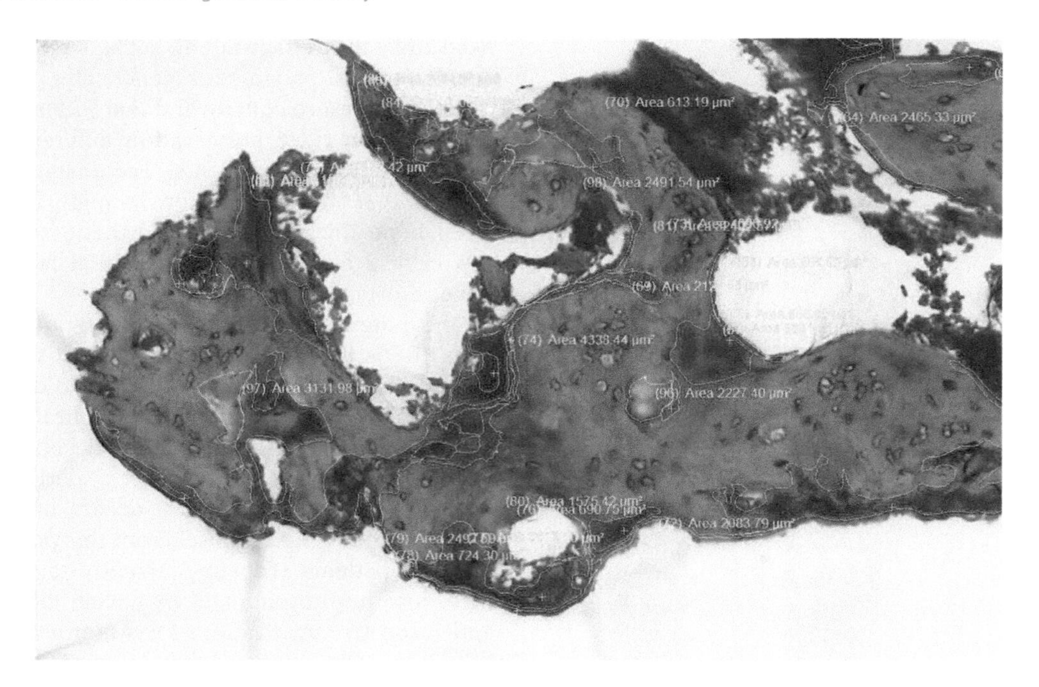

Figure 5.16 Manual tracing of the individual tissue components of the bone at highest magnification using Stream Essentials software (Olympus).

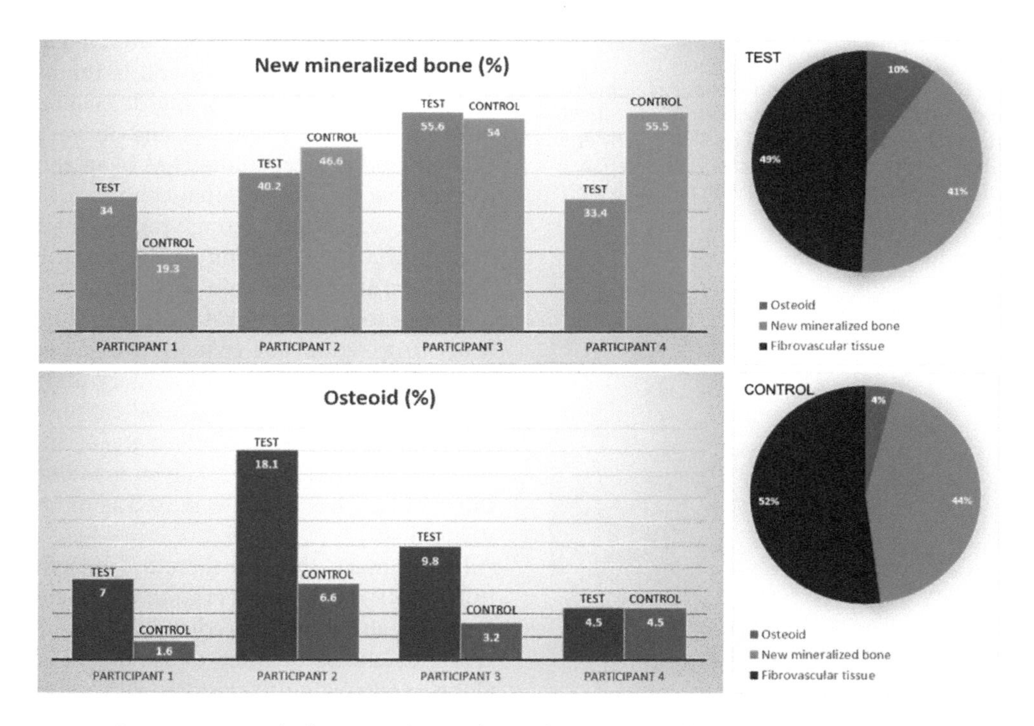

Figure 5.17 Comparative results for PRF and control sites, for mineralized bone and osteoid measured (bar graphs). Newly formed bone to fibrovascular tissue ratios for PRF and control sites (pie charts). Source: Du Toit *et al.* 2016 [53]. Reproduced with permission of Quintessence Publishing Co., Inc.

in the alveolar socket are still observed irrespective of the preservation attempt or material used. It is also further noted that a cost/benefit analysis would greatly favor PRF's use versus more commonly utilized and more costly bone grafts and/or barrier membranes frequently utilized. PRF is furthermore anti-bacterial due to its leukocyte content, reduces postoperative surgical extraction pain, and infection. Future research aimed at utilizing the low-speed centrifugation concept are needed to further evaluate if an increase in leukocyte number and growth factor release from PRF scaffolds may further translate into further clinical benefit.

References

1 Schropp L, Kostopoulos L, Wenzel A. Bone healing following immediate versus delayed placement of titanium implants into extraction sockets: a prospective clinical study. The International journal of oral & maxillofacial implants. 2003;18(2):189–99.
2 Botticelli D, Persson LG, Lindhe J, Berglundh T. Bone tissue formation adjacent to implants placed in fresh extraction sockets: an experimental study in dogs. Clinical oral implants research. 2006;17(4):351–8.
3 Johnson K. A study of the dimensional changes occurring in the maxilla after tooth extraction.—Part I. Normal healing. Australian Dental Journal. 1963;8(5): 428–33.
4 Morjaria KR, Wilson R, Palmer RM. Bone healing after tooth extraction with or without an intervention: a systematic review of randomized controlled trials. Clinical implant dentistry and related research. 2014;16(1):1–20.
5 Mammoto A, Connor KM, Mammoto T, Yung CW, Huh D, Aderman CM, et al. A mechanosensitive transcriptional mechanism that controls angiogenesis. Nature. 2009;457(7233):1103–8.
6 Mörmann W, Ciancio SG. Blood supply of human gingiva following periodontal surgery: a fluorescein angiographic study. Journal of periodontology. 1977;48(11): 681–92.
7 Choukroun J, Adda F, Schoeffler C, Vervelle A. Une opportunité en paro-implantologie: le PRF. Implantodontie. 2001;42(55):e62.
8 Araújo MG, Lindhe J. Dimensional ridge alterations following tooth extraction. An experimental study in the dog. Journal of clinical periodontology. 2005;32(2): 212–8.
9 Scala A, Lang NP, Schweikert MT, Oliveira JA, Rangel-Garcia I, Botticelli D. Sequential healing of open extraction sockets. An experimental study in monkeys. Clinical oral implants research. 2014;25(3):288–95.
10 Chappuis V, Engel O, Reyes M, Shahim K, Nolte LP, Buser D. Ridge alterations post-extraction in the esthetic zone: a 3D analysis with CBCT. Journal of dental research. 2013;92(12 Suppl):195s–201s.
11 Brkovic BM, Prasad HS, Konandreas G, Milan R, Antunovic D, Sandor GK, et al. Simple preservation of a maxillary extraction socket using beta-tricalcium phosphate with type I collagen: preliminary clinical and histomorphometric observations. Journal (Canadian Dental Association). 2008;74(6):523–8.
12 Brkovic BM, Prasad HS, Rohrer MD, Konandreas G, Agrogiannis G, Antunovic D, et al. Beta-tricalcium phosphate/type I collagen cones with or without a barrier membrane in human extraction socket healing: clinical, histologic, histomorphometric, and immunohistochemical evaluation. Clinical oral investigations. 2012;16(2):581–90.
13 Mardas N, Chadha V, Donos N. Alveolar ridge preservation with guided bone regeneration and a synthetic bone substitute or a bovine-derived xenograft: a randomized, controlled clinical trial.

Clinical oral implants research. 2010; 21(7):688–98.
14 Wallace S. Histomorphometric and 3D Cone-Beam Computerized Tomographic Evaluation of Socket Preservation in Molar Extraction Sites Using Human Particulate Mineralized Cancellous Allograft Bone With a Porcine Collagen Xenograft Barrier: A Case Series. The Journal of oral implantology. 2015;41(3):291–7.
15 Bayat M, Momen Heravi F, Mahmoudi M, Bahrami N. Bone Reconstruction following Application of Bone Matrix Gelatin to Alveolar Defects: A Randomized Clinical Trial. International journal of organ transplantation medicine. 2015;6(4): 176–81.
16 Mardas N, D'Aiuto F, Mezzomo L, Arzoumanidi M, Donos N. Radiographic alveolar bone changes following ridge preservation with two different biomaterials. Clinical oral implants research. 2011;22(4):416–23.
17 Coomes AM, Mealey BL, Huynh-Ba G, Barboza-Arguello C, Moore WS, Cochran DL. Buccal bone formation after flapless extraction: a randomized, controlled clinical trial comparing recombinant human bone morphogenetic protein 2/absorbable collagen carrier and collagen sponge alone. Journal of periodontology. 2014;85(4):525–35.
18 Fiorellini JP, Howell TH, Cochran D, Malmquist J, Lilly LC, Spagnoli D, et al. Randomized study evaluating recombinant human bone morphogenetic protein-2 for extraction socket augmentation. Journal of periodontology. 2005;76(4):605–13.
19 Misch CM. The use of recombinant human bone morphogenetic protein-2 for the repair of extraction socket defects: a technical modification and case series report. The International journal of oral & maxillofacial implants. 2010;25(6):1246–52.
20 Wallace SC, Pikos MA, Prasad H. De novo bone regeneration in human extraction sites using recombinant human bone morphogenetic protein-2/ACS: a clinical, histomorphometric, densitometric, and 3-dimensional cone-beam computerized tomographic scan evaluation. Implant dentistry. 2014;23(2):132–7.
21 Miron RJ, Saulacic N, Buser D, Iizuka T, Sculean A. Osteoblast proliferation and differentiation on a barrier membrane in combination with BMP2 and TGFbeta1. Clinical oral investigations. 2013;17(3): 981–8.
22 De Risi V, Clementini M, Vittorini G, Mannocci A, De Sanctis M. Alveolar ridge preservation techniques: a systematic review and meta-analysis of histological and histomorphometrical data. Clinical oral implants research. 2015;26(1):50–68.
23 Jambhekar S, Kernen F, Bidra AS. Clinical and histologic outcomes of socket grafting after flapless tooth extraction: a systematic review of randomized controlled clinical trials. J Prosthet Dent. 2015;113(5):371–82.
24 Moraschini V, Barboza ED. Quality assessment of systematic reviews on alveolar socket preservation. International journal of oral and maxillofacial surgery. 2016.
25 Spagnoli D, Choi C. Extraction socket grafting and buccal wall regeneration with recombinant human bone morphogenetic protein-2 and acellular collagen sponge. Atlas of the oral and maxillofacial surgery clinics of North America. 2013;21(2): 175–83.
26 Tan WL, Wong TL, Wong MC, Lang NP. A systematic review of post-extractional alveolar hard and soft tissue dimensional changes in humans. Clinical oral implants research. 2012;23 Suppl 5:1–21.
27 Kotsakis G, Chrepa V, Marcou N, Prasad H, Hinrichs J. Flapless alveolar ridge preservation utilizing the "socket-plug" technique: clinical technique and review of the literature. The Journal of oral implantology. 2014;40(6):690–8.
28 MacBeth N, Trullenque-Eriksson A, Donos N, Mardas N. Hard and soft tissue changes following alveolar ridge preservation: a systematic review. Clinical oral implants research. 2016.

29 Botticelli D, Berglundh T, Lindhe J. Hard-tissue alterations following immediate implant placement in extraction sites. J Clin Periodontol. 2004;31(10):820–8.
30 Hammerle CH, Chen ST, Wilson TG, Jr. Consensus statements and recommended clinical procedures regarding the placement of implants in extraction sockets. The International journal of oral & maxillofacial implants. 2004;19 Suppl: 26–8.
31 Quirynen M, Van Assche N, Botticelli D, Berglundh T. How does the timing of implant placement to extraction affect outcome? The International journal of oral & maxillofacial implants. 2007;22 Suppl:203–23.
32 Schwartz-Arad D, Chaushu G. Placement of implants into fresh extraction sites: 4 to 7 years retrospective evaluation of 95 immediate implants. Journal of periodontology. 1997;68(11):1110–6.
33 Huys LW. Replacement therapy and the immediate post-extraction dental implant. Implant dentistry. 2001;10(2):93–102.
34 Polizzi G, Grunder U, Goene R, Hatano N, Henry P, Jackson WJ, et al. Immediate and delayed implant placement into extraction sockets: a 5-year report. Clinical implant dentistry and related research. 2000; 2(2):93–9.
35 Becker W, Dahlin C, Lekholm U, Bergstrom C, van Steenberghe D, Higuchi K, et al. Five-year evaluation of implants placed at extraction and with dehiscences and fenestration defects augmented with ePTFE membranes: results from a prospective multicenter study. Clinical implant dentistry and related research. 1999;1(1):27–32.
36 Araujo MG, Sukekava F, Wennstrom JL, Lindhe J. Ridge alterations following implant placement in fresh extraction sockets: an experimental study in the dog. J Clin Periodontol. 2005;32(6):645–52.
37 Botticelli D, Renzi A, Lindhe J, Berglundh T. Implants in fresh extraction sockets: a prospective 5-year follow-up clinical study. Clinical oral implants research. 2008; 19(12):1226–32.
38 Kan JY, Rungcharassaeng K, Sclar A, Lozada JL. Effects of the facial osseous defect morphology on gingival dynamics after immediate tooth replacement and guided bone regeneration: 1-year results. Journal of oral and maxillofacial surgery : official journal of the American Association of Oral and Maxillofacial Surgeons. 2007;65(7 Suppl 1):13–9.
39 Chen ST, Beagle J, Jensen SS, Chiapasco M, Darby I. Consensus statements and recommended clinical procedures regarding surgical techniques. The International journal of oral & maxillofacial implants. 2009;24 Suppl:272–8.
40 Chen ST, Darby IB, Reynolds EC, Clement JG. Immediate implant placement postextraction without flap elevation. Journal of periodontology. 2009;80(1): 163–72.
41 Lee CT, Chiu TS, Chuang SK, Tarnow D, Stoupel J. Alterations of the bone dimension following immediate implant placement into extraction socket: systematic review and meta-analysis. Journal of clinical periodontology. 2014; 41(9):914–26.
42 Iocca O, Farcomeni A, Pardinas-Lopez S, Talib HS. Alveolar Ridge Preservation after tooth extraction: a Bayesian Network meta-analysis of grafting materials efficacy on prevention of bone height and width reduction. Journal of clinical periodontology. 2016.
43 Hauser F, Gaydarov N, Badoud I, Vazquez L, Bernard JP, Ammann P. Clinical and histological evaluation of postextraction platelet-rich fibrin socket filling: a prospective randomized controlled study. Implant dentistry. 2013;22(3): 295–303.
44 Girish Rao S, Bhat P, Nagesh KS, Rao GH, Mirle B, Kharbhari L, et al. Bone regeneration in extraction sockets with autologous platelet rich fibrin gel. Journal of maxillofacial and oral surgery. 2013; 12(1):11–6.

45 Hoaglin DR, Lines GK. Prevention of localized osteitis in mandibular third-molar sites using platelet-rich fibrin. International journal of dentistry. 2013;2013:875380.

46 Suttapreyasri S, Leepong N. Influence of platelet-rich fibrin on alveolar ridge preservation. The Journal of craniofacial surgery. 2013;24(4):1088–94.

47 Das S, Jhingran R, Bains VK, Madan R, Srivastava R, Rizvi I. Socket preservation by beta-tri-calcium phosphate with collagen compared to platelet-rich fibrin: A clinico-radiographic study. European journal of dentistry. 2016;10(2):264–76.

48 Anwandter A, Bohmann S, Nally M, Castro AB, Quirynen M, Pinto N. Dimensional changes of the post extraction alveolar ridge, preserved with Leukocyte- and Platelet Rich Fibrin: A clinical pilot study. Journal of dentistry. 2016;52:23–9.

49 Temmerman A, Vandessel J, Castro A, Jacobs R, Teughels W, Pinto N, et al. The use of leucocyte and platelet-rich fibrin in socket management and ridge preservation: a split-mouth, randomized, controlled clinical trial. Journal of clinical periodontology. 2016;43(11):990–9.

50 Bilginaylar K, Uyanik LO. Evaluation of the effects of platelet-rich fibrin and piezosurgery on outcomes after removal of impacted mandibular third molars. The British journal of oral & maxillofacial surgery. 2016;54(6):629–33.

51 Eshghpour M, Dastmalchi P, Nekooei AH, Nejat A. Effect of platelet-rich fibrin on frequency of alveolar osteitis following mandibular third molar surgery: a double-blinded randomized clinical trial. Journal of oral and maxillofacial surgery : official journal of the American Association of Oral and Maxillofacial Surgeons. 2014;72(8):1463–7.

52 Hatakeyama I, Marukawa E, Takahashi Y, Omura K. Effects of platelet-poor plasma, platelet-rich plasma, and platelet-rich fibrin on healing of extraction sockets with buccal dehiscence in dogs. Tissue engineering Part A. 2014;20(3-4): 874–82.

53 Du Toit J, Siebold A, Dreyer A, Gluckman H. Choukroun Platelet-Rich Fibrin as an Autogenous Graft Biomaterial in Preimplant Surgery: Results of a Preliminary Randomized, Human Histomorphometric, Split-Mouth Study. The International journal of periodontics & restorative dentistry. 2016;36 Suppl: s75–86.

54 Miron RJ, Fujioka-Kobayashi M, Bishara M, Zhang Y, Hernandez M, Choukroun J. Platelet-Rich Fibrin and Soft Tissue Wound Healing: A Systematic Review. Tissue engineering Part B, Reviews. 2016.

6

Maxillary Sinus Floor Elevation in the Atrophic Posterior Maxillae: Anatomy, Principles, Techniques, Outcomes, and Complications

Alberto Monje, Hom-Lay Wang, and Richard J. Miron

Abstract

Over 30 years have now passed since the first maxillary sinus floor elevation procedure was performed. While a great deal of improvement has been made regarding surgical techniques, armamentarium utilized, and selected choice of biomaterials, it remains a procedure associated with numerous potential risks for complication. Therefore, it is imperative that the treating clinician be familiar with anatomical features and anomalies of the maxillary sinus cavity. This chapter highlights the anatomical considerations, dimensions, and vascularization of the maxillary sinus. Furthermore, the rate of Schneiderian membrane perforation with various surgical instruments is reported with discussion over the risk of acute and chronic infection as well as other post-surgical complications.

Highlights

- Surgical techniques for maxillary sinus floor elevation procedures
- Anatomical considerations of the maxillary sinus
- Maxillary sinus dimensions and vascularization
- Rate of Schneiderian membrane perforation with various surgical instruments
- Risk of acute and chronic infection
- Post-surgical complications

6.1 Introduction

Oral rehabilitation in the posterior maxilla often represents a challenge due to the centripetal resorption after tooth extraction as a consequence of trauma or periodontal disease [1]. Early findings showed that while in the maxilla the alveolar process resorbs upward and inward due to the direction and inclination of the roots, there is an outward resorption in the mandible where the ridge progressively becomes wider and flatter [2]. Furthermore, it was demonstrated that the edentulous ridge shifts toward a position closer to the palatal aspect having greater impact in the molar and premolar sites where greater and faster resorption is seen in the maxilla when compared to the mandible [3]. More recent observations have elucidated that following tooth extraction, 50% of the dimension may be lost as a consequence of the remodeling phenomena [4]. In addition to this, sinus pneumatization is an inevitable outcome associated with aging and tooth loss [5]. Therefore, maxillary sinus floor elevation (MSFE) has become a routinely performed procedure for the rehabilitation of the posterior maxillary edentulous sextants.

Platelet Rich Fibrin in Regenerative Dentistry: Biological Background and Clinical Indications, First Edition.
Edited by Richard J. Miron and Joseph Choukroun.

6.2 Anatomical considerations

In order to understand and address intra- and post-operative complications, anatomy must be thoroughly studied. Certainly, with the recent advancements made with three-dimensional (3D) radiographic tools, such as cone-beam computed tomography (CBCT), anatomical features can more easily be detected and investigated (Figure 6.1) [6]. Nonetheless, the surgeon must be aware of the common maxillary sinus anatomical structure to safely approach MSFE.

6.2.1 Embryologic development

The maxillary sinus cavity is the first parasal sinus to develop with a continuous growing pattern during mixed dentition. While at birth its volume is 6–8 cm^3, during deciduous dentition it extends laterally to the infraorbital canal (4 years old) and toward the

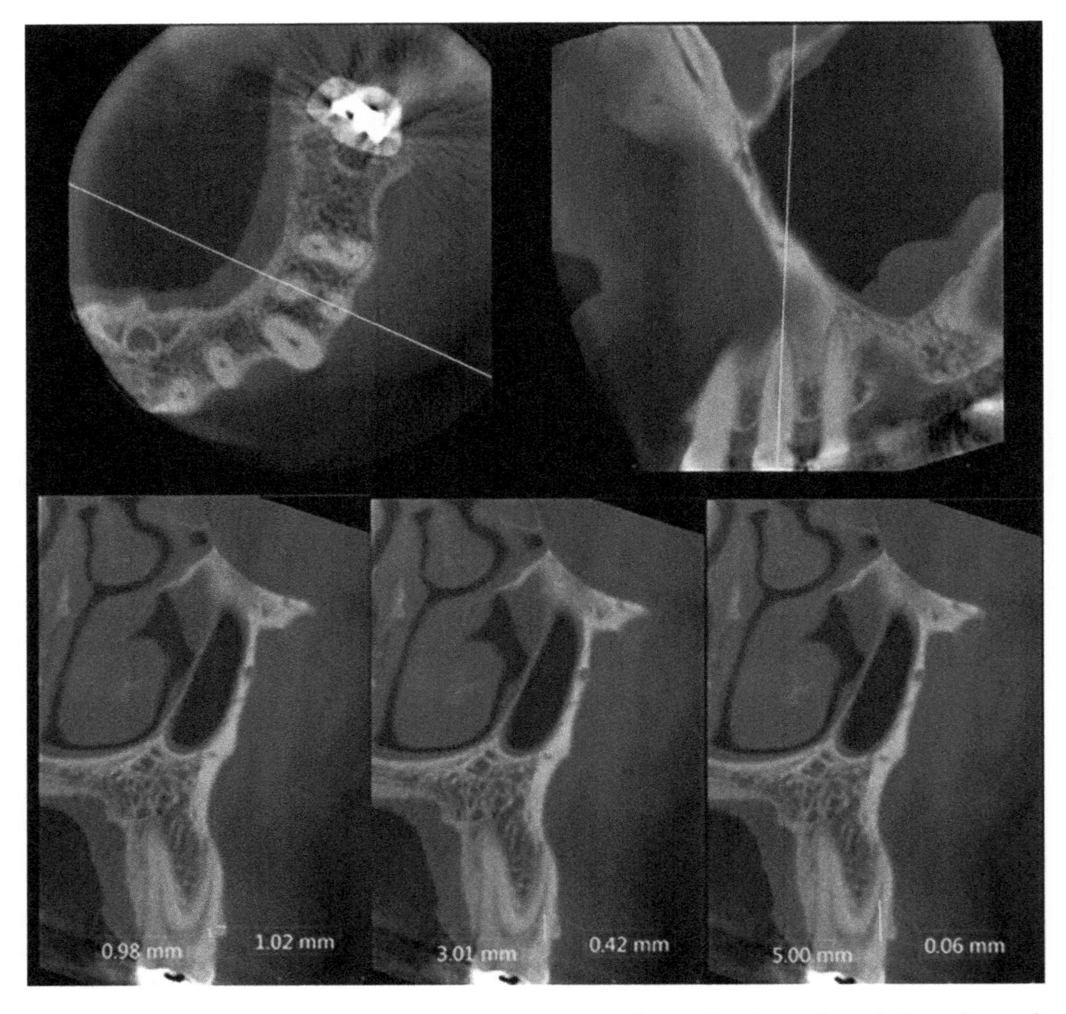

Figure 6.1 CBCT Evaluation of ideal tooth root. Individual, ideal reference line drawn through the mid-root of the tooth from apical to coronal (upper portion of view above). Magnified buccolingual slice of tooth root with measurements made at 1 mm, 3 mm, and 5 mm from the crest of bone perpendicular to the PDL space (lower portion of view above). Source: Temple *et al.* 2016 [6]. Reproduced with permission of John Wiley & Sons.

maxillary bone (9 years old). Moreover, when the dentition shifts to permanent dentition, a further pneumatization occurs to 4 to 5 mm below the floor of the nasal cavity [7], which may continue up to the second decade of life for females and the third for males [8].

6.2.2 Maxillary sinus dimension

The maxillary sinus is a quadrangular pyramidal cavity with its base in the medial nasal wall and the apex being located at the lateral aspect of the zygomatic process (Figure 6.2) [9]. Its height ranges between 36 to 45 mm counting with a width of 25 to 35 mm [10] and a volume of 15.859 mm^3 and 24.043 mm^3 on males and females, respectively [8]. More recent findings from cone beam–computed tomography studies have found that the maxillary sinus width is greater at molar than premolar sites [11], and that it presents with a more acute palato-nasal recess at the premolar than at the molar sites [12]. In addition, it has been shown that due to the zygomatic process, the higher the lateral wall is evaluated, the thicker the bony structure [13].

Certainly, various factors may influence the maxillary sinus dimensions. For instance, a positive association was found between age, body height and weight with enlargement of the maxillary sinus cavity [14]. In this sense, it was shown that mean volume was 1.5 times greater in males than in females [8]. Moreover, the presence of deviated nasal septa and the interzygomatic buttress distance might potentially impact sinus dimensions [14,15]. A positive correlation was also observed between the residual ridge height with the lateral wall thickness and the maxillary sinus width [13].

6.2.3 Vascularization

While the maxillary is densely vascularized in young individuals, the blood vessels gradually reduce with age [16]. The vasculature of the maxillary sinus is mainly supplied through three main branches: the infraorbital artery (IOA), the lateral nasal artery and the posterior superior alveolar artery (PSAA) (Figures 6.3, 6.4, and 6.5) [17]. The latter has a mean caliper of 1.3 to 2 mm and runs caudally on the outside of the convexity of the maxillary tuberosity and is in close contact with the periostium [18]. It was found that the anastomoses could be identified in the intraosseous artery but can only be visualized in the cone-beam computer tomography

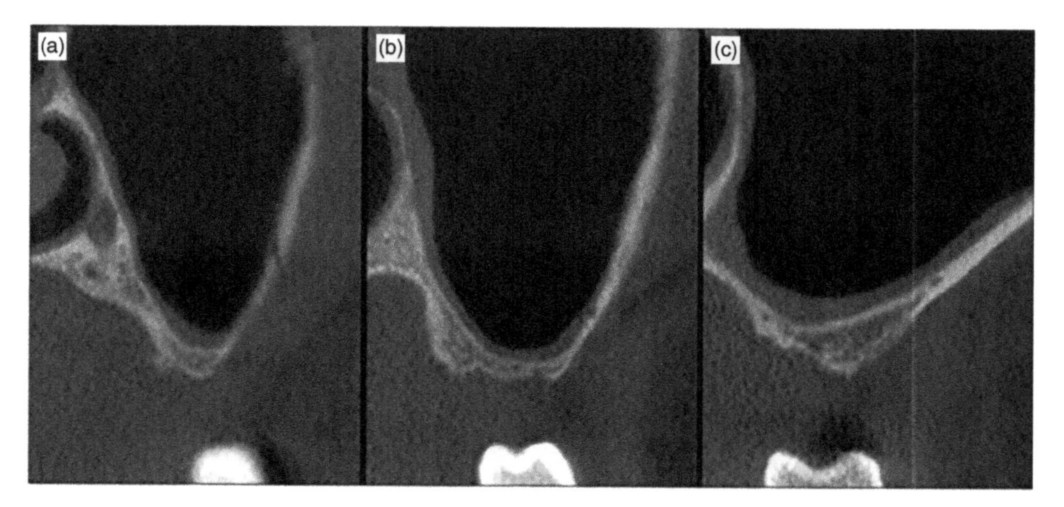

Figure 6.2 Cone beam–computed tomography (CBCT) images of representative sinuses those separately belong to narrow (a), average (b), and wide (c) sinus groups. Source: Teng *et al.* 2016 [9]. Reproduced with permission of John Wiley & Sons.

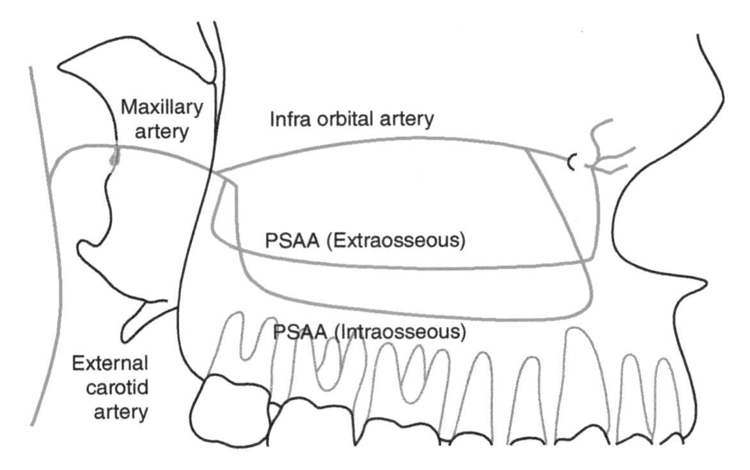

Figure 6.3 Schematic diagram demonstrating an anastomosis of the PSAA and infraorbital artery at the maxillary sinus lateral wall. Source: Danesh-Sani *et al.* 2016 [17]. Reproduced with permission of John Wiley & Sons.

scans 53% of the time [19]. The IOA has a similar caliper and it frequently originates from the maxillary artery at a similar level to the PSAA. It enters the maxillary sinus through the infraorbital fissure and runs through the infraorbital canal supplying anterior and posterior branches [18]. Some of these anastomoses along with the dental branch of the PSAA, vascularize the Schneiderian membrane on the buccal side from anterior to posterior [18].

6.2.4 Lining membrane

The maxillary sinus is lined by a respiratory mucous membrane characterized by a

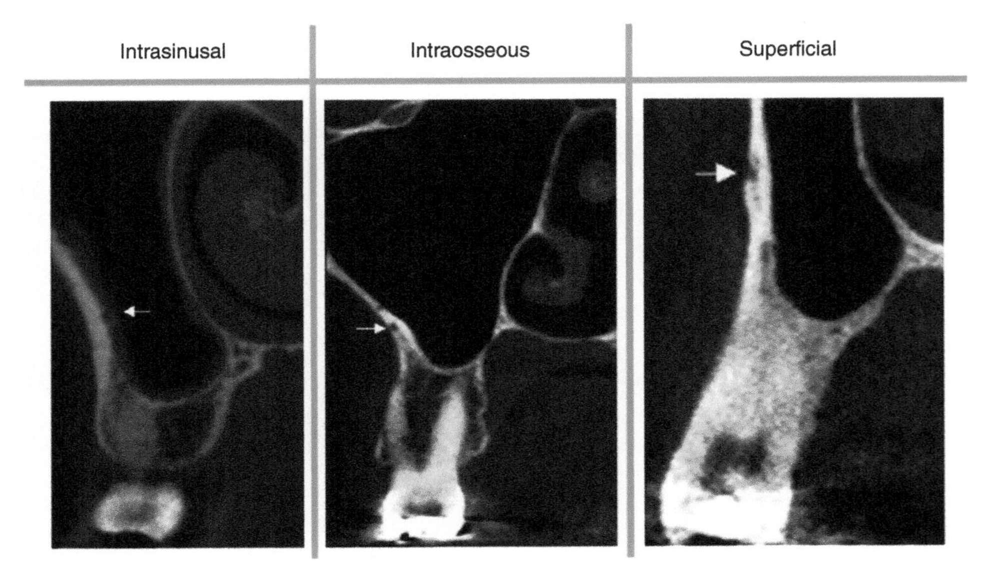

Figure 6.4 Transverse view of the CBCT scan of a sinus showing PSAA below the Schneiderian membrane (intrasinusal), inside the bone (intraosseous), and on the outer cortex of the lateral sinus wall (superficial). Source: Danesh-Sani *et al.* 2016 [17]. Reproduced with permission of John Wiley & Sons.

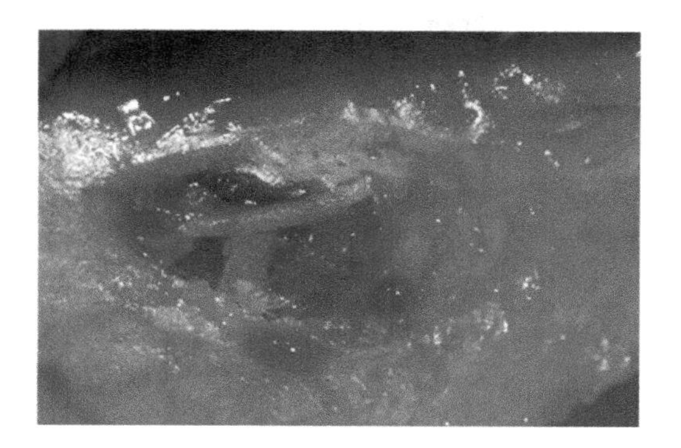

Figure 6.5 Visible posterior superior maxillary artery during sinus lifting procedure. (Figure provided courtesy of Prof. Pablo Galindo-Moreno).

pseudostratified, ciliated, columnar epithelium resting on a basement membrane (Figure 6.6) [20,21]. This membrane is thinner than the nasal membrane having a single layer of epithelium over a lamina propria composed by a superficial loose connective tissue over a more compact layer [22]. A mucoperiosteal layer is observed between the deep layer of the lamina propria and the periosteum [22]. In addition, the Schneiderian membrane is composed of basal cells, goblet cells, and ciliated cells [23]. While basal cells can differentiate into ciliated or goblet cells [24], goblet cells are mucin-secretory cells and this mucus is moved by the cilia of ciliated cells against gravity toward the ostium draining into the nasal cavity [25]. Moreover, connective tissue cells, collagen bundles, and elastic fibers can be found in the lamina propria. Recent findings have pointed that its thickness is on average 1 mm [21]; nevertheless, its evaluation using CBCT might overestimate the Schneiderian thickness by 2.5 to 2.6 times [21,26]. Along these lines, it is also important to note that factors such as smoking, gingival phenotype, or periodontal disease have shown strong associations with Schneiderian membrane thickness [27,28].

Furthermore, tearing of the Schneiderian membrane may potentially lead to post-operative infection. In a mechanical in vitro study it was shown that perforation occurred when a mean tension of 7.3 N/mm^2 was applied [29]. Additionally, it was demonstrated that it could be stretched to 132.6% of its original size in one-dimensional elongation, and to 124.7% in two-dimensional elongation [29]. Moreover, the mean modulus of elasticity was found to be 0.058 gigapascals (GPa). Clinical studies have also pointed to the importance of Schneiderian membrane thickness on perforation as it was hypothesized that thicker membranes may be less prone to tearing during access instrumentation and lifting, and could endure stronger compressing forces to allow more grafting material insertion [30]. As such, clinical findings have revealed that membrane perforation occurs less frequently when the Schneiderian membrane thickness is 1 to 1.5 mm in thickness for the lateral approach and 2 mm in thickness for the crestal approach [31,32].

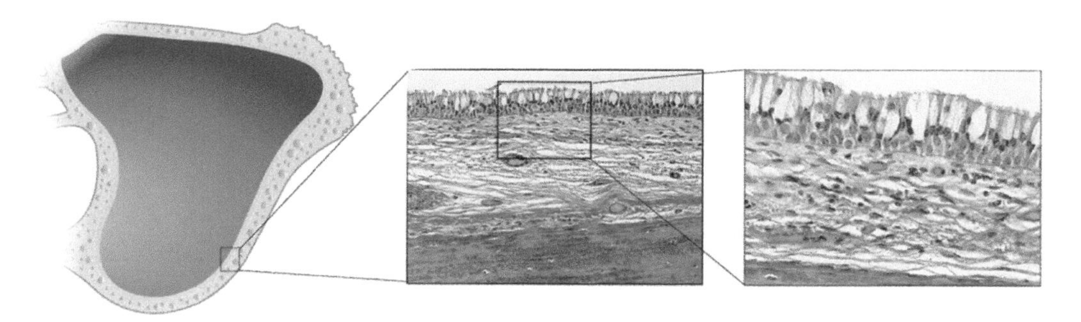

Figure 6.6 Depiction and histologic slide (Masson trichrome staining) of a Schneiderian membrane at X20 and X40. Source: Monje *et al.* 2016 [21]. Reproduced with permission of the American Academy of Periodontology.

6.2.5 Sinus septa

Another relevant anatomical feature are the sinus septa due to their association with membrane perforation. Primary septa are embryologically derived whereas secondary septa are the result of bone remodeling after tooth extraction [33,34]. The overall incidence of septa is 28.4% (24.5% and 17.2% unilateral and bilateral, respectively) and their height ranges from 3.55 mm to 9.2 mm [35]. The most common orientation is in mediolateral direction being taller medially and the most common location is the first molar area [36].

6.3 Biological principles

MSFE was initially described using autogenous marrow to promote new bone formation for adequate anchorage of the fixtures [37]. Recent advances in material sciences along with the exhaustive knowledge in bone biology illustrate the quintessence in regenerative dentistry, especially for MSFE. This fact allows the predictable reconstruction of a robust biological structure mimicking native tissues that may withstand occlusal forces transmitted during mastication in the posterior maxilla. Understanding the principles for regeneration, the maxillary sinus cavity represents a contained cavity where angiogenesis should not be a drawback due to the large number of vessels supplying this area. In this sense, the supply from the adjacent walls together with the Schneiderian membrane to the avascular scaffold with oxygen and nutrients is required for cell growth and differentiation [38,39]. Numerous growth factors, such as vascular endothelial growth factor (VEGF), fibroblastic growth factor (FGF), some subgroups of the β-transforming growth factor family (TGFβ), transcriptional factors to induce hypoxia (HIF), angioproteins (Ang-1), hepatocyte growth factor (HGF), bone morphogenetic protein (BMP), platelet-derived growth factor (PDGF), insulin-like derived growth factors (IGF-1, IGF-2), and neurotrophins growth factors (NGF) are involved in the process of bone regeneration [40–42]. Moreover, the stability of the clot must be granted in the maxillary sinus owing to the cavity containment.

In addition, the Schneiderian membrane has also been shown to possess reparative potential by means of mesenchymal progenitor cells that could be induced to express alkaline phosphatase, BMP-2, osteopontin, osteonectin, and osteocalcin and to mineralize their extracellular matrix [43]. Although the number of progenitor cells is deemed low, this might provide a plausible biological rationale for (1) the newly formed bone even in graftless MSFE procedures [44] and (2) the higher vital bone formation in perforated Schneiderian membranes [45]. Along these lines, it was demonstrated that, unlike for guided bone regeneration, the placement of a barrier membrane on the lateral aspect of the access window does not positively impact neither newly tissue characteristics nor implant survival [46].

Last but not least, space creation must be warrantied. Accordingly, Schneiderian membrane elevation must be carefully performed, detachment from all walls being a requirement. This has shown to be more challenging and risky in the presence of a high septa [47] or acute palato-nasal recess angulations [12] (Figure 6.7). The ultimate goal is to

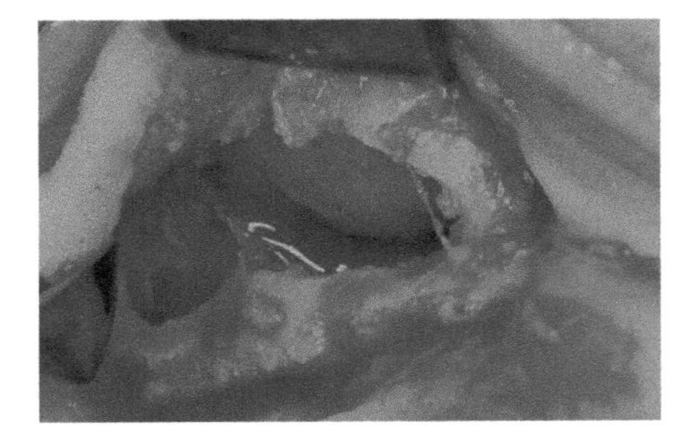

Figure 6.7 Presence of high primary septa induces a higher chance of Schneiderian membrane performation. (Figure provided courtesy of Prof. Pablo Galindo-Moreno).

attain free-tension and thus avoiding its collapse. This will ensure a proper hard tissue compartment.

6.4 Surgical techniques

Since the description of sinus augmentation as a feasible technique following the Caldwell-Luc approach to achieve sufficient bone height in the posterior atrophic maxilla, a myriad of modifications has been reported in the literature. As aforementioned, the MSFE via lateral window approach was introduced by Tatum at an Alabama conference on Implant Dentistry and later published by Boyne and James [37,48]. Briefly, it consisted of an osteotomy (antrostomy) on the lateral aspect of the maxillary sinus with a round bur to create a U-shape trap door to obtain access into the antrum and thereafter using autologous bone to graft the site (Figure 6.8). In the pursuit of reaching less invasiveness and thus, higher patient satisfaction/lower morbidity, the crestal approach was proposed by Summers [49]. Herein, it was claimed that by using a sequence of osteotomes it was feasible to reconstruct the atrophic maxilla vertically and horizontally and to achieve implant primary stability during the same surgery, shortening and simplifying the therapy. It must be highlighted that residual ridge height is the most common determinant regarding the decision making to select the appropriate approach [50].

Nowadays, a large variety of modifications have been introduced to both modalities. This is mainly a consequence of advancements in material sciences. For instance, early findings observed that by using a rotatory bur for the lateral window osteotomy, the likelihood of Schneiderian membrane perforation ranged from 0% to 58.3% with a mean value of 19.5% [51]. On the contrary,

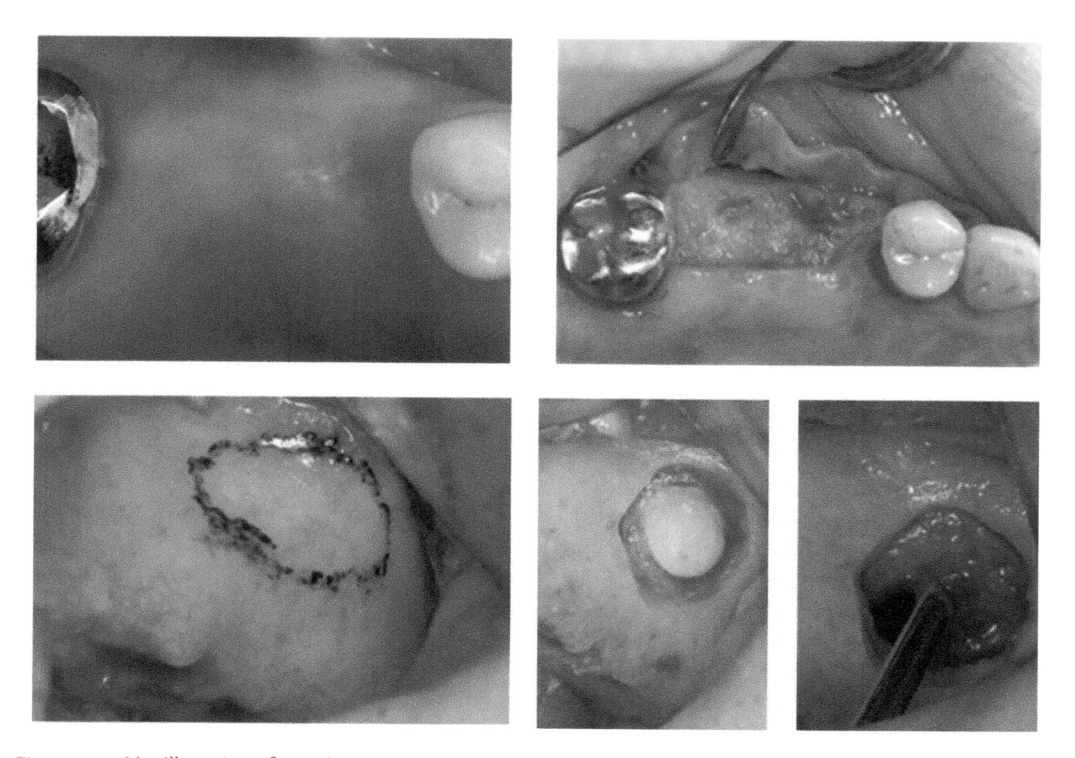

Figure 6.8 Maxillary sinus floor elevation performed via lateral wall approach in the presence of a moderately pneumatized ridge where implant primary stability could be achieved. (Case performed by Dr. Alberto Monje).

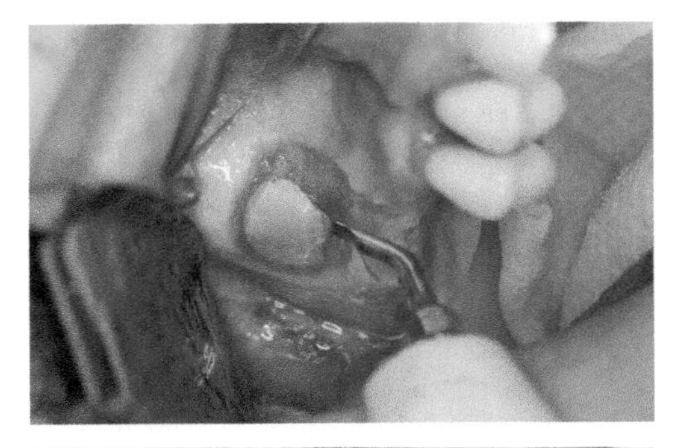

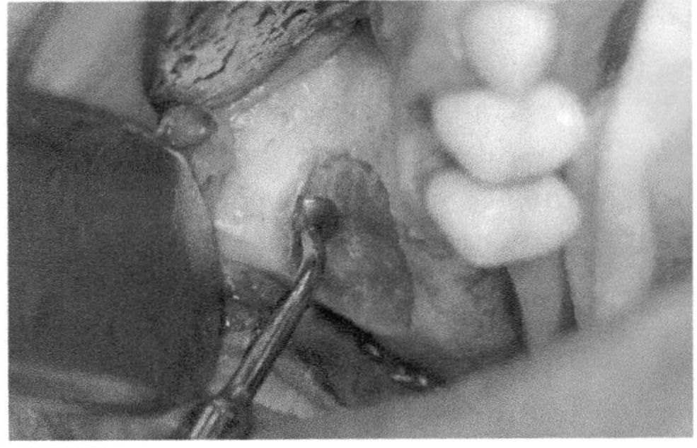

Figure 6.9 Use of piezo-electric surgery devices has improved the ability for clinicians to reduce complications associated with sinus augmentation procedures utilizing a lateral approach. (Clinical images courtesy of Dr. Michael A. Pikos).

novel devices such as piezoelectric using ultrasound technology have shown to reduce to 7% Schneiderian membrane perforation (Figure 6.9) [52,53]. Alike, a Bayesian network study has demonstrated that by using a minimally invasive piezoelectric instruments, only 6% of membrane perforation occurred [54]. Likewise, air driven sonic instruments have shown to reduce to 7.5% the likelihood of perforation [55]. These improvements are not surprising since the main advantages of these instruments are soft-tissue protection, decreased excessive bleeding by avoiding artery perforation as well as better visibility [56]. Furthermore, a reamer tool was developed to perform the procedure in an efficient manner. A report showed that the use of the drill recently significantly shorten the surgical time (11.1 versus 15.1 minutes) as well as minimized membrane perforation rate (8% versus 32%) when compared to conventional rotatory instruments [56]. Another study found that indeed Schneiderian membrane perforation could be minimized to 0% using the same tool if the lateral wall thickness was <1.25 mm [57].

A more recent novelty that was brought to market for MSFE was the use of a balloon to reach Schneiderian membrane and assist in its lifting thereby avoiding tearing/perforation, particularly in areas where there is adjacent dentition to the edentulous site. Other advantages to this technique is the need for a smaller lateral window, and minimal incision and mucoperiosteal flap reflection [58]. Moreover, this technique has also been applied during the crestal approach to gently lift the Schneiderian membrane (Figure 6.10) [59]. Indeed, it has been demonstrated to be effective for lifting the membrane achieving comparable bone gain to the osteotome approach and involving a low risk of complications [60]. Nevertheless, the main drawback of this technique is that if membrane perforation does occur, it cannot be controlled and in such a case, the perforation cannot be addressed due to the lack of visibility. Therefore, even though results seem to be promising, its use is limited to low risk cases (i.e., no presence of septa or other inconvenient anatomical features).

Recently, a classification containing three main categories has been proposed to overcome maxillary complications derived from the presence, orientation and number of maxillary septa. Interestingly, it was proposed than when the septum is ≤6 mm high, a wall-off/wall-gone technique could be used; nonetheless when the septum is >6 mm, it is very difficult to bypass a septum with such a height from only one side of it and hence, a two-access approach should be carried out to minimize Schneiderian membrane perforation [61].

6.5 Clinical outcomes

MSFE has been shown to be effective by means of bone gain and implant survival/

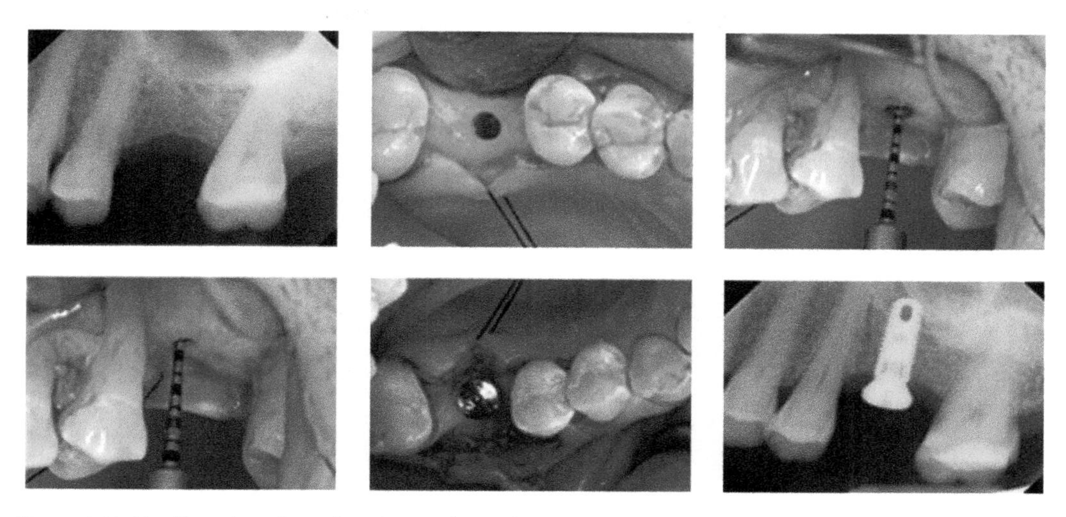

Figure 6.10 Maxillary sinus floor elevation performed via crestal approach in the presence of a maxillary sinus slightly pneumatized. (Case performed by Dr. Alberto Monje).

success in the long term. Indeed, if uneventful healing is completed, early success is warrantied. The long-term stability of the peri-implant tissues are therefore mainly dependent on other modifiable and non-modifiable factors (i.e., smoking, occlusion, oral hygiene or infection) [62]. Due to the continuous development and improvements of bone biomaterials, clinical trials of implants placed after MSFE are continuously being published and consequently, systematic reviews aiming at presenting the current state of the art. Data from these high scientific evidence showed that in the early 2000s implant survival was on average 91.8% [63], while more recent quantitative assessments indicate an increase to 97.2% [64,65]. True is to note that higher implant survival predictability as available residual bone increases <5 mm: 96% (80%–100%), and (2) >4 mm 99% (97%–100%) [66]. This fact is of crucial importance in MSFE via crestal approach where implant survival was found to be 96% or higher when pretreatment bone height was 5 mm but only 85.7% when it was <4 mm [67].

Regarding peri-implant bone stability, a clinical retrospective study reported that for maxillary reconstruction involving bilateral MSFE, implant survival was 100% with only 1.4 mm of marginal bone loss 15 years after loading [68]. Therefore, MSFE represents a predictable option to restore the posterior atrophic maxilla. Nonetheless, other alternatives such as short or tilted implants might lead to higher patient satisfaction since they are subject to less complications and a shorter treatment protocols.

6.6 Surgical and post-surgical complications

In order to avoid potential complications, the surgeon must be aware of the anatomical features described previously (Table 6.1). Complications related to MSFE most frequently include but are not limited to:

- Schneiderian membrane perforation
- Acute and chronic infection
- Hemorrhage
- Sinus oro-antral communication/fistula
- Implant migration into the maxillary sinus cavity
- Alterations in the voice quality

6.6.1 Schneiderian membrane perforation

Schneiderian membrane perforation is indeed the most common intra-operative

Table 6.1 Complications related to MSFE.

Risk indicators	Complication	Level of risk	Diagnostic method	Clinical recommendation
Maxillary sinus septa	Schneiderian membrane perforation	+++	CBCT	• Large access window to enhance visibility and instrument accessibility/ manipulation • Two-window approach to by-pass the septa
Schneiderian membrane thickening	Schneiderian membrane perforation	+	CBCT	• Gentle management of the Schneiderian membrane
Posterior superior alveolar artery	Hemorrhage	++	CBCT	• The use of ultrasonic instruments or scrappers to access the sinus cavity • In case of vassal perforation, prompt suture or coagulation must be carried out
Palato-nasal recess	Schneiderian membrane perforation	++	CBCT	• Carefully management of the Schneiderian membrane to lift it in acute palato-nasal recesses
Acute or chronic infection	Schneiderian membrane perforation	++	CBCT	• Broad-spectrum antibiotics should be the primary choice • Referral to the otolaryngologist (ENT) if does not remit
Alveolar ridge density	Implant failure/implant migration to the maxillary sinus cavity	++	Implant torque/ Implant stability (ISQ)/CBCT	• Achieve proper primary stability • Leading the implant loading approach according to the ISQ value • If ISQ is <60, follow a two-stage approach and submerge it.
Alveolar ridge height	Implant failure/implant migration to the maxillary sinus cavity	++	CBCT	• In <5 mm alveolar ridge height, simultaneous implant placement is not advocated
Smoking	Schneiderian membrane perforation/early-late implant failure	+++	Oral communication	• Smoking cessation counseling prior to MSFE procedure
Poor plaque control	Post-surgical infection	++	Plaque-index	• Prior to treatment plan fro MSFE, plaque index must be <15% to 20%
Adjacent tooth infection	Post-surgical maxillary sinus infection	++	CBCT	• Infection control must be managed and healed prior to MSFE

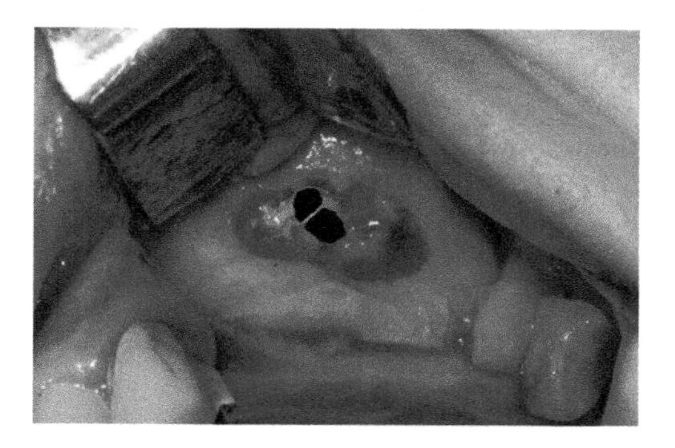

Figure 6.11 Medium size Schneiderian membrane perforation (5 to 10 mm). (Clinical image courtesy of Prof. Pablo Galindo-Moreno).

complication when performing MSFE. Schneiderian membrane perforation rate has dramatically decreased from over the last decade due to novel tools such as piezoelectric (7%) or reamer (12.5%) devices.

It has been observed that certain anatomical features such as presence of septa together with operator inexperience might negatively be associated with higher perforation rates (Figure 6.11). Although it has not been shown in an evidence-based manner that Schneiderian membrane thickness is significantly related to perforation, it has been suggested that very thin or very thick membranes may be more susceptible to tear due to their elasticity properties (Monje *et al.*, 2016a).

It is important to note that Schneiderian membrane perforation may lead to post-operative infection, jeopardizing the stability of the viability/stability of the graft and/or the implant. Furthermore, if abundant grafting material access within the lining membrane is found, there is a higher risk for ostium obliteration, impeding adequate drainage and triggering an adverse foreign body reaction.

Its management is crucial for the success of the regenerative therapy. Although it remains a matter of controversy, small perforations (<5 mm) seem straightforward to treat. Accordingly, it could either be self-folded under a tension-free Schneiderian membrane release or a biodegradable (i.e., collagen) membrane could be placed. In this sense, platelet rich fibrin (PRF) represents a promising autogenous material to be placed as a substitute of allogeneic or xenogeneic barrier membranes (discussed in the following chapter). In addition, this might offer an alternative to further promote angiogenesis at implant site development in the maxillary sinus. When Schneiderian membrane perforation is >5 mm but <10 mm, more controversy is found in the literature due to the increased difficulty to manage [69]. Again, a larger autogenous or heterogonous barrier membrane would be advocated. Contrarily, in the presence of a larger membrane perforation, the surgical outcome could be compromised and thus, it may be wise to abort and attempt a second stage surgery at >3 months once the membrane is healed [70]. In the meantime, the clinician could identify the triggering factor and better address this issue in a subsequent attempt.

6.6.2 Acute or chronic infections

As previously stated, Schneiderian membrane perforation may lead to post-operative infection. This might occur via retrograde infection of the biomaterial or displacement of the grafting material within the lining membrane. In order to address this issue, the clinician must diagnose whether the infection is acute or chronic in nature. While typically acute infections last 4 weeks, chronic infections have been described as being a minimum of 12 weeks. Nevertheless, both present with consistent and similar symptoms: suppuration, nasal congestion, facial pressure-like feeling, and anosmia. Acute sinusitis presents with a lack/reduced permeability of the airflow, whereas chronic sinusitis displays thickening of the Schneiderian membrane and demonstrates histologically the presence of epithelial damage including impairment of the cilia function, absence of cilia and epithelial erosion [71,72].

Sinus pathology is a frequent finding and the inflammatory sinus condition is the most common disease among the paranasal sinuses [25]. Some reports have noted that

40% of patients scheduled for sinus augmentation report some sinus pathology. Others have reported a 45.1% sinus pathology among patients undergoing implant therapy [73,74]. Mucosal thickening higher than 5 mm was reported in 56.5% of the patients, presence of polyps in 28.2%, and partial or complete sinus opacification in 15.4% of cases [74]. Therefore, these findings seem to indicate that after MSFE, a period of time must pass to accurately diagnose the potential presence of pathology.

The etiology of chronic sinusitis is multifactorial: anatomical issues, developmental disorders, bacterial, or viral infections, among others [75]. In this sense, CBCT rather than two-dimensional radiographic tools result in high specific detection of pathology and/or irritant that may be triggering an inflammatory reaction.

Regarding to treatment, broad-spectrum antibiotics should be the primary choice. If these are not effective in treating the pathology, the biomaterial must then be retrieved and the MSFE procedure should restart following 6 months of total clearance. The clinician may also consider a referral to the otolaryngologist (ENT) with the goal of promoting ostium permeability and fostering an aerobic bacterial and fungal environment.

6.6.3 Hemorrhage

Excessive hemorrhage might occur as a consequence of damage to the double anastomosis of the PSAA or due to the damage to the arterial complex of the basal membrane of the Schneiderian membrane. Therefore, the osteotomy to obtain access to the maxillary sinus antrum must be performed under cautiousness in the presence of PSAA and IOA anastomoses. The reported rate of incidence has been reported in the range of 0% to 47% according to radiographic and cadaver studies [76,77]. It is generally located 18 to 19 mm above the ridge crest, although it is case-dependent and 20% may even be located at the 16 mm level, particularly in severely atrophic posterior maxillae. Once again, this fact highlights the importance of pre-operative three-dimensional radiographic evaluation. The diameter is commonly <2 mm in 95.7% of the cases, whereas 4.3% of the cases have a reported size >2 mm but it is actually <3 mm. In these scenarios, the situation should be managed by applying hemostatic materials to reduce excessive bleeding [77]. If on the contrary, the artery is >3 mm and is damaged, obliteration must be carried out with sutures.

Since this complication must be given remarkable importance owing to the threat that represents to the unprepared clinician, prevention must be exercised. As such, CBCT should be advocated for every MSFE case in order to better understand the vascular network and thus, reducing the risk of complication. Moreover, ultrasonic technology (i.e., piezosurgery) should be utilized to avoid undesired trauma to the arterial complex.

6.6.4 Implant migration

Implant migration to the maxillary and the ethmoid sinuses represents an uncommon post-operative complication [78,79]. Several theories have been proposed to explain this fact such as changes in the intrasinusal and nasal pressures, autoimmune reaction to the implant or inadequate occlusal loading triggering a loss of osseointegration and thus, migrating into the sinus cavity. An interesting study found out that 73.3% of sites that did not receive any biomaterial to increase available bone height experienced implant migration. Moreover, it was elucidated that cylindrical and narrow implants in scenarios of lesser residual ridge height (5 mm to 6.9 mm) were more prone to have migrations into the maxillary sinus cavity [80]. In this context, it is noteworthy to mention that higher implant primary stability in the posterior atrophic maxilla via drilling protocol modifications favor more optimal results since this area presents with less bone density [81,82].

6.7 Conclusion

Although, maxillary sinus floor elevation has been widely explored in the last three decades, it is essential that the treating clinician be aware of the anatomy, risks, and complications associated with maxillary sinus floor elevation procedures. As such, anatomical features of the maxillary sinus including the maxillary sinus dimensions, size of the lining membrane, and features of the sinus septa are all factors affecting the rate of complication. More recently, the development of novel surgical instrumentation including piezoelectric devices has drastically lowered the rate of perforation of the Schneiderian membrane by improving surgical handling. Nevertheless, the treating physician must be aware and responsible for managing subsequent potential complications that may nevertheless occur including Schneiderian membrane perforation, acute and chronic infection, hemorrhage, sinus oro-antral communication/fistula, implant migration into the maxillary sinus cavity, as well as alterations in the voice quality. This chapter highlights the importance of utilizing three-dimensional radiographic analysis (cone-beam computed tomography) thereby minimizing the risk of complication and improving patient outcomes/satisfaction. As advancements in radiography, surgical instrumentation, and bone biomaterials continue to evolve, it is imperative that the treating clinician be well educated with this changing field in order to further improve treatment outcomes and reduce the risk and frequency of complications associated with MSFE treatment protocols.

References

1 Pietrokovski J, Massler M. Alveolar ridge resorption following tooth extraction. J Prosthet Dent. 1967;17(1):21–7.
2 Swenson HM, Hudson JR. Roentgenographic examination of edentulous patients. The Journal of prosthetic dentistry. 1967;18(4):304–7.
3 Pietrokovski J, Massler M. Alveolar ridge resorption following tooth extraction. The Journal of prosthetic dentistry. 1967;17(1): 21–7.
4 Schropp L, Wenzel A, Kostopoulos L, Karring T. Bone healing and soft tissue contour changes following single-tooth extraction: a clinical and radiographic 12-month prospective study. The International journal of periodontics & restorative dentistry. 2003;23(4):313–23.
5 van den Bergh JP, ten Bruggenkate CM, Disch FJ, Tuinzing DB. Anatomical aspects of sinus floor elevations. Clin Oral Implants Res. 2000;11(3):256–65.
6 Temple KE, Schoolfield J, Noujeim ME, Huynh-Ba G, Lasho DJ, Mealey BL. A cone beam computed tomography (CBCT) study of buccal plate thickness of the maxillary and mandibular posterior dentition. Clinical oral implants research. 2016;27(9):1072–8.
7 Scuderi AJ, Harnsberger HR, Boyer RS. Pneumatization of the paranasal sinuses: normal features of importance to the accurate interpretation of CT scans and MR images. AJR American journal of roentgenology. 1993;160(5):1101–4.
8 Jun BC, Song SW, Park CS, Lee DH, Cho KJ, Cho JH. The analysis of maxillary sinus aeration according to aging process; volume assessment by 3-dimensional reconstruction by high-resolutional CT scanning. Otolaryngology–head and neck surgery: official journal of American Academy of Otolaryngology-Head and Neck Surgery. 2005;132(3):429–34.
9 Teng M, Cheng Q, Liao J, Zhang X, Mo A, Liang X. Sinus Width Analysis and New Classification with Clinical Implications for Augmentation. Clinical implant

dentistry and related research. 2016;18(1): 89–96.
10 van den Bergh JP, ten Bruggenkate CM, Disch FJ, Tuinzing DB. Anatomical aspects of sinus floor elevations. Clinical oral implants research. 2000;11(3):256–65.
11 Chan HL, Suarez F, Monje A, Benavides E, Wang HL. Evaluation of maxillary sinus width on cone-beam computed tomography for sinus augmentation and new sinus classification based on sinus width. Clinical oral implants research. 2014;25(6):647–52.
12 Chan HL, Monje A, Suarez F, Benavides E, Wang HL. Palatonasal recess on medial wall of the maxillary sinus and clinical implications for sinus augmentation via lateral window approach. Journal of periodontology. 2013;84(8):1087–93.
13 Monje A, Catena A, Monje F, Gonzalez-Garcia R, Galindo-Moreno P, Suarez F, et al. Maxillary sinus lateral wall thickness and morphologic patterns in the atrophic posterior maxilla. Journal of periodontology. 2014;85(5):676–82.
14 Ariji Y, Kuroki T, Moriguchi S, Ariji E, Kanda S. Age changes in the volume of the human maxillary sinus: a study using computed tomography. Dento maxillo facial radiology. 1994;23(3):163–8.
15 Gencer ZK, Ozkiris M, Okur A, Karacavus S, Saydam L. The possible associations of septal deviation on mastoid pneumatization and chronic otitis. Otology & neurotology: official publication of the American Otological Society, American Neurotology Society [and] European Academy of Otology and Neurotology. 2013;34(6):1052–7.
16 Soikkonen K, Wolf J, Hietanen J, Mattila K. Three main arteries of the face and their tortuosity. The British journal of oral & maxillofacial surgery. 1991;29(6):395–8.
17 Danesh-Sani SA, Movahed A, ElChaar ES, Chong Chan K, Amintavakoli N. Radiographic Evaluation of Maxillary Sinus Lateral Wall and Posterior Superior Alveolar Artery Anatomy: A Cone-Beam Computed Tomographic Study. Clinical implant dentistry and related research. 2016.
18 Solar P, Geyerhofer U, Traxler H, Windisch A, Ulm C, Watzek G. Blood supply to the maxillary sinus relevant to sinus floor elevation procedures. Clinical oral implants research. 1999;10(1):34–44.
19 Elian N, Wallace S, Cho SC, Jalbout ZN, Froum S. Distribution of the maxillary artery as it relates to sinus floor augmentation. The International journal of oral & maxillofacial implants. 2005;20(5): 784–7.
20 Rehl RM, Balla AA, Cabay RJ, Hearp ML, Pytynia KB, Joe SA. Mucosal remodeling in chronic rhinosinusitis. American journal of rhinology. 2007;21(6):651–7.
21 Monje A, Diaz KT, Aranda L, Insua A, Garcia-Nogales A, Wang HL. Schneiderian Membrane Thickness and Clinical Implications for Sinus Augmentation: A Systematic Review and Meta-Regression Analyses. Journal of periodontology. 2016;87(8):888–99.
22 Stierna P, Carlsoo B. Histopathological observations in chronic maxillary sinusitis. Acta oto-laryngologica. 1990;110(5-6): 450–8.
23 Mogensen C, Tos M. Quantitative histology of the maxillary sinus. Rhinology. 1977;15(3):129–40.
24 Oughlis S, Lessim S, Changotade S, Bollotte F, Poirier F, Helary G, et al. Development of proteomic tools to study protein adsorption on a biomaterial, titanium grafted with poly(sodium styrene sulfonate). Journal of chromatography B, Analytical technologies in the biomedical and life sciences. 2011;879(31):3681–7.
25 Bell GW, Joshi BB, Macleod RI. Maxillary sinus disease: diagnosis and treatment. British dental journal. 2011;210(3): 113–8.
26 Insua A, Monje A, Chan HL, Zimmo N, Shaikh L, Wang HL. Accuracy of Schneiderian membrane thickness: a cone-beam computed tomography analysis with histological validation. Clinical oral implants research. 2016.

27 Aimetti M, Massei G, Morra M, Cardesi E, Romano F. Correlation between gingival phenotype and Schneiderian membrane thickness. The International journal of oral & maxillofacial implants. 2008;23(6): 1128–32.
28 Yilmaz HG, Tozum TF. Are gingival phenotype, residual ridge height, and membrane thickness critical for the perforation of maxillary sinus? Journal of periodontology. 2012;83(4):420–5.
29 Pommer B, Unger E, Suto D, Hack N, Watzek G. Mechanical properties of the Schneiderian membrane in vitro. Clinical oral implants research. 2009;20(6):633–7.
30 Garcia-Denche JT, Wu X, Martinez PP, Eimar H, Ikbal DJ, Hernandez G, et al. Membranes over the lateral window in sinus augmentation procedures: a two-arm and split-mouth randomized clinical trials. Journal of clinical periodontology. 2013; 40(11):1043–51.
31 Lin YH, Yang YC, Wen SC, Wang HL. The influence of sinus membrane thickness upon membrane perforation during lateral window sinus augmentation. Clinical oral implants research. 2015.
32 Wen SC, Lin YH, Yang YC, Wang HL. The influence of sinus membrane thickness upon membrane perforation during transcrestal sinus lift procedure. Clinical oral implants research. 2015;26(10): 1158–64.
33 Krennmair G, Ulm C, Lugmayr H. Maxillary sinus septa: incidence, morphology and clinical implications. Journal of cranio-maxillo-facial surgery: official publication of the European Association for Cranio-Maxillo-Facial Surgery. 1997;25(5):261–5.
34 Lugmayr H, Krennmair G, Holzer H. [The morphology and incidence of maxillary sinus septa]. RoFo: Fortschritte auf dem Gebiete der Rontgenstrahlen und der Nuklearmedizin. 1996;165(5):452–4.
35 Kim MJ, Jung UW, Kim CS, Kim KD, Choi SH, Kim CK, et al. Maxillary sinus septa: prevalence, height, location, and morphology. A reformatted computed tomography scan analysis. Journal of periodontology. 2006;77(5):903–8.
36 Pommer B, Ulm C, Lorenzoni M, Palmer R, Watzek G, Zechner W. Prevalence, location and morphology of maxillary sinus septa: systematic review and meta-analysis. Journal of clinical periodontology. 2012;39(8):769–73.
37 Boyne PJ, James RA. Grafting of the maxillary sinus floor with autogenous marrow and bone. Journal of oral surgery. 1980;38(8):613–6.
38 King TW, Brey EM, Youssef AA, Johnston C, Patrick CW, Jr. Quantification of vascular density using a semiautomated technique for immunostained specimens. Anal Quant Cytol Histol. 2002;24(1):39–48.
39 Buser D, Dula K, Belser U, Hirt HP, Berthold H. Localized ridge augmentation using guided bone regeneration. 1. Surgical procedure in the maxilla. The International journal of periodontics & restorative dentistry. 1993;13(1):29–45.
40 Madeddu P. Therapeutic angiogenesis and vasculogenesis for tissue regeneration. Experimental physiology. 2005;90(3): 315–26.
41 Miron RJ, Zhang YF. Osteoinduction: a review of old concepts with new standards. Journal of dental research. 2012;91(8): 736–44.
42 Saghiri MA, Asatourian A, Garcia-Godoy F, Sheibani N. The role of angiogenesis in implant dentistry part II: The effect of bone-grafting and barrier membrane materials on angiogenesis. Medicina oral, patologia oral y cirugia bucal. 2016;21(4): e526–37.
43 Srouji S, Kizhner T, Ben David D, Riminucci M, Bianco P, Livne E. The Schneiderian membrane contains osteoprogenitor cells: in vivo and in vitro study. Calcified tissue international. 2009; 84(2):138–45.
44 Thor A, Sennerby L, Hirsch JM, Rasmusson L. Bone formation at the maxillary sinus floor following simultaneous elevation of the mucosal lining and implant installation without graft material: an evaluation of

20 patients treated with 44 Astra Tech implants. Journal of oral and maxillofacial surgery: official journal of the American Association of Oral and Maxillofacial Surgeons. 2007;65(7 Suppl 1):64–72.
45 Froum SJ, Khouly I, Favero G, Cho SC. Effect of maxillary sinus membrane perforation on vital bone formation and implant survival: a retrospective study. Journal of periodontology. 2013;84(8): 1094–9.
46 Suarez-Lopez Del Amo F, Ortega-Oller I, Catena A, Monje A, Khoshkam V, Torrecillas-Martinez L, et al. Effect of barrier membranes on the outcomes of maxillary sinus floor augmentation: a meta-analysis of histomorphometric outcomes. The International journal of oral & maxillofacial implants. 2015;30(3): 607–18.
47 von Arx T, Fodich I, Bornstein MM, Jensen SS. Perforation of the sinus membrane during sinus floor elevation: a retrospective study of frequency and possible risk factors. The International journal of oral & maxillofacial implants. 2014;29(3): 718–26.
48 Tatum H, Jr. Maxillary and sinus implant reconstructions. Dental clinics of North America. 1986;30(2):207–29.
49 Summers RB. A new concept in maxillary implant surgery: the osteotome technique. Compendium. 1994;15(2):152, 4-6, 8 passim; quiz 62.
50 Wang HL, Katranji A. ABC sinus augmentation classification. The International journal of periodontics & restorative dentistry. 2008;28(4):383–9.
51 Pjetursson BE, Tan WC, Zwahlen M, Lang NP. A systematic review of the success of sinus floor elevation and survival of implants inserted in combination with sinus floor elevation. Journal of clinical periodontology. 2008;35(8 Suppl):216–40.
52 Rickert D, Vissink A, Slater JJ, Meijer HJ, Raghoebar GM. Comparison between conventional and piezoelectric surgical tools for maxillary sinus floor elevation. A randomized controlled clinical trial. Clinical implant dentistry and related research. 2013;15(2):297–302.
53 Wallace SS, Mazor Z, Froum SJ, Cho SC, Tarnow DP. Schneiderian membrane perforation rate during sinus elevation using piezosurgery: clinical results of 100 consecutive cases. The International journal of periodontics & restorative dentistry. 2007;27(5):413–9.
54 Merli M, Moscatelli M, Mariotti G, Pagliaro U, Bernardelli F, Nieri M. A minimally invasive technique for lateral maxillary sinus floor elevation: a Bayesian network study. Clinical oral implants research. 2014.
55 Weitz DS, Geminiani A, Papadimitriou DE, Ercoli C, Caton JG. The incidence of membrane perforation during sinus floor elevation using sonic instruments: a series of 40 cases. The International journal of periodontics & restorative dentistry. 2014;34(1):105–12.
56 Kazancioglu HO, Tek M, Ezirganli S, Mihmanli A. Comparison of a novel trephine drill with conventional rotary instruments for maxillary sinus floor elevation. The International journal of oral & maxillofacial implants. 2013;28(5): 1201–6.
57 Monje A, Monje-Gil F, Burgueno M, Gonzalez-Garcia R, Galindo-Moreno P, Wang HL. Incidence of and Factors Associated with Sinus Membrane Perforation During Maxillary Sinus Augmentation Using the Reamer Drilling Approach: A Double-Center Case Series. The International journal of periodontics & restorative dentistry. 2016;36(4):549–56.
58 Soltan M, Smiler DG. Antral membrane balloon elevation. The Journal of oral implantology. 2005;31(2):85–90.
59 Kfir E, Kfir V, Mijiritsky E, Rafaeloff R, Kaluski E. Minimally invasive antral membrane balloon elevation followed by maxillary bone augmentation and implant fixation. The Journal of oral implantology. 2006;32(1):26–33.
60 Chan HL, Oh TJ, Fu JH, Benavides E, Avila-Ortiz G, Wang HL. Sinus

augmentation via transcrestal approach: a comparison between the balloon and osteotome technique in a cadaver study. Clinical oral implants research. 2013;24(9): 985–90.

61 Wen SC, Chan HL, Wang HL. Classification and management of antral septa for maxillary sinus augmentation. The International journal of periodontics & restorative dentistry. 2013;33(4):509–17.

62 Chambrone L, Preshaw PM, Ferreira JD, Rodrigues JA, Cassoni A, Shibli JA. Effects of tobacco smoking on the survival rate of dental implants placed in areas of maxillary sinus floor augmentation: a systematic review. Clinical oral implants research. 2014;25(4):408–16.

63 Wallace SS, Froum SJ. Effect of maxillary sinus augmentation on the survival of endosseous dental implants. A systematic review. Annals of periodontology/the American Academy of Periodontology. 2003;8(1):328–43.

64 Del Fabbro M, Wallace SS, Testori T. Long-Term Implant Survival in the Grafted Maxillary Sinus: A Systematic Review. Int J Periodont Rest. 2013;33(6):773–+.

65 Duttenhoefer F, Souren C, Menne D, Emmerich D, Schon R, Sauerbier S. Long-Term Survival of Dental Implants Placed in the Grafted Maxillary Sinus: Systematic Review and Meta-Analysis of Treatment Modalities. PloS one. 2013;8(9).

66 Rios HF, Avila G, Galindo P, Bratu E, Wang HL. The influence of remaining alveolar bone upon lateral window sinus augmentation implant survival. Implant dentistry. 2009;18(5):402–12.

67 Rosen PS, Summers R, Mellado JR, Salkin LM, Shanaman RH, Marks MH, et al. The bone-added osteotome sinus floor elevation technique: multicenter retrospective report of consecutively treated patients. The International journal of oral & maxillofacial implants. 1999;14(6): 853–8.

68 Urban IA, Monje A, Lozada JL, Wang HL. Long-term Evaluation of Peri-implant Bone Level after Reconstruction of Severely Atrophic Edentulous Maxilla via Vertical and Horizontal Guided Bone Regeneration in Combination with Sinus Augmentation: A Case Series with 1 to 15 Years of Loading. Clinical implant dentistry and related research. 2016.

69 Hernandez-Alfaro F, Torradeflot MM, Marti C. Prevalence and management of Schneiderian membrane perforations during sinus-lift procedures. Clinical oral implants research. 2008;19(1):91–8.

70 Watelet JB, Demetter P, Claeys C, Cauwenberge P, Cuvelier C, Bachert C. Wound healing after paranasal sinus surgery: neutrophilic inflammation influences the outcome. Histopathology. 2006;48(2):174–81.

71 Anselmo-Lima WT, Ferreira MD, Valera FC, Rossato M, de Mello VR, Demarco RC. Histological evaluation of maxillary sinus mucosa after functional endoscopic sinus surgery. American journal of rhinology. 2007;21(6):719–24.

72 Pawankar R, Nonaka M. Inflammatory mechanisms and remodeling in chronic rhinosinusitis and nasal polyps. Current allergy and asthma reports. 2007;7(3): 202–8.

73 Beaumont C, Zafiropoulos GG, Rohmann K, Tatakis DN. Prevalence of maxillary sinus disease and abnormalities in patients scheduled for sinus lift procedures. Journal of periodontology. 2005;76(3):461–7.

74 Manji A, Faucher J, Resnik RR, Suzuki JB. Prevalence of maxillary sinus pathology in patients considered for sinus augmentation procedures for dental implants. Implant dentistry. 2013;22(4):428–35.

75 Chan HL, Wang HL. Sinus pathology and anatomy in relation to complications in lateral window sinus augmentation. Implant dentistry. 2011;20(6):406–12.

76 Solar P, Geyerhofer U, Traxler H, Windisch A, Ulm C, Watzek G. Blood supply to the maxillary sinus relevant to sinus floor elevation procedures. Clinical oral implants research. 1999;10(1):34–44.

77 Rosano G, Taschieri S, Gaudy JF, Weinstein T, Del Fabbro M. Maxillary sinus vascular anatomy and its relation to sinus lift surgery. Clinical oral implants research. 2011;22(7):711–5.

78 Bakhshalian N, Sim YC, Nowzari H, Cha HS, Ahn KM. Accidental Migration of a Dental Implant into the Ethmoid Sinus following a Transalveolar Sinus Elevation Procedure. Clinical implant dentistry and related research. 2015;17(2):360–4.

79 Galindo P, Sanchez-Fernandez E, Avila G, Cutando A, Fernandez JE. Migration of implants into the maxillary sinus: Two clinical cases. Int J Oral Max Impl. 2005; 20(2):291–5.

80 Galindo-Moreno P, Padial-Molina M, Avila G, Rios HF, Hernandez-Cortes P, Wang HL. Complications associated with implant migration into the maxillary sinus cavity. Clinical oral implants research. 2012; 23(10):1152–60.

81 Monje A, Monje F, Gonzalez-Garcia R, Suarez F, Galindo-Moreno P, Garcia-Nogales A, et al. Influence of Atrophic Posterior Maxilla Ridge Height on Bone Density and Microarchitecture. Clinical implant dentistry and related research. 2015;17(1):111–9.

82 Monje A, Gonzalez-Garcia R, Monje F, Chan HL, Galindo-Moreno P, Suarez F, et al. Microarchitectural Pattern of Pristine Maxillary Bone. Int J Oral Max Impl. 2015; 30(1):125–32.

7

Maxillary Sinus Floor Elevation Procedures with Platelet Rich Fibrin: Indications and Clinical Recommendations

Richard J. Miron, Michael A. Pikos, and Hom-Lay Wang

Abstract

An array of bone biomaterials have now been utilized to regenerate the atrophic maxillary sinus. While bone substitutes with or without collagen barrier membranes have most commonly been utilized, more recently, the development of a second generation platelet concentrates (platelet rich fibrin; PRF) has been investigated. Attempts were first made to determine whether PRF could be utilized alone to replace conventional biomaterials by 100% autologous blood-derived fibrin scaffolds. Following 10 years of clinical testing, reports now show that PRF can be utilized as a sole grafting material but more frequently should be combined with bone grafting particles to improve their space maintenance as well as angiogenic potential within the sinus cavity. Interestingly, PRF has also been frequently utilized for the repair of Schneiderian membrane perforations and investigated for window closure following maxillary sinus floor elevation utilizing the lateral approach. While this chapter highlights the clinical studies that have been performed to date utilizing PRF for maxillary sinus floor elevation procedures, conservative clinical recommendations are provided with indications supporting its effective use for sinus grafting procedures.

Highlights

- The use of PRF as a sole grafting material
- Anatomical considerations for utilizing PRF as a sole grafting material
- Use of PRF in combination with bone grafting materials for sinus elevation procedures
- Use of PRF for repair of Schneiderian membrane perforation
- Use of PRF to close the lateral window

7.1 Introduction

The use of platelet rich fibrin (PRF) derived from human blood has now been extensively utilized in regenerative dentistry due to its ability to increase angiogenesis via the release of autologous growth factors [1]. While these factors are not necessarily osteoinductive, they support new blood vessel formation by the release of vascular endothelial growth factor (VEGF), the most potent pro-angiogenic growth factor [2]. Due to these biological advantages, PRF has been investigated during sinus floor elevation procedures [3]. As expressed in the previous chapter, the alveolar ridge undergoes various changes over time and most notably following tooth loss where bone is rapidly resorbed due to loss of compressive force (Chapter 6). While bone-grafting materials are most commonly utilized, over the past decade, an array of investigations have been performed utilizing PRF either alone or in

Platelet Rich Fibrin in Regenerative Dentistry: Biological Background and Clinical Indications, First Edition.
Edited by Richard J. Miron and Joseph Choukroun.

combination with a bone substitute material. In 2006, Choukroun *et al.* demonstrated that PRF could be successfully combined with a bone grafting material with the hypothesis that its angiogenic potential could further facilitate new bone formation in the maxillary sinus following a lateral window approach [4]. While its direct effect was not compared to bone-grafting material alone in a randomized, controlled clinical study, it was hypothesized that by adding pro-angiogenic growth factors into the maxillary sinus where blood flow is reduced, bone cell migration from the maxillary sinus bony walls could be increased, thereby speeding the ability for osteoblasts to form new bone.

Interestingly, more recently the use of PRF has been utilized alone as a sole grafting material during sinus lifting procedures either using the lateral or crestal approach as discussed later in this chapter. While original studies were performed investigating PRF even in extreme cases with limited crestal bone volume, conservative approaches have more recently been recommended to reduce the potential risk of failure later discussed.

Nowadays, the utilization of PRF has three relevant areas of practice with documented evidence supporting its use. As previously stated, PRF has been utilized alone or in combination with bone grafts to augment lost or missing bone during maxillary sinus floor elevation procedures. More recently, PRF has also been utilized either to repair Schneiderian membrane tears, or to close the bony window following lateral sinus augmentation procedures. Below we demonstrate case reports and documented evidence from the literature supporting its use in each of the indications presented below.

7.2 PRF as a sole grafting material during sinus lifting procedures

A variety of bone-grafting materials have been utilized to date to augment lost or missing bone as a result of pneumatization of the sinus [5,6]. One of the main focuses of research has addressed the question whether or not PRF could be utilized as a sole grafting material during sinus floor elevation procedures. While most of these studies demonstrate the use of PRF in case reports, various studies have shown that PRF alone could lead to increases in new bone formation around implants (Figures 7.1 and 7.2). For this approach to be successful, it is an absolute requirement that implants be placed simultaneously. This is because the use of an implant by itself will act as a space creator to provide needed space for bone to ingrow. So far, studies have supported the notion that implants can be placed alone with no use of biomaterials. So long as a blood clot is formed around the implant surface, new bone formation will follow [7–9].

Although the addition of PRF to bone grafting materials is more common and generally the accepted standard to regenerate missing bone in the sinus resulting in high rates of success, several authors have demonstrated that its use could be utilized to promote bone healing with vertical bone height gain reported at 7.52 mm [10], 10.1 mm [11], and 10.4 mm [12] between the sinus floor and the top of the alveolar ridge following augmentation with PRF alone. Although no controls were utilized in these studies, the results demonstrate that PRF alone could be used as a treatment modality and no implants were lost at 6 months, 1 year, and 6 years in their respective studies [10–12]. In total, eight studies have now followed a similar approach utilizing PRF as a sole grafting material (Table 7.1). While some authors have suggested that its use alone may be a valid treatment option for the majority of maxillary sinus floor elevation procedures, a lack of controls and limited data regarding patient inclusion and characterization of the sinuses were made available. In this sense, it is crucial to understand that the treatment outcome that these studies applied was primarily radiographic bone gain and consequently, it can only be speculated that the formation of new bone is better ascertained with histologic analysis.

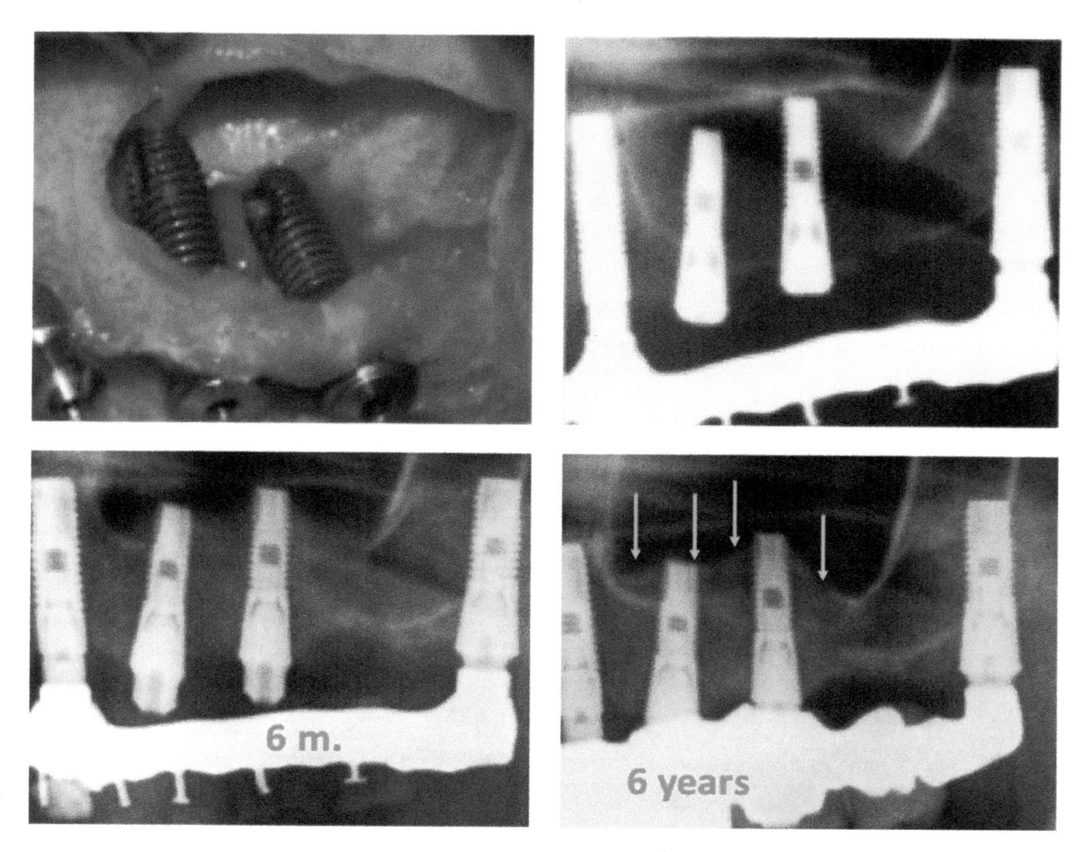

Figure 7.1 Sinus augmentation procedure performed with PRF utilized as a sole grafting material. Following implant placement, sinus cavity filled with PRF alone. X-rays taken at day 0, following 6 months, and following 6 years of healing. Notice the appreciable amount of new bone formation when PRF was utilized alone. Case performed by Dr. Alain Simonpieri.

Due to the preferred osteoconductive properties of bone substitute materials, it is more common to recommend the combination of PRF with a bone-grafting material for sinus floor elevation [13–16]. While few studies have compared PRF in combination with bone graft to bone graft alone, they have generally reported improvements in new bone formation as determined by the study endpoints, and the majority of these studies report the possibility of shortening the overall healing period when PRF is utilized [13–16]. A systematic review investigating the use of PRF for sinus elevation procedures published in 2015 found that of 290 initial clinical publications searched on the topic of PRF, only 8 met the inclusion criteria with half not utilizing controls or other biomaterials to compared results [17]. Furthermore, the major described limitation reported was the great heterogeneity regarding the surgical technique utilized (osteotome versus lateral window approach), time of implant placement (simultaneous versus delayed), outcomes measures, biopsy analysis and follow-up period [17]. Therefore, based on the results obtained and the limited comparative studies, to this day it remains difficult to assess the "ideal" treatment protocol utilizing PRF for sinus lifting procedures. Nevertheless, the use of PRF has been shown to lead to improvements in bone regeneration even when utilized alone as depicted in Figures 7.1 and 7.2. It remains

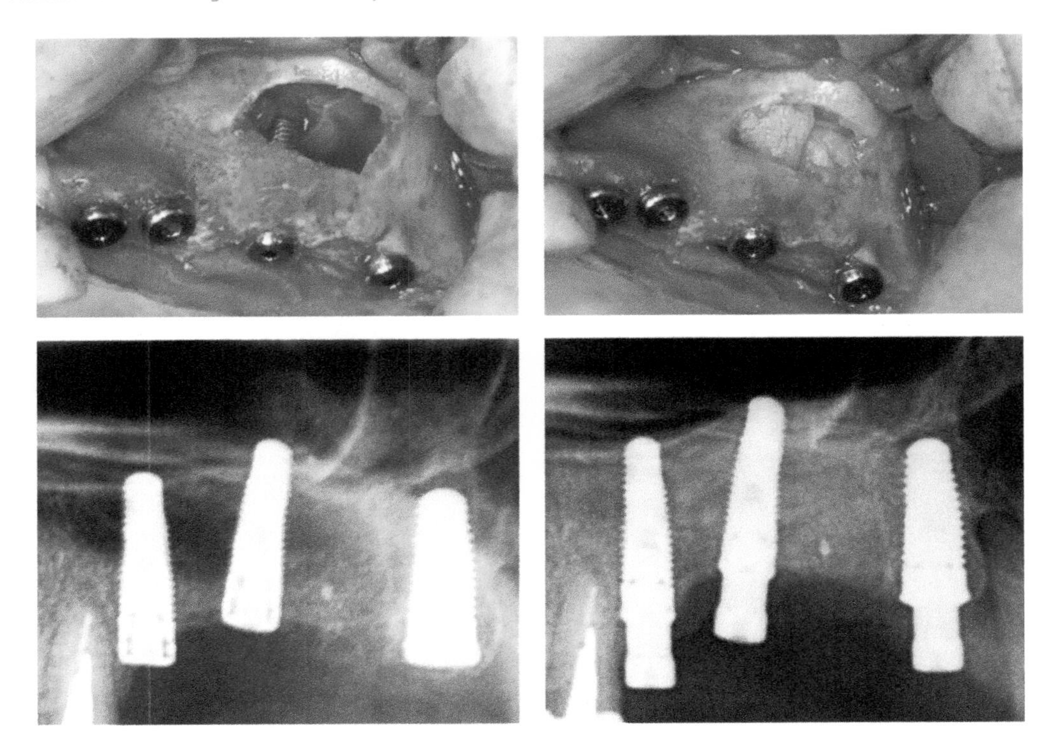

Figure 7.2 Sinus augmentation procedure performed with PRF utilized as a sole grafting material. Once again, notice the appreciable amount of new bone formation taking place around these implants. Case performed by Dr. Alain Simonpieri.

Table 7.1 Use of platelet rich fibrin (PRF) utilized as a sole grafting material for sinus lift augmentation procedures.

Diss *et al.* (2008); OOOE	Osteotome sinus floor elevation using Choukroun's platelet rich fibrin as grafting material: a 1-year prospective pilot study with microthreaded implants.
Mazor *et al.* (2009); JPerio	Sinus floor augmentation with simultaneous implant placement using Choukroun's platelet rich fibrin as the sole grafting material: a radiologic and histologic study at 6 months.
Simonpieri *et al.* (2011); Implant Dent.	Simultaneous sinus-lift and implantation using microthreaded implants and leukocyte- and platelet rich fibrin as sole grafting material: a 6-year experience.
Tajima *et al.* (2013); IJOMI	Evaluation of sinus floor augmentation with simultaneous implant placement using platelet rich fibrin as sole grafting material.
Jeong *et al.* (2014); J Craniomaxillofac Surg	Simultaneous sinus lift and implantation using platelet rich fibrin as sole grafting material.
Zhao *et al.* (2015); J Formos Med Assoc.	Clinical application of platelet rich fibrin as the sole grafting material in maxillary sinus augmentation.
Aoki *et al.* (2016); Case Rep Dent.	Sinus augmentation by platelet rich fibrin alone: a report of two cases with histological examinations.
Kanayama *et al.* (2016); Implant Dent.	Crestal approach to sinus floor elevation for atrophic maxilla using platelet rich fibrin as the only grafting material: a 1-year prospective study.

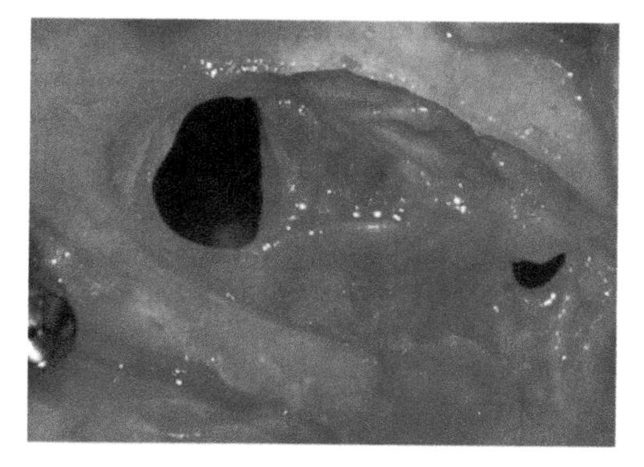

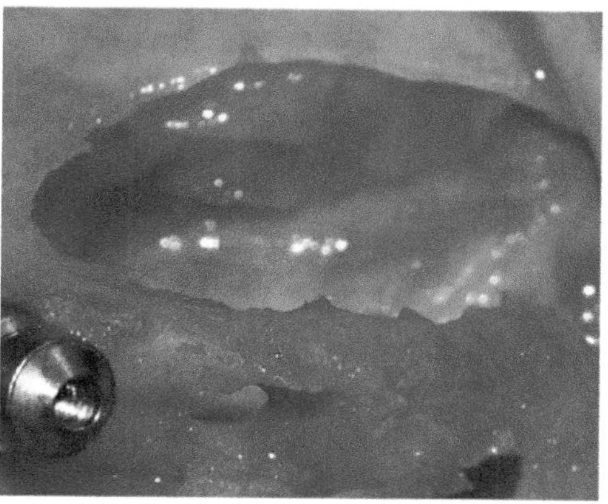

Figure 7.3 Large Schneiderian membrane perforation covered with a double layer of PRF membranes. Case performed by Dr. Alain Simonpieri.

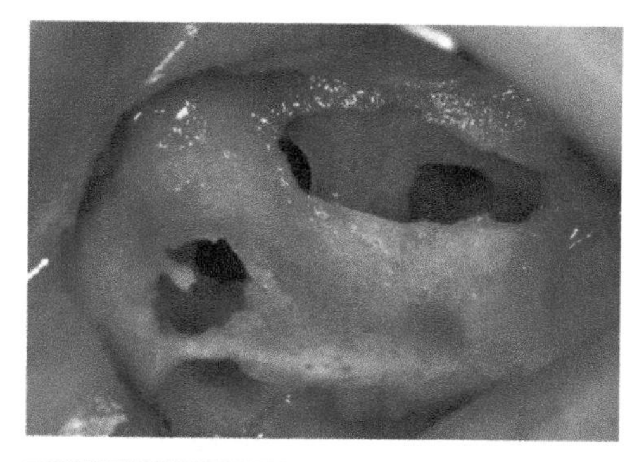

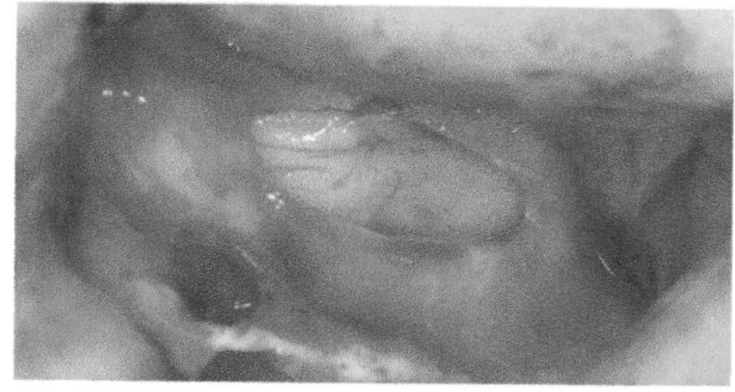

Figure 7.4 Another large Schneiderian membrane perforation covered with a double layer of PRF membranes. Case performed by Dr. Alain Simonpieri.

prominent that much further research be performed to support the predictability of its use.

Interestingly, in 2010, Avila *et al.* published an article titled: "The Influence of the Bucco-Palatal Distance on Sinus Augmentation Outcomes" [18]. In that study, it was found that the width of the bucco-palatal distance had a major impact on new bone formation for lateral sinus augmentation procedures performed with an allograft. Narrow sinuses regenerated with a higher percentage of new bone formation when compared to wide sinuses. For these reasons, it has been generally recommended by many clinicians that wide sinuses (>15 mm) should not be regenerated utilizing PRF alone (due to its limited bone-inducing capacity) and should thereby be combined with a bone-grafting material when sinus regeneration is extensive [18]. For narrow sinuses (<10 mm), PRF alone may be utilized. While no study has thus far investigated the bucco-palatal distance for regenerated sinuses utilizing PRF alone, these guidelines provide a conservative protocol when used as a sole grafting material for sinus lifting procedures.

7.3 PRF for the repair of Schneiderian membranes

A second use of PRF during sinus lifting procedures has been for the repair of Schneiderian membranes (Figure 7.3). It has been shown that generally 20% of sinus lifts (most commonly lateral window) report a Schneiderian membrane perforation [19,20]. Typically, these are covered with absorbable collagen barrier membranes with simultaneous implant placement or implant placement following a 4- to 6-month healing period [19–21]. Interestingly, a second-generation

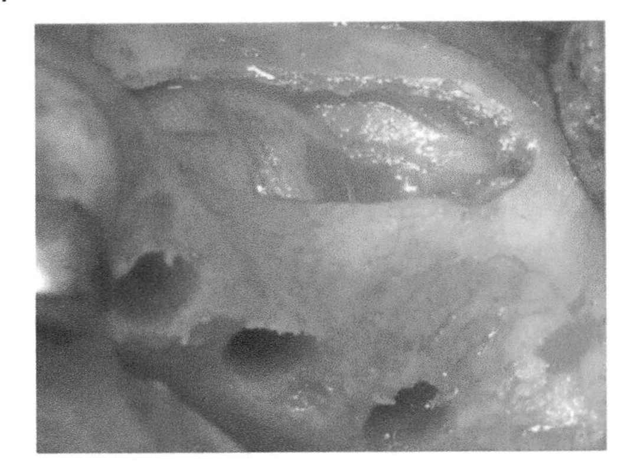

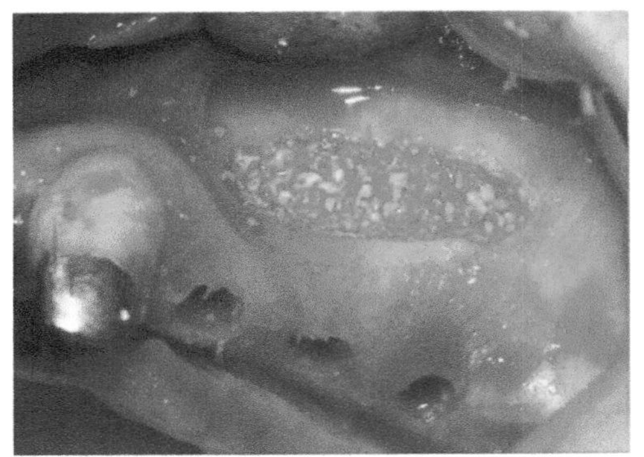

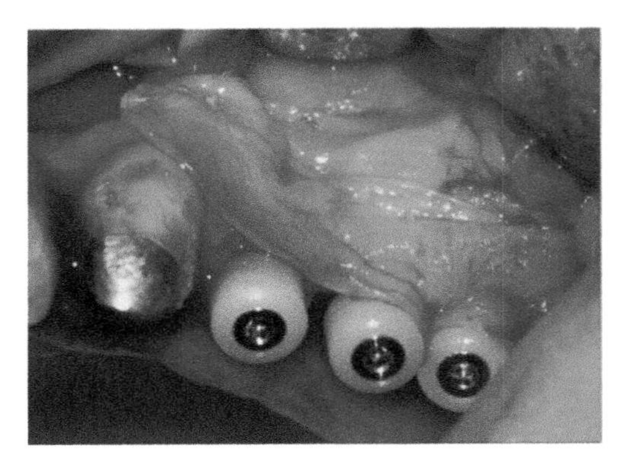

Figure 7.5 Lateral window sinus augmentation procedure performed with two PRF membranes utilized to protect the Schneiderian membrane, followed by allograft placement and lateral window closure with PRF. Case performed by Dr. Alain Simonpieri.

platelet concentrate has been shown to act as an available material to be placed over Schneiderian membrane perforations due to its 100% biocompatible source [4,22,23]. Figure 7.4 illustrates a case of a perforation of the Schneiderian membrane treated with PRF alone. These cases are treated with PRF alone, whereby the consistency of the membrane allows the PRF membrane to act slightly as a sticky fibrin matrix able to rapidly repair perforations and allow subsequent placement of bone grafts and implants when needed. Generally, it is recommended that any perforation should be utilized in a double layering technique to cover tears 3 mm in size predictably. For larger perforations, PRF can be utilized either alone or in combination with a collagen barrier membrane depending on the clinician's preferences. Two PRF membranes are always recommended to be placed overtop of tears to assure adequate coverage and extend the resorption period of 10 to 14 days typically seen when PRF is utilized as a membrane alone.

7.4 PRF for the closure of the lateral maxillary access window

PRF has also been utilized to cover the lateral maxillary window in two studies [24,25]. In a first study, Gassling *et al.* utilized a split mouth design to investigate 12 sinuses from six patients requiring bilateral sinus floor augmentation treated with a two-stage surgical approach. The sinuses were grafted with autologous bone and bone-substitute material (Bio-Oss®) mixed in a 1:1 ratio covered with either 1) a PRF membrane or a 2) conventional collagen membrane (Bio-Gide®). Five months later, threaded titanium dental implants were inserted and bone specimens were harvested with a trephine burr and evaluated histomorphometrically. Mean vital bone formation after 5 months was reported at 17.0% and 17.2%, for the PRF and collagen sites, respectively. The mean residual bone-substitute was 15.9% and 17.3% for PRF and collagen groups, respectively. No local complications, such as dehiscence or membrane exposure were detected at either sites in any of the treated patients and all implants reached primary stability. The conclusion

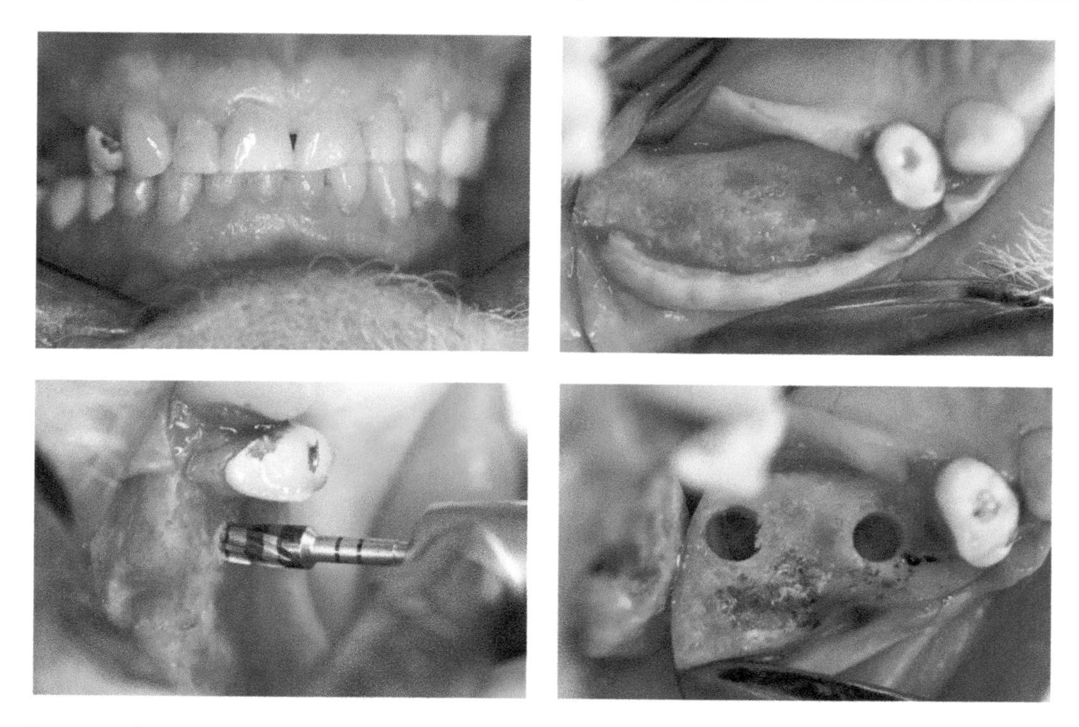

Figure 7.6 Case presentation of a sinus lifting procedure performed in the maxillary right quadrant. Case performed by Dr. Michael A. Pikos.

from this first study was that the coverage of the lateral sinus window could be achieved equally with either PRF or absorbable collagen membrane resulting in a similar amount of vital bone formation and residual bone-substitute [25].

Similarly, in a second nearly identical study, Bosshardt *et al.* evaluated in humans the amount of new bone after sinus floor elevation with a synthetic bone substitute material consisting of nanocrystalline hydroxyapatite embedded in a highly porous silica gel matrix [24]. A collagen membrane (group 1) or a PRF membrane (group 2) was placed over the bony window. After healing periods between 7 and 11 months, 16 biopsy specimens were harvested with a trephine bur during implant bed preparation. For group 1, the amount of new bone, residual graft material, and soft tissue was reported at 28.7% ± 5.4%, 25.5% ± 7.6%, and 45.8% ± 3.2%, respectively. For group 2, the values were 28.6% ± 6.90%, 25.7% ± 8.8%, and 45.7% ± 9.3%, respectively. All differences between groups 1 and 2 were not statistically significant. In conclusion, there was no differences between PRF membranes over the non-cross-linked collagen membranes [24].

Therefore, and based on these two reports, it may be concluded that sinus windows may be closed with PRF as a low-cost, completely autogenous membrane with no reported statistical differences to standard commonly utilized collagen membranes (Figure 7.5).

7.5 Discussion and future outlook

The available literature to date has demonstrated that PRF can safely be utilized during sinus lifting procedures and facilitates angiogenesis due to the local release of blood-derived growth factors. It has also been concluded in numerous reports that

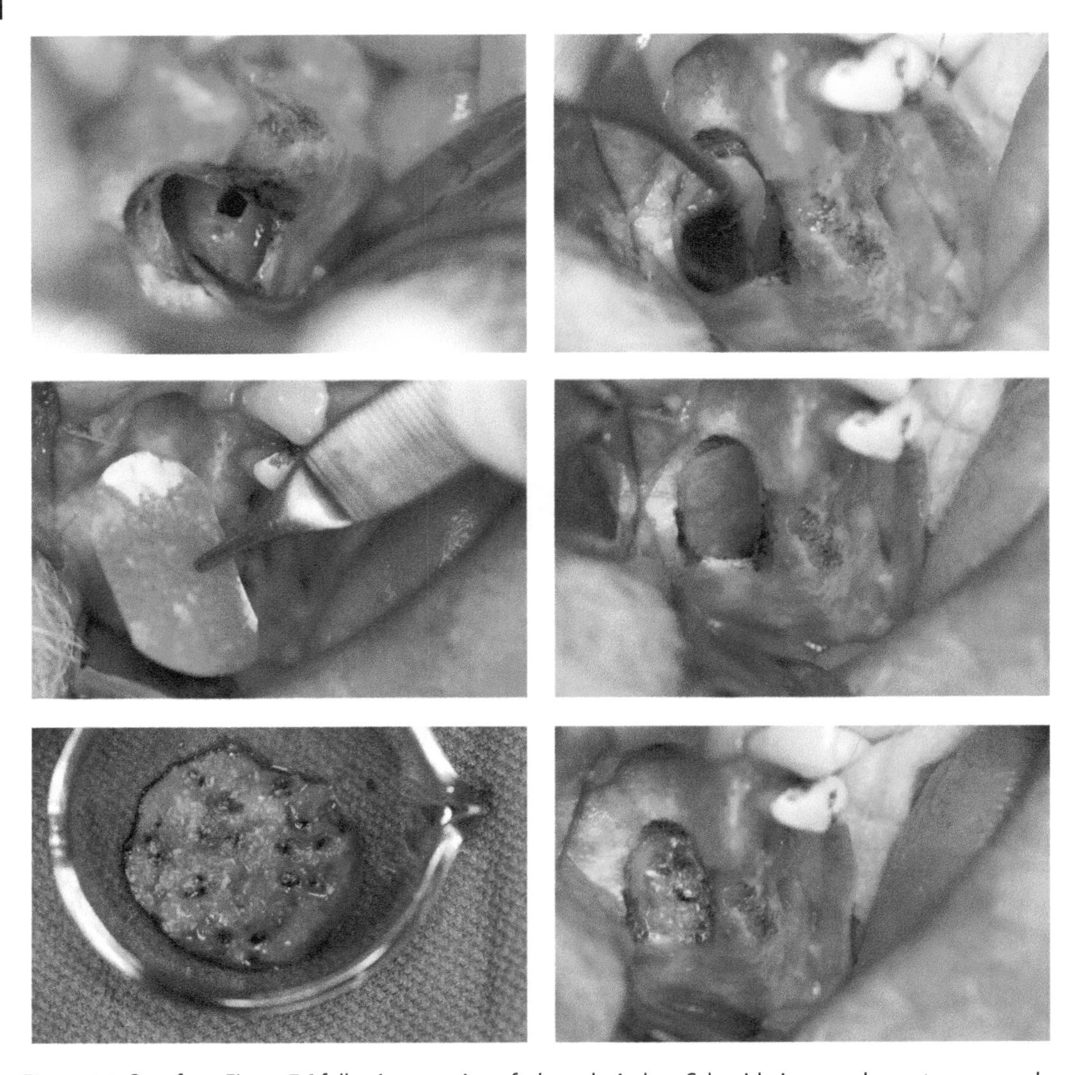

Figure 7.7 Case from Figure 7.6 following opening of a lateral window. Schneiderian membrane tear covered with PRF membranes followed by a collagen barrier membrane. Thereafter, bone-grafting material was mixed with PRF and placed inside the sinus. Case performed by Dr. Michael A. Pikos.

it may further be utilized alone as a sole grafting material to augment missing bone (although caution is recommended for wide sinuses due to the lack of containment), has the ability to be utilized for the repair of perforated Schneiderian membranes, and can be utilized to close a lateral window during sinus augmentation procedures as efficiently as collagen barrier membranes. Noteworthy, however, is that future research is absolutely essential to better understand and characterize the potential of PRF specifically during the bone regenerative process. It remains interesting to point out that data from other chapters have demonstrated that PRF has been shown to limit dimensional changes post extraction when utilized alone, but has limited additional benefit when combined with a bone-grafting materials during guided bone regeneration (GBR) procedures. Therefore, the mechanisms by which PRF is able to improve bone formation around implants

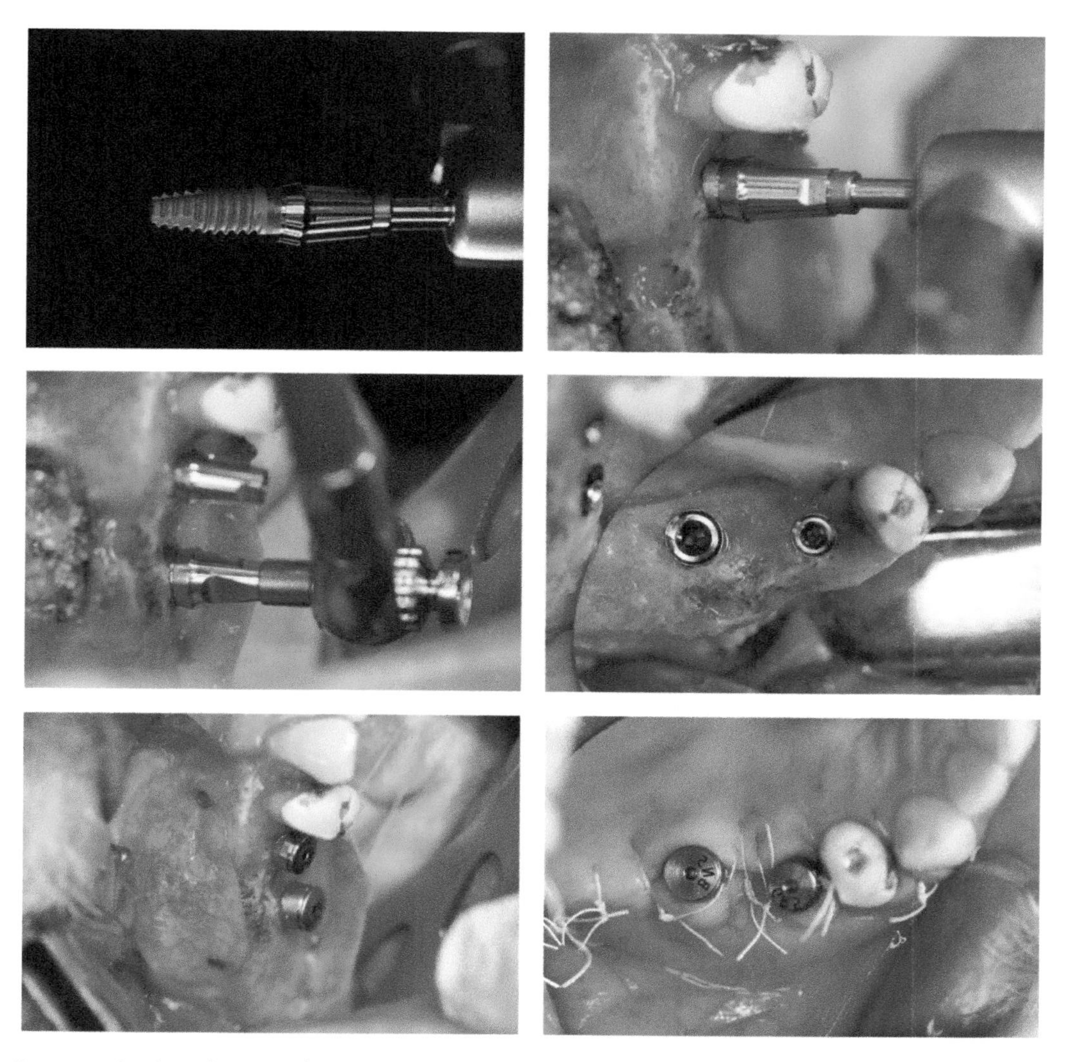

Figure 7.8 Implant placement from case presented in Figures 7.6 and 7.7 following sinus augmentation procedure performed with PRF and a bone grafting material. Case performed by Dr. Michael A. Pikos.

during sinus lifting procedures remains to be investigated. Based on these findings, it may be hypothesized that PRF is able to increase blood flow into the sinus cavity via the release of potent growth factors, however, its exact role remains inconclusive. Nevertheless, PRF may be utilized to protect the Schneiderian membrane from damage caused by implant placement and for these reasons has been an additional beneficial tool during sinus lifting procedures both via a crestal approach where PRF plugs can be utilized prior to implant placement to minimize the chance of implant damage to the Schneiderian membrane.

One prominent area of research that also requires a great deal of further investigation is to determine the dimensional width whereby PRF can be utilized as a sole grafting material as opposed to combined with a bone graft. Case 1 presents a large sinus regenerated via a lateral approach utilizing PRF with a grafting material (Figures 7.6–7.8). Similarly, Case 2 also depicts a conservative approach whereby the sinus is regenerated by

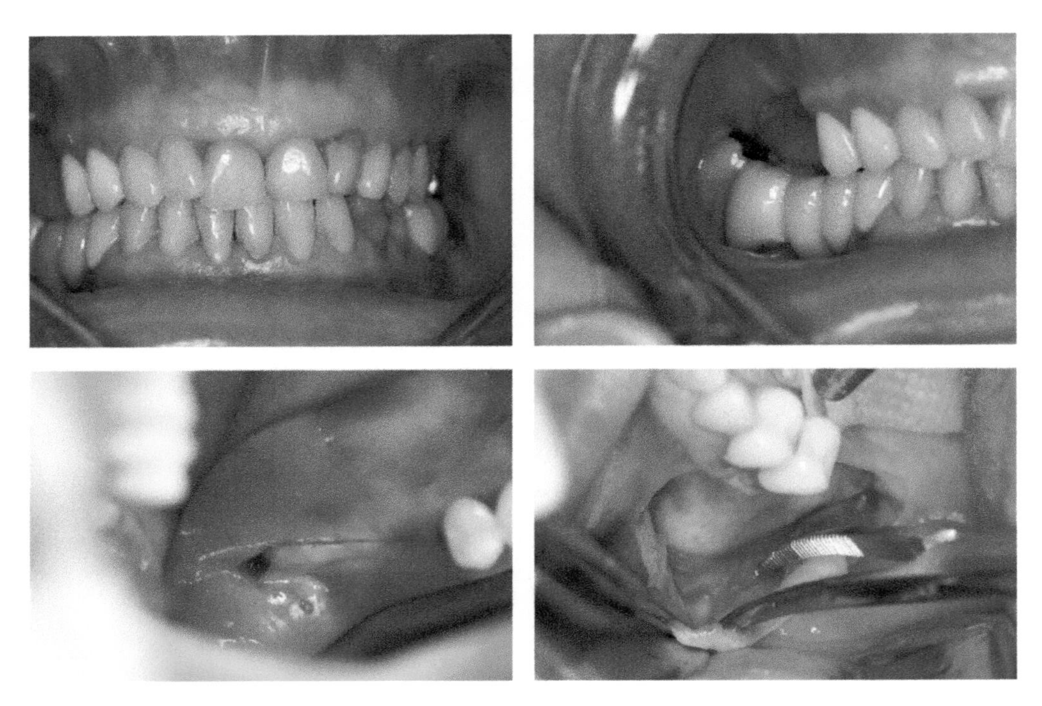

Figure 7.9 Case presentation of a sinus lifting procedure performed in the maxillary right quadrant with extensive bone loss. Case performed by Dr. Michael A. Pikos.

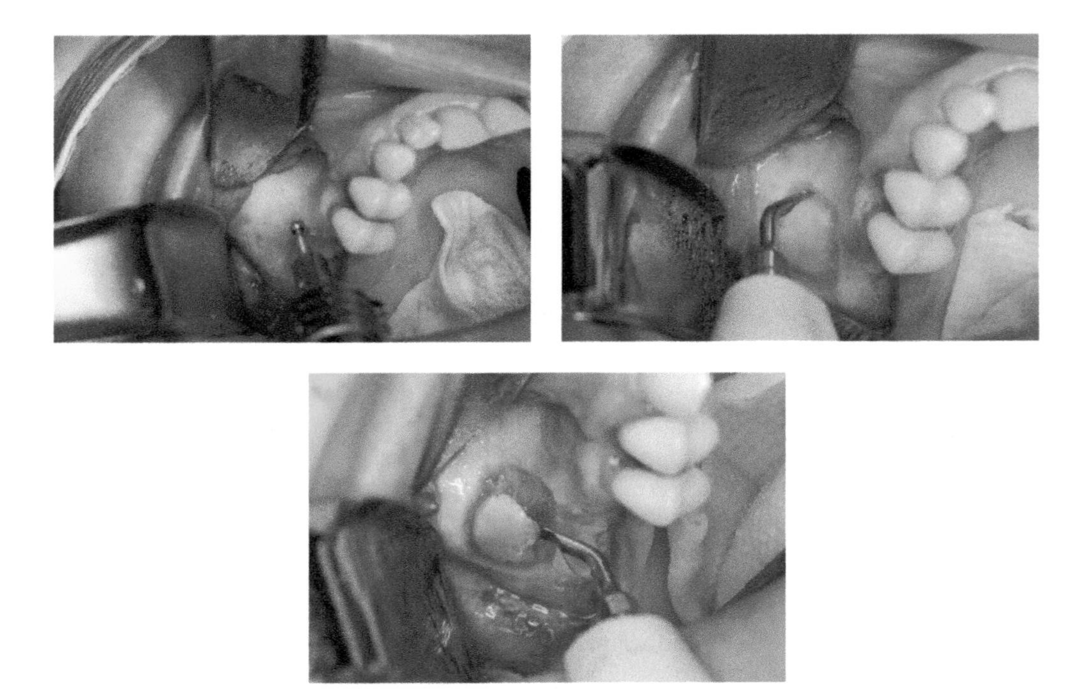

Figure 7.10 Opening of the sinus cavity via a lateral approach using piezo instrumentation. Case performed by Dr. Michael A. Pikos.

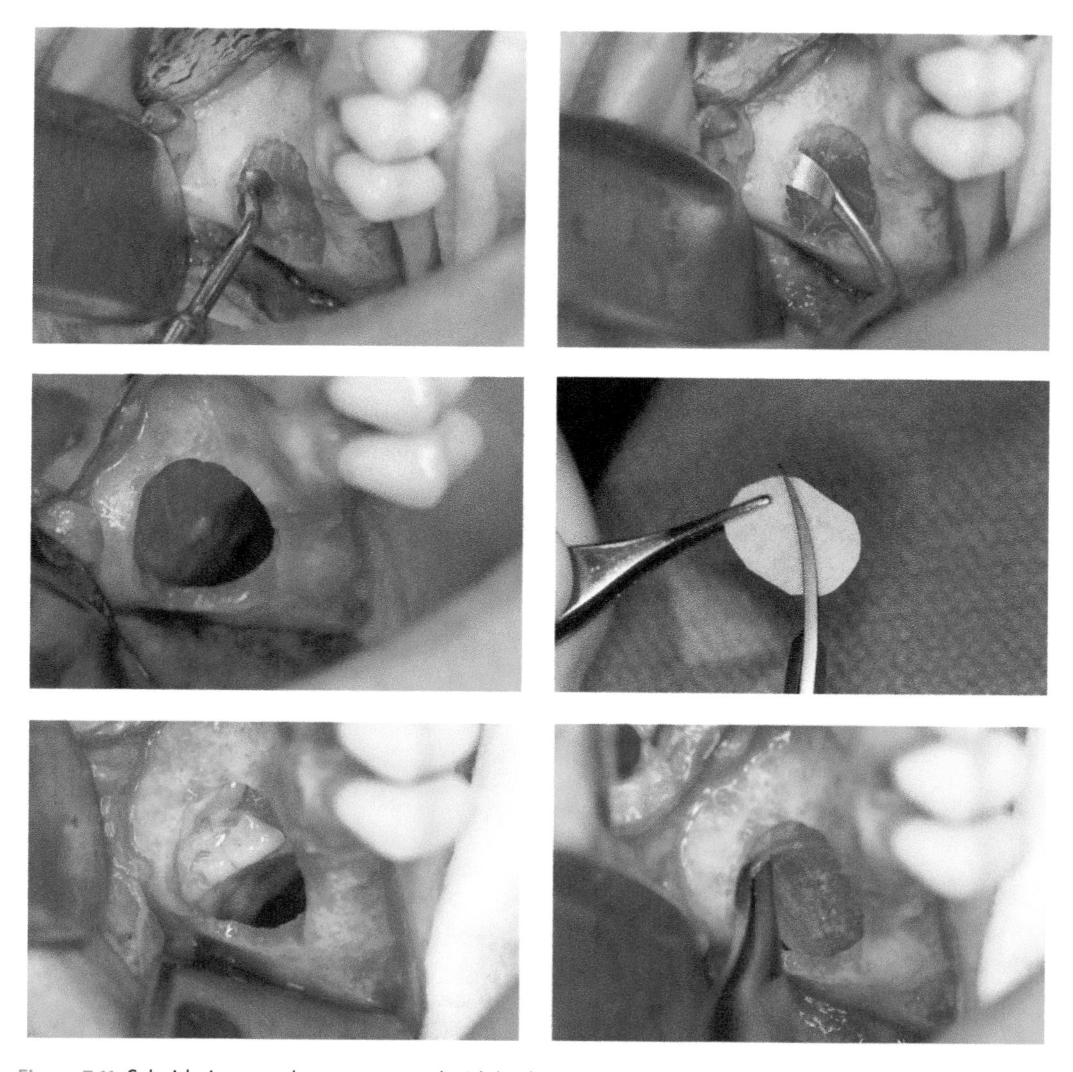

Figure 7.11 Scheiderian membrane protected with both PRF in combination with a collagen membrane. Case performed by Dr. Michael A. Pikos.

combining PRF with a bone grafting material (Figures 7.9–7.14). Clinical researchers have suggested that a bucco-palatal width of more than 15 mm of the sinus absolutely necessitates the additional use of bone grafting materials, whereas a sinus width of <10 mm can be predictably augmented with PRF alone. Nevertheless, proper characterization of when to utilize PRF alone versus in combination with a bone grafting material is lacking. Thus, future research is necessary.

While PRF has been shown to act as a more suitable autogenous biomaterial for the repair of the Schneiderian membrane, it is generally recommended that two PRF membranes are always utilized to assure enough thickness/stability over the initial healing period. Nevertheless, with Schneiderian membrane perforation being reported around 20% in multiple studies, clinicians may utilize PRF as a low-cost completely natural way to repair tears without the associated higher costs of

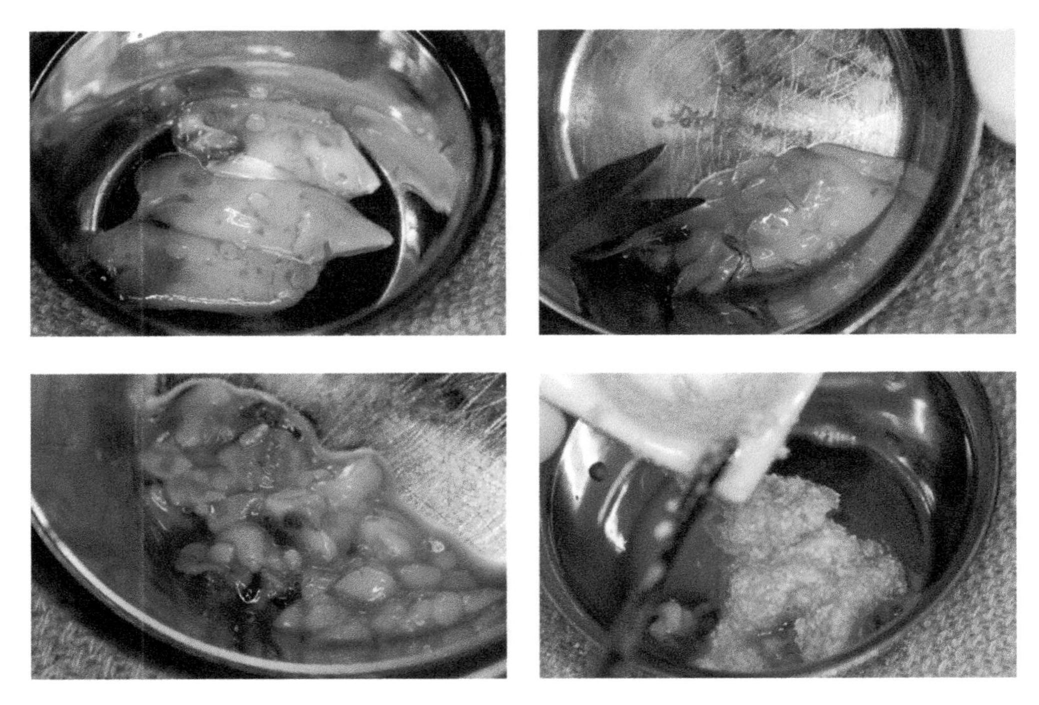

Figure 7.12 Three PRF membranes cut and mixed with a bone-grafting material (Case in Figures 7.10–7.14). Case performed by Dr. Michael A. Pikos.

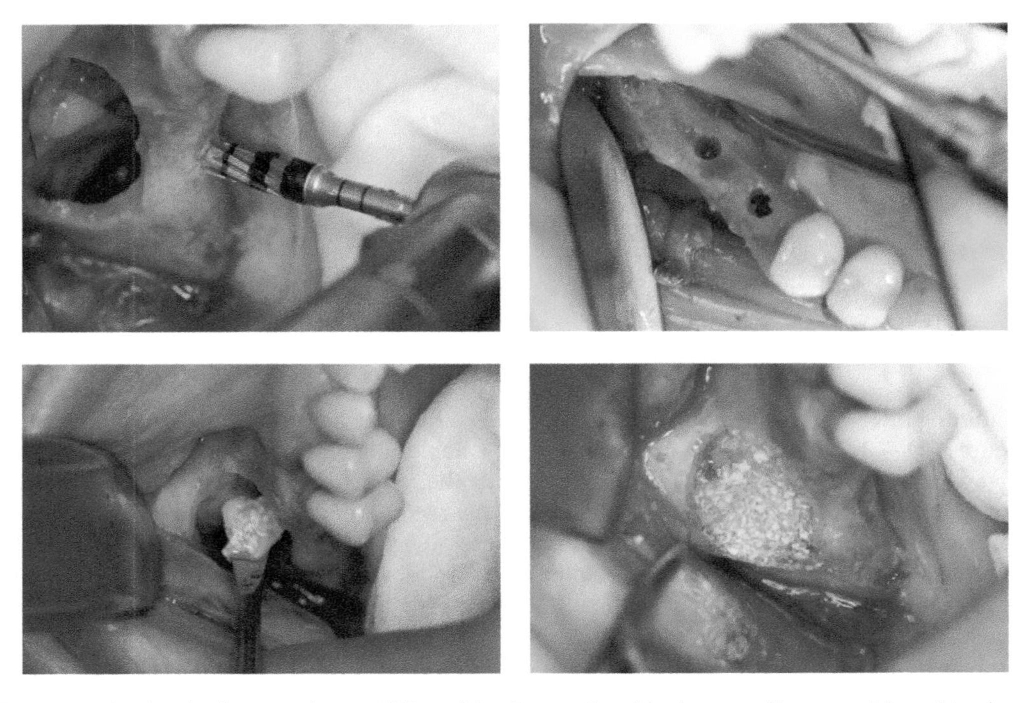

Figure 7.13 Implant bed preparation and filling of the sinus cavity with a bone grafting material combined with PRF from case presented in Figures 7.9–7.14. Case performed by Dr. Michael A. Pikos.

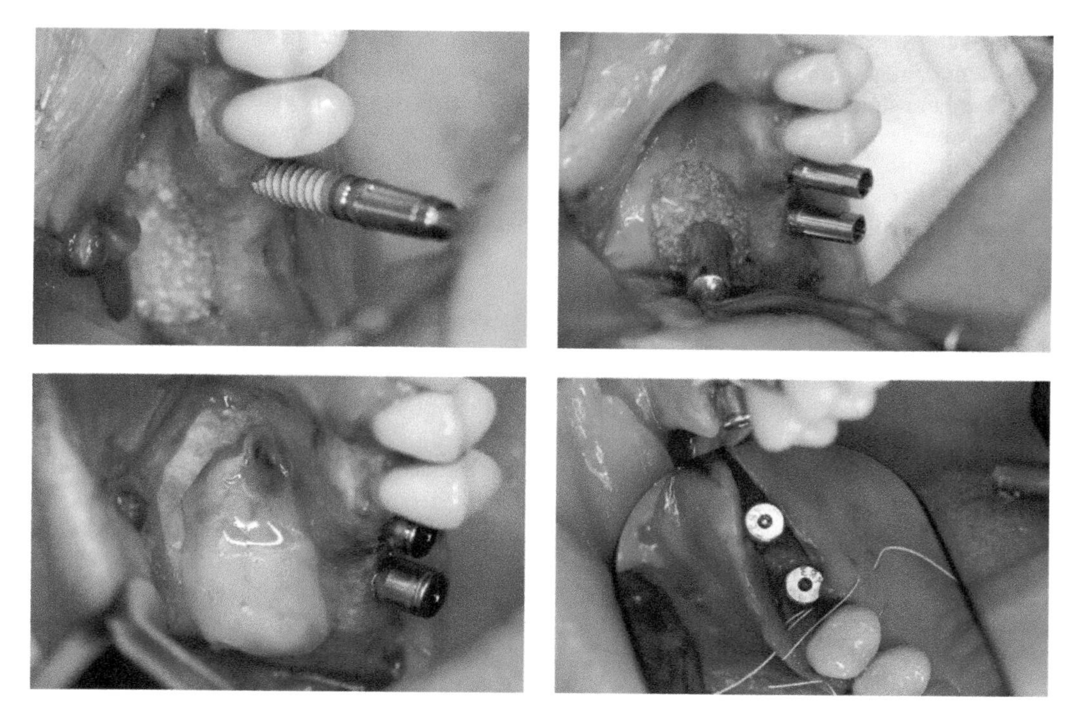

Figure 7.14 Implant placement followed by coverage of the lateral window with PRF membranes. Case performed by Dr. Michael A. Pikos.

utilizing a collagen barrier membrane. Furthermore, since PRF is 100% autologous, a foreign body reaction is not present as with the use of collagen-derived barrier membranes from bovine or porcine sources and therefore healing is expected to be more uneventful. In conclusion, PRF may therefore be recommended as a safe and efficient low-cost biomaterial for sinus augmentation procedures.

References

1 Kobayashi E, Fluckiger L, Fujioka-Kobayashi M, Sawada K, Sculean A, Schaller B, et al. Comparative release of growth factors from PRP, PRF, and advanced-PRF. Clinical oral investigations. 2016.

2 Leach JK, Kaigler D, Wang Z, Krebsbach PH, Mooney DJ. Coating of VEGF-releasing scaffolds with bioactive glass for angiogenesis and bone regeneration. Biomaterials. 2006;27(17): 3249–55.

3 Simonpieri A, Choukroun J, Del Corso M, Sammartino G, Ehrenfest DMD. Simultaneous sinus-lift and implantation using microthreaded implants and leukocyte-and platelet-rich fibrin as sole grafting material: a six-year experience. Implant dentistry. 2011;20(1):2–12.

4 Choukroun J, Diss A, Simonpieri A, Girard M-O, Schoeffler C, Dohan SL, et al. Platelet-rich fibrin (PRF): a second-generation platelet concentrate. Part V: histologic evaluations of PRF effects on bone allograft maturation in sinus lift. Oral Surgery, Oral Medicine, Oral Pathology, Oral Radiology, and Endodontology. 2006;101(3):299–303.

5 Nkenke E, Stelzle F. Clinical outcomes of sinus floor augmentation for implant placement using autogenous bone or bone substitutes: a systematic review. Clinical oral implants research. 2009;20(s4):124–33.
6 Wallace SS, Froum SJ. Effect of maxillary sinus augmentation on the survival of endosseous dental implants. A systematic review. Annals of periodontology. 2003; 8(1):328–43.
7 Chen T-W, Chang H-S, Leung K-W, Lai Y-L, Kao S-Y. Implant placement immediately after the lateral approach of the trap door window procedure to create a maxillary sinus lift without bone grafting: a 2-year retrospective evaluation of 47 implants in 33 patients. Journal of Oral and Maxillofacial Surgery. 2007;65(11):2324–8.
8 Lambert F, Léonard A, Drion P, Sourice S, Layrolle P, Rompen E. Influence of space-filling materials in subantral bone augmentation: blood clot vs. autogenous bone chips vs. bovine hydroxyapatite. Clinical oral implants research. 2011;22(5): 538–45.
9 Thor A, Sennerby L, Hirsch JM, Rasmusson L. Bone formation at the maxillary sinus floor following simultaneous elevation of the mucosal lining and implant installation without graft material: an evaluation of 20 patients treated with 44 Astra Tech implants. Journal of Oral and Maxillofacial Surgery. 2007;65(7):64–72.
10 Tajima N, Ohba S, Sawase T, Asahina I. Evaluation of sinus floor augmentation with simultaneous implant placement using platelet-rich fibrin as sole grafting material. The International journal of oral & maxillofacial implants. 2013;28(1):77–83.
11 Mazor Z, Horowitz RA, Del Corso M, Prasad HS, Rohrer MD, Dohan Ehrenfest DM. Sinus floor augmentation with simultaneous implant placement using Choukroun's platelet-rich fibrin as the sole grafting material: a radiologic and histologic study at 6 months. J Periodontol. 2009;80(12):2056–64.
12 Simonpieri A, Choukroun J, Del Corso M, Sammartino G, Dohan Ehrenfest DM. Simultaneous sinus-lift and implantation using microthreaded implants and leukocyte- and platelet-rich fibrin as sole grafting material: a six-year experience. Implant dentistry. 2011;20(1):2–12.
13 Inchingolo F, Tatullo M, Marrelli M, Inchingolo AM, Scacco S, Inchingolo AD, et al. Trial with Platelet-Rich Fibrin and Bio-Oss used as grafting materials in the treatment of the severe maxillar bone atrophy: clinical and radiological evaluations. European review for medical and pharmacological sciences. 2010;14(12): 1075–84.
14 Tatullo M, Marrelli M, Cassetta M, Pacifici A, Stefanelli LV, Scacco S, et al. Platelet Rich Fibrin (P.R.F.) in reconstructive surgery of atrophied maxillary bones: clinical and histological evaluations. International journal of medical sciences. 2012;9(10):872–80.
15 Zhang Y, Tangl S, Huber CD, Lin Y, Qiu L, Rausch-Fan X. Effects of Choukroun's platelet-rich fibrin on bone regeneration in combination with deproteinized bovine bone mineral in maxillary sinus augmentation: a histological and histomorphometric study. Journal of cranio-maxillo-facial surgery: official publication of the European Association for Cranio-Maxillo-Facial Surgery. 2012; 40(4):321–8.
16 Choukroun J, Diss A, Simonpieri A, Girard MO, Schoeffler C, Dohan SL, et al. Platelet-rich fibrin (PRF): a second-generation platelet concentrate. Part V: histologic evaluations of PRF effects on bone allograft maturation in sinus lift. Oral surgery, oral medicine, oral pathology, oral radiology, and endodontics. 2006; 101(3):299–303.
17 Ali S, Bakry SA, Abd-Elhakam H. Platelet-Rich Fibrin in Maxillary Sinus Augmentation: A Systematic Review. The Journal of oral implantology. 2015;41(6): 746–53.
18 Avila G, Wang H-L, Galindo-Moreno P, Misch CE, Bagramian RA, Rudek I, et al. The influence of the bucco-palatal distance

on sinus augmentation outcomes. Journal of periodontology. 2010;81(7):1041–50.
19 Hernández-Alfaro F, Torradeflot MM, Marti C. Prevalence and management of Schneiderian membrane perforations during sinus-lift procedures. Clinical oral implants research. 2008;19(1):91–8.
20 Schwartz-Arad D, Herzberg R, Dolev E. The prevalence of surgical complications of the sinus graft procedure and their impact on implant survival. Journal of periodontology. 2004;75(4):511–6.
21 Becker ST, Terheyden H, Steinriede A, Behrens E, Springer I, Wiltfang J. Prospective observation of 41 perforations of the Schneiderian membrane during sinus floor elevation. Clinical oral implants research. 2008;19(12):1285–9.
22 Mazor Z, Horowitz RA, Del Corso M, Prasad HS, Rohrer MD, Dohan Ehrenfest DM. Sinus floor augmentation with simultaneous implant placement using Choukroun's platelet-rich fibrin as the sole grafting material: a radiologic and histologic study at 6 months. Journal of periodontology. 2009;80(12):2056–64.
23 Toffler M, Toscano N, Holtzclaw D. Osteotome-mediated sinus floor elevation using only platelet-rich fibrin: an early report on 110 patients. Implant dentistry. 2010;19(5):447–56.
24 Bosshardt DD, Bornstein MM, Carrel J-P, Buser D, Bernard J-P. Maxillary sinus grafting with a synthetic, nanocrystalline hydroxyapatite-silica gel in humans: histologic and histomorphometric results. International Journal of Periodontics & Restorative Dentistry. 2014;34(2).
25 Gassling V, Purcz N, Braesen J-H, Will M, Gierloff M, Behrens E, et al. Comparison of two different absorbable membranes for the coverage of lateral osteotomy sites in maxillary sinus augmentation: a preliminary study. Journal of Cranio-Maxillofacial Surgery. 2013;41(1): 76–82.

8

Use of Platelet Rich Fibrin for the Treatment of Muco-Gingival Recessions: Novel Improvements in Plastic Aesthetic Surgery Utilizing The Fibrin Assisted Soft Tissue Promotion (FASTP) Technique

Alexandre-Amir Aalam and Alina Krivitsky Aalam

Abstract

The use of platelet rich fibrin (PRF) has been utilized for a wide variety of procedures in both the medical and dental fields. Results from many randomized clinical trials have now pointed to its marked ability to promote soft-tissue wound healing where PRF has been documented to facilitate wound closure and speed regeneration of muco-gingival recessions. Within this chapter, a systematic review of the various clinical studies utilizing PRF for recession coverage procedures is presented. Furthermore, a new surgical concept is introduced following years of clinical experience with PRF described as the "Fibrin Assisted Soft Tissue Promotion" FASTP technique.

Highlights

- PRF for the regeneration of soft-tissue healing
- Early studies using PRF for the treatment of gingival recessions
- Systematic review of the randomized clinical trials using PRF for gingival recessions
- Presentation of the Fibrin Assisted Soft Tissue Promotion (FASTP) technique

8.1 Introduction

Periodontal plastic surgery plays an ever-growing role in modern dentistry due to the increasing demand for optimal aesthetics. In the United States, reports have now shown that by the age of 60, 90% of the population will have at least one tooth with a 1 mm recession with up to 40% of the same population presenting sites with a greater than 3 mm recessions [1–3]. These studies combined with the fact that untreated recessions may worsen the periodontal status necessitates regenerative procedures aimed at augmenting lost tissues. The ultimate outcome of a root coverage procedure is resolution of the defect by providing a thicker keratinized and attached tissue that is esthetically seamless with the neighboring tissue as well as re-establishes the functional attachment apparatus [4].

In the case of multiple adjacent teeth with recessions, there is considerably more avascular exposed roots making the reparative procedure increasingly invasive and less predictable due to the reduced blood supply to the surgical site (Figures 8.1 and 8.2). Multiple periodontal plastic surgical procedures have been proposed to correct

Platelet Rich Fibrin in Regenerative Dentistry: Biological Background and Clinical Indications, First Edition.
Edited by Richard J. Miron and Joseph Choukroun.

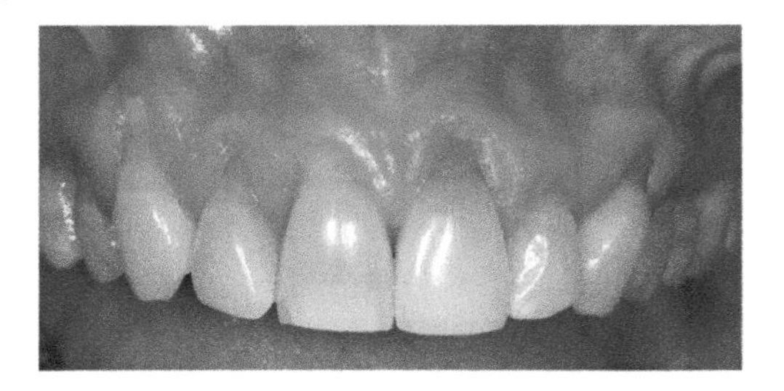

Figure 8.1 **Pre-treatment.** Class 2–3 Miller recessions associated with inflammation and a lack of attached tissue.

these mucogingival deformities and, thus, rebuild the lost attachment apparatus, as well as increase the zone of attached and keratinized tissue required for the long-term maintenance of a healthy dentition [1,2,5,6]. Traditionally, connective tissue grafts from the palate utilized in combination with a pedicle flap (coronal or lateral positioned flap) has been a gold standard treatment for such defects [4,7]. Limiting factors including insufficient amount of connective tissue, patient refusal to harvest within a second surgical site as well as the additional morbidity associated with these invasive procedures have necessitated the use of alternative strategies from autogenous connective tissue grafting [4,7]. For these reasons, a variety of allograft and xenograft dermal tissue substitutes are routinely used in periodontal plastic surgery with various reported clinical outcomes [8,9]. While these substitute materials act as a three-dimensional scaffold that allow "fibro-conduction," the natural healing potential as well as the final long-term stability of keratinized tissues has been controversial.

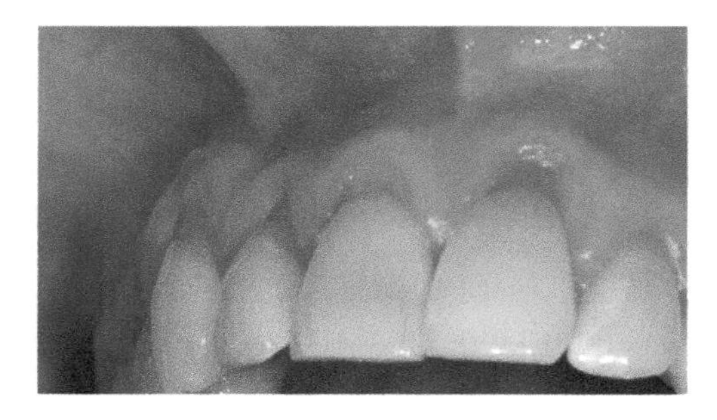

Figure 8.2 **Pre-treatment.** Sectional view showing the advanced severity of the gingival deformity, the canine root prominence and concavities.

Similarly, another strategy has been to employ an enamel matrix derivative product (EMD) derived from porcine origin as a bioactive agent [10]. EMD has been shown to lead to some positive clinical and histological results when combined with a coronally advanced flap procedure to induce periodontal regeneration [10]. While the clinical results are significant when compared to the use of coronally positioned flap alone [7], a lack of evidence comparing EMD to connective or allograft tissue grafts are not reported.

In the last decade, blood-derived biological modifiers have been commonly utilized to enhance hard and soft tissue healing. Platelet rich plasma (PRP) was initially described as a first generation of such platelet concentrates having seen widespread use in the field of maxillofacial surgery [11]. Some of the reported drawbacks included lack of hard-tissue growth factors, poor physical properties, lengthy centrifugation protocols, and rapid release of growth factors [12]. The use of PRP application for root coverage and muco-gingival procedures has therefore not been adapted for routine surgical procedures in the field of periodontology.

In the early 2000s, a new concept was developed by Dr. Joseph Choukroun whereby the removal of anticoagulants from PRP and modifications to centrifugation procedures led to the development of Platelet Rich Fibrin (PRF) [7,13,14]. This second-generation blood derivative was therefore used in the form of a fibrin membrane (also containing leukocytes and growth factors), which has since been utilized for a variety of surgical procedures either alone or in combination with bone graft materials for periodontal regeneration, sinus grafting, and ridge augmentation as highlighted throughout this textbook. Below we describe its use in plastic periodontal surgery for the treatment of gingival recessions.

8.2 Plastic periodontal procedures with PRF

In the early years, limited data existed investigating the use of PRF for the treatment of gingival recessions. In a first study, Aroca *et al.* compared 20 patients treated with a coronally positioned flap with and without PRF membranes. It was found that at 6 months, the PRF group benefited from an increased zone of keratinized tissue but a lower percentage of complete root coverage [15]. Aleksic *et al.* [16] and Jankovic *et al.* [17] compared the use of a connective tissue graft to PRF as a sole graft material for the treatment of Miller class I and II gingival recessions in 19 patients. Following 6 months of healing, no statistical difference was found between the groups when comparing the amount of root coverage and zone of keratinized tissue, thereby supporting the use of PRF for such procedures when compared to the gold standard connective tissue graft. An added advantage of PRF from these studies was that patients reported higher comfort of the procedure and less post-operatory pain since no intra-oral donor site was utilized to harvest CTGs from the palate. Tunali *et al.* further compared PRF versus a connective tissue graft in 20 patients over a 12-month follow-up [18]. Both treatment modalities significantly reduced the amount of recession (76% and 77% respectively) and increased the clinical attachment levels (2.9 m and 3.04 m respectively) to near identical outcomes [18]. In total, 13 studies have now investigated in randomized clinical trials the use of PRF versus other regenerative modalities as highlighted in Table 8.1 [19–31]. In general, the use of PRF has been found to successfully regenerate Miller class 1 and 2 gingival recessions as predictably as CTG, whereas generally Miller class 3 and a limited amount of keratinized tissue have less predictable data supporting the use of PRF alone, due to a limited keratinized tissue dimension.

8.3 Fibro promotion: the basic mechanism of Fibrin-Assisted Soft Tissue Promotion (FASTP) technique

One aspect requiring further research was to determine whether the wound healing benefits associated with PRF were optimized in the field of plastic periodontal aesthetic surgery; specifically as it relates to root coverage procedures. After a comprehensive review of the surgical techniques and clinical applications of PRF, the authors attributed the non-conclusive results to multiple key points requiring further surgical modifications to optimize the clinical outcomes.

One of the major oversights found analyzing the literature is the comparative studies investigating PRF versus a connective tissue graft. Even though they share very similar physical characteristics by both being autologous, the mode of surgical operation and the final product obtained are different.

Naturally, the connective tissue graft harvested from the palate will transfer its genetic expression (keratinization) from the donor site to the recipient site. Karring *et al.* have described this concept in an animal model convincingly [32]. The recipient site has little input in the quality or quantity of the final tissue obtained. We describe this mechanism of action as "Fibro-Genesis."

Interestingly, years of experimenting with PRF revealed that it functions via an increase in fibrin associated with angiogenesis. Naturally, the fibrin is considered as a biological matrix with an increased source of VEGF and growth factors. PRF will therefore promote and induce the formation of neovascularization and new tissues at the recipient site. It thus becomes apparent that the quality of the recipient bed soft tissue is crucial for the

Table 8.1 Effects of PRF on intrabony defect regeneration (PPD = Probing Periodontal Depth; CAL = Clinical Attachment Level; OFD = Open Flap Debridement; PRF = Platelet Rich Fibrin; DFDBA = Demineralized Freeze-Dried Bone Allograft, MF = Metformin; HA = Hydroxyappatite).

Author	Defect #	Healing Time	Groups	ΔPPD (mm)	CAL Gain (mm)	P Value
Thorat (2011)	32	9 months	OFD	3.56	2.13	ΔPPD: <0.01
			OFD + PRF	4.56	3.69	CAL: <0.01
Sharma (2011)	56	9 months	OFD	3.21	2.77	ΔPPD: 0.006
			OFD + PRF	4.55	3.31	CAL: n.s.
Pradeep (2012)	90	9 months	OFD	2.97	2.67	ΔPPD: 0.002
			OFD + PRF	3.90	3.03	GAL: n.s.
Pradeep (2012)	90	9 months	OFD	2.97	2.83	ΔPPD: 0.018
			OFD + PRF	3.77	3.17	GAL: n.s.
Shah (2015)	40	6 months	OFD + DFDBA	3.70	2.97	n.s.
			OFD + PRF	3.67	2.97	
Pradeep (2015)	120	9 months	OFD	3.01	2.96	ΔPPD: <0.001
			OFD + PRF	4.01	4.03	CAL: <0.001 both
			ORF + 1% MF	3.93	3.93	treatment groups
			OFD + 1% MF + PRF	4.9	4.9	
Ajwani (2015)	40	9 months	OFD	1.60	1.3	PPD: <0.001
			OFD + PRF	1.90	1.8	CAL: <0.001
Elgandhy (2015)	40	6 months	OFD + HA	3.42	3.55	PPD: <0.02
			OFD + HA + PRF	3.82	3.9	CAL: <0.027
Agarwal (2016)	60	12 months	OFD +DFDBA	3.60	2.61	PPD: <0.05
			OFD + DFDBA + PRF	4.15	3.73	CAL: <0.05
Panda (2016)	32	9 months	barrier membrane	3.19	3.38	PPD: 0.002
			membrane + PRF	3.88	4.44	CAL = 0.001

procedure to be successful. It goes without saying that if an existing band of keratinized tissue is available, it will further promote the fabrication of more keratinized tissue. If on the contrary, only a loose mucosal non-attached tissue is present, a similar formation of poor quality tissue should be expected. We describe this mechanism of action as "fibro-promotion."

For fibro-promotion to occur, two conditions are needed: "biotensegrity" and "volume." Over extensive clinical experience using PRF, it was observed that these conditions are necessary for augmentation procedures involving the use of any biological bio-modifier. The failure to satisfy either of these two parameters will translate into graft failure minimizing the regenerative potential of PRF and thus resulting in sub-optimal clinical outcomes.

8.3.1 Biotensegrity

The notion of Biotensegrity was introduced by Dr. Ingber DE, physician from Harvard school of medicine, who demonstrated that the positive or negative forces (tension/pressure) generated at the surface of a cell are transferred through the acto-myosin filaments complex through the cytoskeleton and finally transmitted to the nucleus [33]. Therefore, a balance exists between the extra-cellular forces and the intra-cellular compartments. Biotensegrity is the theory that helps to guide force transmission and orchestrate multi-molecular responses to stress at all

Table 8.2 Effects of PRF on root coverage of gingival recessions (CAF = Coronally Advanced Flap; PRF = Platelet Rich Fibrin; EMD = Enamel Matrix Derivative; CTG = Connective Tissue Graft; DLSBF = Double Lateral Sliding Bridge Flap; AM = Amniotic Membrane).

Author	Study Type	Patient #	Healing Period	Treatment Groups	Root Coverage (%)	P Value
Aroca (2009)	Split-mouth; Miller class I or II	20	6 months	CAF CAF + PRF	91.5 80.7	<0.004
Jankovic (2010)	Split-mouth; Miller class I or II	20	12 months	CAF + EMD CAF + PRF	70.5 72.1	n.s.
Aleksic (2010)	Split-mouth; Miller class I or II	19	12 months	CAF + CTG CAF + PRF	88.6 79.9	n.s.
Jankovic (2012)	Split-mouth; Miller class I or II	15	6 months	CAF + CTG CAF + PRF	88.7 92	n.s.
Padma (2013)	Split-mouth; Miller class I or II	15	1, 3, 6 months	CAF CAF + PRF	68.4 100	<0.0001
Eren (2014)	Split-mouth; Miller class I or II	22	6 months	CAF + CTG CAF + PRF	94.2 92.7	n.s.
Tunaliota (2015)	Split-mouth; Miller class I or II	22	12 months	CAF + CTG CAF + PRF	77.4 76.6	n.s.
Thamaraiselvan (2015)	Split-mouth; Miller class I or II	20	3 and 6 months	CAF CAF + PRF	65 74.2	n.s.
Gupta (2015)	Split-mouth; Miller class I or II	26	3 and 6 months	CAF CAF + PRF	86.6 91	n.s.
Keceli (2015)	Split-mouth; Miller class I or II	40	3 and 6 months	CAF + CTG CAF + CTG + PRF	79.9 89.6	<0.05
Dogan (2015)	Split-mouth; Miller class I or II	20	6 months	CAF CAF + PRF	82.1 86.7	n.s.
Rajaram (2015)	Split-mouth; Miller class II	20	12 and 24 months	DLSBF DLSBF + PRF	80 78.8	n.s.
Agarwal (2016)	Split-mouth; Miller class I or II	30	3 and 6 months	CAF CAF + AM CAF + PRF	33 36 56	<0.05

size scales in all organ systems. When the mechanical external forces applied on the cell surface (cell surface mechanoreceptors) are beyond the scope of the intra-cellular tolerance, an alteration in the cytoskeletal structure inside the cell leads to changes in intracellular gene expression changed from their original programmed expression. One of the clinical translational applications of this concept is the impact of flap tension on neo-angiogenesis. Mammoto *et al.* showed convincingly in an animal model that pressure generated from stretching the mucosa of mice significantly reduced the amount of VEGF production and thus a vascular reduction of the flap was observed [34,35]. Shortly afterwards, bone loss was also observed [34,35]. Pini Prato *et al.* confirmed this hypothesis in a randomized controlled clinical study performed by measuring the tension of the coronally advanced flap before suturing (high and low values) and thereafter comparing recession following coronally advanced flap therapy

[36]. The statistical analysis demonstrated that minimal flap tension (ranging from 0.0 to 0.4 g) favored less recession, while higher tension (ranging from 4 to 7 g) was associated with statistically higher recession. This negative impact of flap tension is now generally understood and observed also in the field of maxillofacial bone reconstruction [36]. Leaders in this field attribute the success of vertical bone augmentation procedures to the passive, non-tensile nature of flap closure that result from the maintenance of the cellular integrity of large bone grafting procedures [37].

8.3.2 Volume

In order to generate clinically relevant Fibro-promotion using PRF, a maximum quantity of platelets and leukocytes are needed during harvesting procedures to increase the final quantity of growth factors released. These growth factors are embedded into a tight and well-organized fibrin mesh, which will be released over time following a 10- to 15-day period (resorption rate of the PRF membranes). For this reason, the quality and quantity of soft tissues obtained after surgery is directly related to the amount of fibrin matrix grafted.

Interestingly, Ghanaati *et al.* evaluated the composition of PRF membranes in a quantitative histomorphometric analysis of cell populations and penetration [38]. By utilizing lower centrifugation speeds as highlighted in Chapter 3, a higher percentage of leukocytes and growth factors could be contained within PRF membranes. The totality of these findings correlates well with the author's clinical experience, which have found that by using three to four PRF membranes per pair of teeth, fibro-promotion may be clinically predictable.

8.4 FASTP: the surgical technique

The surgical technique proposed is a simplification of the Vestibular Incision Subperiosteal Technique Access (VISTA)[39] and an improvement of the Tunnel Technique [40].

8.4.1 Incision

The vertical mucosal incision allows a horizontal (mesio-distal) and apico-coronal full thickness flap resulting in a total relaxation and passive coronal displacement of the mucco-gingiva-papillary complex.

8.4.2 Root preparation and decontamination

Root preparation follows the same indications already proposed for periodontal mucco-gingival procedures described below:

- A thorough root preparation is created with a flat or negative root surface allowing for more volume of PRF as well as a lower flap tension leading to minimal PRF membrane resorption (Biotensegrity) (Figure 8.3).
- The root decontamination using 17% EDTA (double application for two minutes) allows the removal of the smear layer created by the root planning/preparation and will enable the collagen fibers of the tome's tubule to be exposed and thus improves the quality of the type of attachment expected (Figure 8.4).

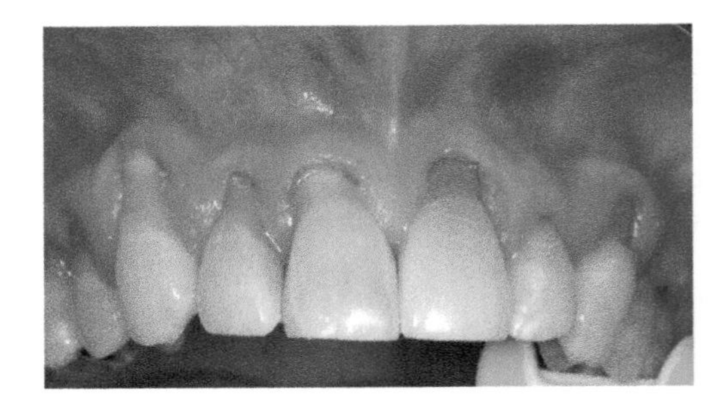

Figure 8.3 **Root preparation.** Achieved with rotary instruments and finished root planning instruments.

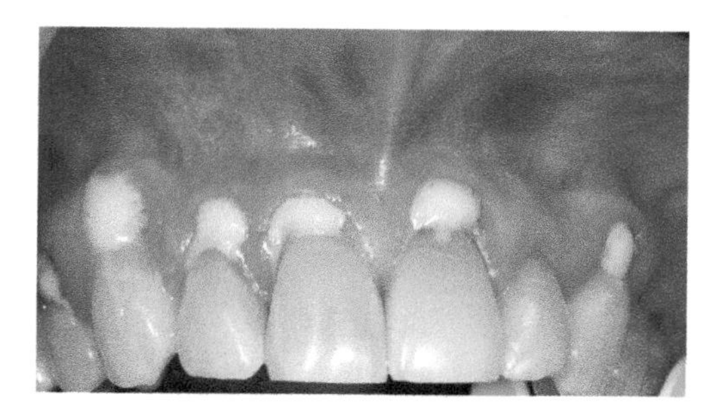

Figure 8.4 **Root decontamination.** EDTA 17% is applied for two minutes. Two rounds of decontaminations are used.

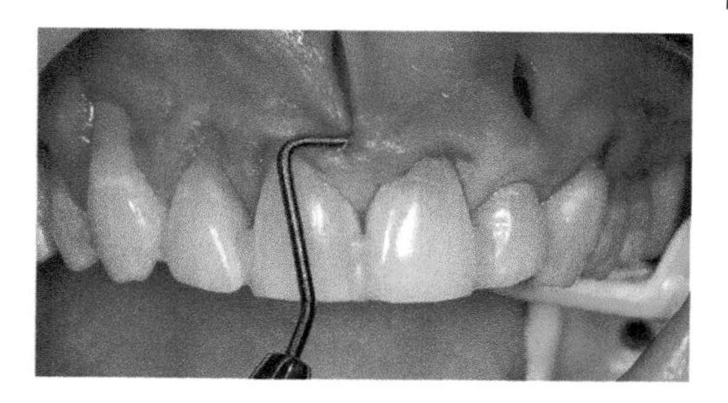

Figure 8.6 **Flap relaxation.** The vertical mucosal full thickness flap allows for a horizontal instrumentation of the flap resulting in a complete flap relaxation and the creation of a space able to hold numerous PRF membranes.

8.4.3 Volume packing

A minimum of three to four membranes per pair of teeth is recommended to enhance clinical outcomes. A "back packing concept" from distal to mesial will provide a homogenous density of PRF membrane volume (Figures 8.5–8.7). As a result of the flap relaxation and dense back packing technique, the flap is displaced physiologically coronally without tension or pull. This tension-free concept is the primary core value of the biotensegrity concept.

8.4.4 Suturing

1. Apical periosteal mattress sutures are the core values of the suturing technique and provides two purposes (Figure 8.8):
   a) Avoids marginal suture tension on the PRF membranes.
   b) Stabilizes and maintains the membranes on the roots surface by avoiding any unwanted displacement of the membranes in the mucosal area.
2. Interproximal vertical sling sutures are used to coronally advance the flap and obtain root coverage without putting any facial pressure on the buccal flap, thus reducing the risk of premature resorption of the PRF membranes (Figure 8.9).

The clinical reproducibility of the root coverage procedure associated with an increase in the zone of keratinized tissue depends on (Figures 8.10–8.12):

1. The comprehensive understanding of the PRF mechanism of action and biological principles.

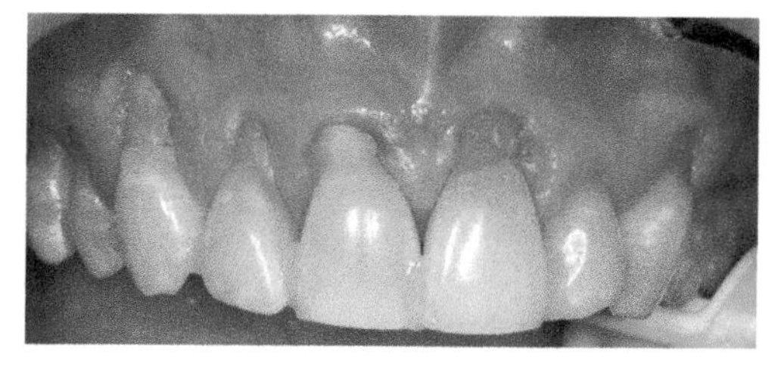

Figure 8.5 Interproximal flowable composite is used without etching or bonding. The curing induces shrinkage of the composite and creates a mechanical lock interproximally. The lack of bonding will ease the removal of the composite once sutures are removed.

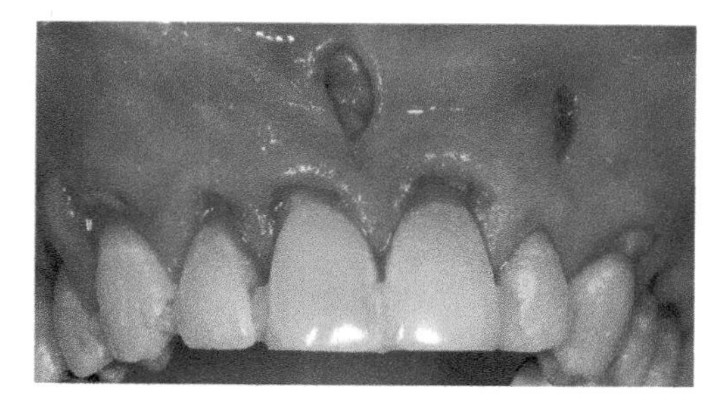

Figure 8.7 **Packing.** Three to four membranes are recommended per pair of teeth. The packing will induce a physiological coronal displacement of the flap. This will assure a passive tensionless closure respecting the laws of biotensegrity.

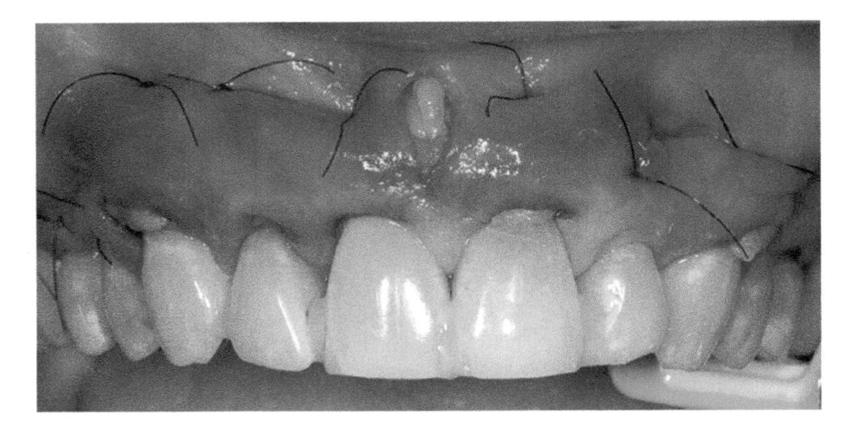

Figure 8.8 **Sutures.** Deep apical mattress is utilized to assist the maintenances of PRF membranes close to the periodontal ligament fibers and immobilize the flap against excessive movement from the muscle of mastication.

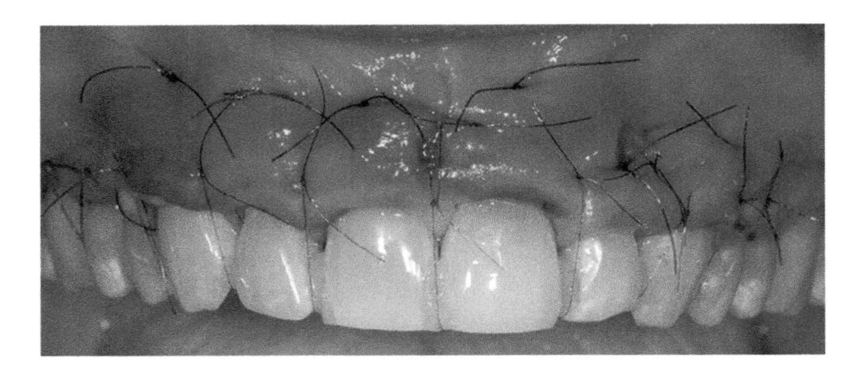

Figure 8.9 **Sutures.** Interproximal vertical sling sutures around the composite tracks the flap coronaly to cover the exposed roots.

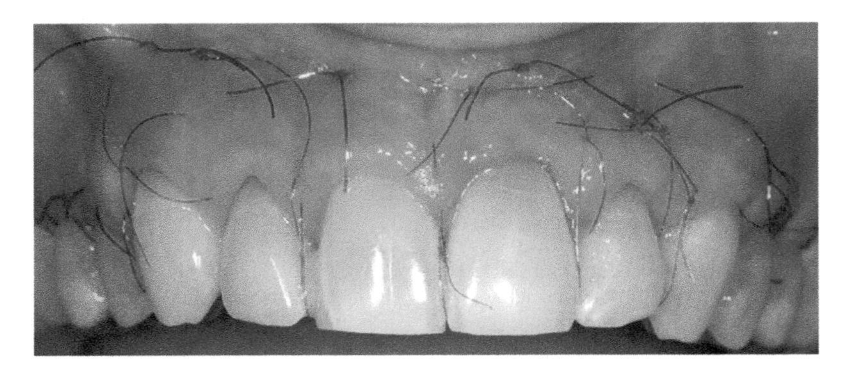

Figure 8.10 **Post-op.** Three weeks post-surgery. Note the amount of root coverage and tissue thickness visible.

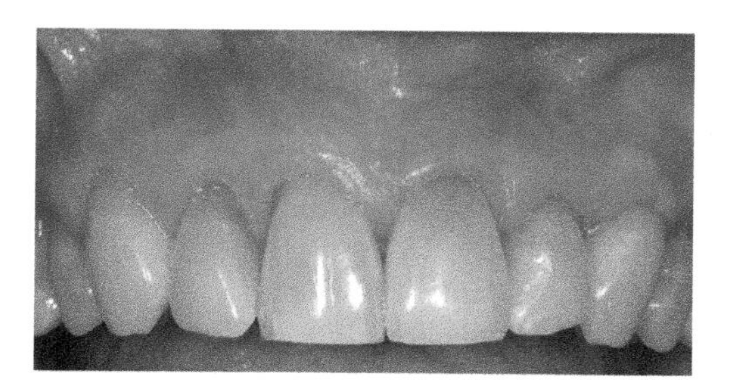

Figure 8.11 **Post-op.** Two years post-operative. Note the amount of vertical root coverage obtained. No pocket depth deeper than 2 mm is measured.

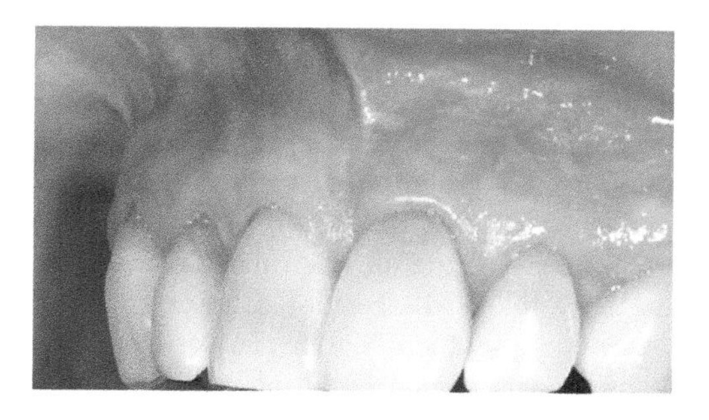

Figure 8.12 **Post-op.** Sectional view at two years post-surgery. Note the amount of three-dimensional soft-tissue fill. The roots are covered; the attached apparatus is restored and the muco-gingival deformity is corrected.

2. The precise execution of the surgical technique that relies heavily on:
   - Flap relaxation
   - Easy access to membrane packing and positioning on roots (volume)
   - Physiological displacement of the flap (biotensegrity)
   - Passive closure without tension

8.5 Conclusion

The use of PRF has been shown to increase the speed and quality of soft-tissue regeneration of gingival recessions. The "FASTP" technique for the purpose of root coverage using PRF is a surgical protocol meant to favor an increase in soft-tissue regeneration of muco-gingival defects. The fundamental concepts of this procedure reside in the understanding of sound biological principles already established in medicine and the clinical translation of such concepts into the clinical arena of dentistry. Although this innovative surgical procedure is still in its infancy, it holds great potential for future clinical and histological studies to validate its long-term use.

References

1 Miller A, Brunelle J, Carlos J, Brown L, Löe H. Oral health of United States adults. The national survey of oral health in US employed adults and seniors. 1985;86:11.

2 Albandar J, Kingman A. Gingival recession, gingival bleeding, and dental calculus in adults 30 years of age and older in the United States, 1988-1994. Journal of periodontology. 1999;70(1):30–43.

3 Sabarinathan J, Prabhu M, Lui LT, Chung V, Lin TS, Chew V, et al. Prevalence of Gingival Recession among the Different Races of Patients Reporting to Penang International Dental College. International Journal of Dental Sciences and Research. 2014;2(4A):1–3.

4 Francetti L, Del Fabbro M, Calace S, Testori T, Weinstein RL. Microsurgical treatment of gingival recession: A controlled clinical study. The International journal of periodontics & restorative dentistry. 2005;25(2):181–8.

5 Oates TW, Robinson M, Gunsolley JC. Surgical therapies for the treatment of gingival recession. A systematic review. Annals of Periodontology. 2003;8(1): 303–20.

6 Chambrone L, Chambrone LA, Frias EGV, Gonzalez MAS, Mancini E, Mendoza G, et al. Rationale for the Surgical Treatment of Single and Multiple Recession-Type Defects. Evidence-Based Periodontal and

Peri-Implant Plastic Surgery: Springer; 2015. p. 45–145.
7 Tatakis DN, Chambrone L, Allen EP, Langer B, McGuire MK, Richardson CR, et al. Periodontal soft tissue root coverage procedures: A consensus report from the AAP Regeneration Workshop. Journal of periodontology. 2015;86(2-s):S52–S5.
8 Jepsen K, Jepsen S, Zucchelli G, Stefanini M, Sanctis M, Baldini N, et al. Treatment of gingival recession defects with a coronally advanced flap and a xenogeneic collagen matrix: a multicenter randomized clinical trial. Journal of clinical periodontology. 2013;40(1):82–9.
9 Sali DD, Pauline George J. Demineralized Freeze Dried Bone Allograft With Amniotic Membrane in the Treatment of Periodontal Intrabony Defects-12 Month Randomized Controlled Clinical Trial. Journal of periodontology. 2016(0):1–18.
10 Miron RJ, Sculean A, Cochran DL, Froum S, Zucchelli G, Nemcovsky C, et al. Twenty years of enamel matrix derivative: the past, the present and the future. Journal of clinical periodontology. 2016;43(8):668–83.
11 Marx RE. Platelet-rich plasma: evidence to support its use. Journal of oral and maxillofacial surgery. 2004;62(4):489–96.
12 Hamdan AAS, Loty S, Isaac J, Bouchard P, Berdal A, Sautier JM. Platelet-poor plasma stimulates the proliferation but inhibits the differentiation of rat osteoblastic cells in vitro. Clinical oral implants research. 2009;20(6):616–23.
13 Choukroun J, Adda F, Schoeffler C, Vervelle A. Une opportunité en paro-implantologie: le PRF. Implantodontie. 2001;42(55):e62.
14 Choukroun J, Diss A, Simonpieri A, Girard M-O, Schoeffler C, Dohan SL, et al. Platelet-rich fibrin (PRF): a second-generation platelet concentrate. Part IV: clinical effects on tissue healing. Oral Surgery, Oral Medicine, Oral Pathology, Oral Radiology, and Endodontology. 2006;101(3):e56–e60.
15 Aroca S, Keglevich T, Barbieri B, Gera I, Etienne D. Clinical evaluation of a modified coronally advanced flap alone or in combination with a platelet-rich fibrin membrane for the treatment of adjacent multiple gingival recessions: a 6-month study. Journal of periodontology. 2009;80(2):244–52.
16 Aleksić Z, Janković S, Dimitrijević B, Divnić-Resnik T, Milinković I, Leković V. [The use of platelet-rich fibrin membrane in gingival recession treatment]. Srpski arhiv za celokupno lekarstvo. 2009; 138(1-2):11–8.
17 Jankovic S, Aleksic Z, Klokkevold P, Lekovic V, Dimitrijevic B, Barrie Kenney E, et al. Use of platelet-rich fibrin membrane following treatment of gingival recession: a randomized clinical trial. International Journal of Periodontics and Restorative Dentistry. 2012;32(2):165.
18 Tunalı M, Özdemir H, Arabacı T, Gürbüzer B, Pikdöken ML, Fıratlı E. Clinical evaluation of autologous platelet-rich fibrin in the treatment of multiple adjacent gingival recession defects: a 12-month study. International Journal of Periodontics & Restorative Dentistry. 2015;35(1).
19 Agarwal SK, Jhingran R, Bains VK, Srivastava R, Madan R, Rizvi I. Patient-centered evaluation of microsurgical management of gingival recession using coronally advanced flap with platelet-rich fibrin or amnion membrane: A comparative analysis. European journal of dentistry. 2016;10(1): 121–33.
20 Aleksic Z, Jankovic S, Dimitrijevic B, Divnic-Resnik T, Milinkovic I, Lekovic V. [The use of platelet-rich fibrin membrane in gingival recession treatment]. Srpski arhiv za celokupno lekarstvo. 2010;138 (1-2):11–8.
21 Aroca S, Keglevich T, Barbieri B, Gera I, Etienne D. Clinical evaluation of a modified coronally advanced flap alone or in combination with a platelet-rich fibrin membrane for the treatment of adjacent multiple gingival recessions: a 6-month study. Journal of periodontology. 2009; 80(2):244–52.

22 Dogan SB, Dede FO, Balli U, Atalay EN, Durmuslar MC. Concentrated growth factor in the treatment of adjacent multiple gingival recessions: a split-mouth randomized clinical trial. Journal of clinical periodontology. 2015;42(9):868–75.
23 Eren G, Atilla G. Platelet-rich fibrin in the treatment of localized gingival recessions: a split-mouth randomized clinical trial. Clinical oral investigations. 2014;18(8): 1941–8.
24 Gupta S, Banthia R, Singh P, Banthia P, Raje S, Aggarwal N. Clinical evaluation and comparison of the efficacy of coronally advanced flap alone and in combination with platelet rich fibrin membrane in the treatment of Miller Class I and II gingival recessions. Contemporary clinical dentistry. 2015;6(2):153–60.
25 Jankovic S, Aleksic Z, Klokkevold P, Lekovic V, Dimitrijevic B, Kenney EB, et al. Use of platelet-rich fibrin membrane following treatment of gingival recession: a randomized clinical trial. The International journal of periodontics & restorative dentistry. 2012;32(2):e41–e50.
26 Jankovic S, Aleksic Z, Milinkovic I, Dimitrijevic B. The coronally advanced flap in combination with platelet-rich fibrin (PRF) and enamel matrix derivative in the treatment of gingival recession: a comparative study. The European journal of esthetic dentistry : official journal of the European Academy of Esthetic Dentistry. 2010;5(3):260–73.
27 Keceli HG, Kamak G, Erdemir EO, Evginer MS, Dolgun A. The Adjunctive Effect of Platelet-Rich Fibrin to Connective Tissue Graft in the Treatment of Buccal Recession Defects: Results of a Randomized, Parallel-Group Controlled Trial. Journal of periodontology. 2015;86(11):1221–30.
28 Padma R, Shilpa A, Kumar PA, Nagasri M, Kumar C, Sreedhar A. A split mouth randomized controlled study to evaluate the adjunctive effect of platelet-rich fibrin to coronally advanced flap in Miller's class-I and II recession defects. Journal of Indian Society of Periodontology. 2013;17(5):631–6.
29 Rajaram V, Thyegarajan R, Balachandran A, Aari G, Kanakamedala A. Platelet Rich Fibrin in double lateral sliding bridge flap procedure for gingival recession coverage: An original study. Journal of Indian Society of Periodontology. 2015;19(6):665–70.
30 Thamaraiselvan M, Elavarasu S, Thangakumaran S, Gadagi JS, Arthie T. Comparative clinical evaluation of coronally advanced flap with or without platelet rich fibrin membrane in the treatment of isolated gingival recession. Journal of Indian Society of Periodontology. 2015;19(1):66–71.
31 Tunaliota M, Ozdemir H, Arabaciota T, Gurbuzer B, Pikdoken L, Firatli E. Clinical evaluation of autologous platelet-rich fibrin in the treatment of multiple adjacent gingival recession defects: a 12-month study. The International journal of periodontics & restorative dentistry. 2015;35(1):105–14.
32 Karring T, Lang N, Löe H. The role of gingival connective tissue in determining epithelial differentiation. Journal of periodontal research. 1975;10(1):1–11.
33 Ingber DE. Tensegrity-based mechanosensing from macro to micro. Progress in biophysics and molecular biology. 2008;97(2):163–79.
34 Mammoto T, Jiang A, Jiang E, Mammoto A. Platelet rich plasma extract promotes angiogenesis through the angiopoietin1-Tie2 pathway. Microvascular research. 2013;89:15–24.
35 Mammoto A, Connor KM, Mammoto T, Yung CW, Huh D, Aderman CM, et al. A mechanosensitive transcriptional mechanism that controls angiogenesis. Nature. 2009;457(7233):1103–8.
36 Pini Prato G, Pagliaro U, Baldi C, Nieri M, Saletta D, Cairo F, et al. Coronally advanced flap procedure for root coverage. Flap with tension versus flap without tension: a randomized controlled clinical study. Journal of periodontology. 2000;71(2):188–201.

37 Marx RE, Shellenberger T, Wimsatt J, Correa P. Severely resorbed mandible: predictable reconstruction with soft tissue matrix expansion (tent pole) grafts. Journal of oral and maxillofacial surgery. 2002;60(8):878–88.

38 Ghanaati S, Booms P, Orlowska A, Kubesch A, Lorenz J, Rutkowski J, et al. Advanced platelet-rich fibrin: a new concept for cell-based tissue engineering by means of inflammatory cells. The Journal of oral implantology. 2014;40(6):679–89.

39 Zadeh HH. Minimally invasive treatment of maxillary anterior gingival recession defects by vestibular incision subperiosteal tunnel access and platelet-derived growth factor BB. International Journal of Periodontics and Restorative Dentistry. 2011;31(6):653.

40 Stimmelmayr M, Allen EP, Gernet W, Edelhoff D, Beuer F, Schlee M, et al. Treatment of Gingival Recession in the Anterior Mandible Using the Tunnel Technique and a Combination Epithelialized-Subepithelial Connective Tissue Graft–A Case Series. International Journal of Periodontics & Restorative Dentistry. 2011;31(2).

9

Use of Platelet Rich Fibrin for Periodontal Regeneration/Repair of Intrabony and Furcation Defects

Richard J. Miron, Brian L. Mealey, and Hom-Lay Wang

Abstract

Over the past 20 years, an increasing trend has been observed in periodontology whereby the regeneration of intrabony and furcation defects has been accomplished by means of biological agents and growth factors. These followed a series of pioneering studies utilizing barrier membranes, which first established the concept of guided tissue regeneration (GTR) with/without various bone-grafting materials. Growth factors and biological agents were then introduced as potential regenerative agents for intrabony and furcation defects roughly 20 years ago following the introduction of recombinant human platelet derived growth factor (PDGF) and enamel matrix derivative (EMD). Similarly, an entire field of platelet concentrates including platelet rich plasma (PRP) and platelet rich fibrin (PRF) have all been investigated for tissue regeneration of periodontal defects. With the advancements made in platelet formulations over the past decade, PRF has recently been introduced and utilized as a supra-physiological concentration of autologous growth factors without necessitating the use of anticoagulants. The additional fibrin network has further been shown to serve as a space-making provisional matrix supporting angiogenesis and blood clot formation within periodontal pockets. This chapter focuses on over 20 randomized clinical trials investigating the use of PRF for intrabony and furcation defect regeneration/repair. We further highlight comparative studies demonstrating that this low-cost regenerative modality reduces periodontal pocket depths and increases clinical attachment levels when utilized either alone or in combination with other periodontal biomaterials.

Highlights

- What is true periodontal regeneration?
- Why is periodontal regeneration more difficult than bone regeneration?
- What are the currently available treatment modalities supporting periodontal regeneration on the market?
- What do the randomized clinical trials utilizing PRF for intrabony defect regeneration demonstrate?
- How does PRF compare to current standards in the field?
- Future research direction of PRF for periodontal regeneration?

9.1 Introduction

The periodontium is a complex functional unit derived from several tissues responsible

Platelet Rich Fibrin in Regenerative Dentistry: Biological Background and Clinical Indications, First Edition.
Edited by Richard J. Miron and Joseph Choukroun.

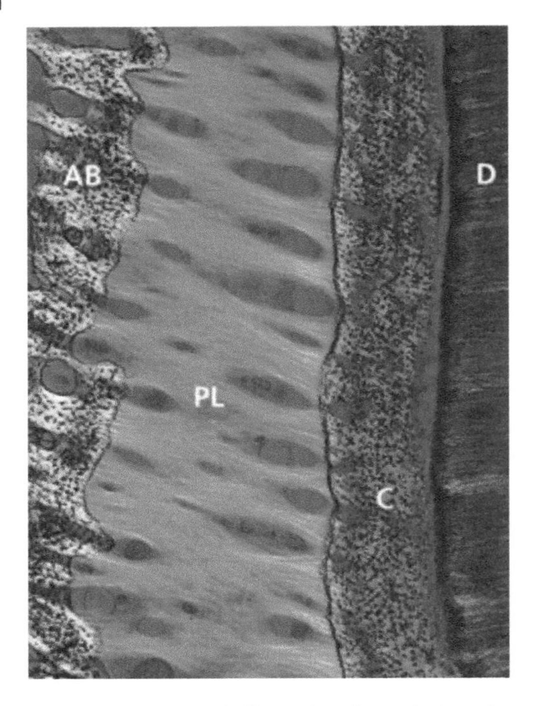

Figure 9.1 Micrograph illustrating the periodontal ligament (PL) with its collagen fiber bundles spanning between the root covered with cementum (C) and the alveolar bone (AB). D, dentin. Undecalcified ground section, unstained and viewed under polarized light. Source: Bosshardt *et al.* 2015 [2]. Reproduced with permission of John Wiley & Sons.

for the connection of teeth with their surrounding bone. This is accomplished by collagen Sharpey's fibers that span from the root cementum through the periodontal ligament and attach to bundle alveolar bone (Figure 9.1) [1,2]. The periodontium provides a flexible defense system with various host cells responsible for the maintenance and structural integrity of the tooth apparatus. It has been well described in the literature that failure to prevent infection by periodontal pathogens may cause gingivitis and without treatment may lead to the development of periodontitis and the eventual loss of periodontal structures [1].

Periodontal disease is one of the most prevalent diseases known to man. It begins as a superficial inflammation of the gingiva without attachment or bone loss (gingivitis) and later progresses to attachment loss with subsequent bone destruction (periodontitis). Results investigating the distribution of the disease from a national survey conducted in the United States found that over 47% of the adult population was affected [3]. Furthermore, it was found that 38.5% of the population had either a moderate or severe case of periodontitis. This finding is most alarming as the disease is characterized with an exponentially more difficult resolution and regeneration once advanced progression has taken place.

Treatment of periodontal disease has now been deemed of utmost importance. Surveys and epidemic studies have shown that periodontitis plays a role in a number of systemic diseases including cardiovascular diseases (heart attack/stroke), diabetes, obesity, and premature births, amongst others [4]. It, therefore, becomes vital that dental practitioners and healthcare providers alike be aware of the disease progression and more research be put into regeneration of these tissues that have been lost due to periodontal disease [5–7]. Since true periodontal regeneration comprises not only the regeneration of the periodontal ligament, but also the surrounding alveolar bone, cementum, and also the overlying soft tissues including new connective and epithelial tissues, complete periodontal regeneration remains but a desired end goal, with much future research still necessary to fulfill these criteria predictably. Therefore, the aim of this chapter is to present research that has been conducted over the years including uses of barrier membranes and bone grafting materials. We then highlight how growth factors and biological agents have more recently become a preferred choice for intrabony and furcation defect regeneration. Lastly, platelet concentrates are described with a large focus on the number of randomized clinical trials that now support the use of platelet rich fibrin (PRF) for the repair/regeneration of intrabony and furcation defects.

9.2 Role of barrier membranes in periodontal regeneration

The use of barrier membranes for guided tissue regeneration (GTR) represents one of the first modalities adapted for periodontal regeneration. It was originally believed that in order to optimize periodontal regeneration, cells from periodontal ligament and alveolar bone should be exclusively separated from the overlaying soft tissues (epithelium or fibrous connective tissue) in order to allow repopulation of the periodontal defects (Figure 9.2). In 1982, Nyman *et al.* first introduced this concept using a cellulose acetate laboratory filter by Millipore to act as a barrier separating periodontal structures from overlaying soft tissues [8]. Today, a variety of barrier membranes derived from several sources have been developed with a number of necessities including biocompatibility with host tissues, space-making characteristics, mechanical strength, and ideal degradation properties all being requirements for GTR treatment of periodontal intrabony or furcation defects.

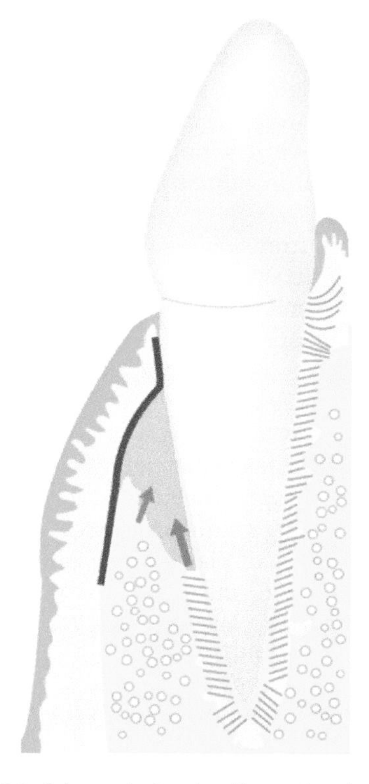

Figure 9.2 Schematic drawing illustrating the principle of guided tissue regeneration. A barrier membrane is used to form a secluded space with the aim to prevent the apical growth of gingival cells and allow cells from the periodontal ligament and alveolar bone to repopulate the space under the membrane. (Courtesy of DD Bosshardt).
Source: Bosshardt *et al.* 2015 [2]. Reproduced with permission of John Wiley & Sons.

Although findings from initial studies utilizing barrier membranes confirmed greater clinical attachment levels [9], a second surgery was required to remove the membrane and was shown to compromise some of the beneficial effects obtained during the regenerative procedure [10]. These drawbacks often outweighed the positive benefits and for these reasons, collagen absorbable membranes have since been developed [11]. Today a wide variety of resorbable barrier membranes are available, with various reported degradation rates and fabrication sources most suitable for the clinician's preferences. Still, complete periodontal regeneration is not possible utilizing barrier membranes alone.

9.3 Role of bone-grafting materials in periodontal regeneration

Much can be dedicated to the role and improvements in bone-grafting materials over the years. Originally, grafts were developed to serve as a passive, structural supporting network with the main criteria being biocompatibility, but advancements made in the field of tissue engineering have introduced a large array of materials, each possessing various advantages and disadvantages. The global market has now surpassed 3 billion U.S. dollars per year and as the population ages, the number of bone-grafting procedures for diseases such as osteoporosis, arthritis, tumors, or trauma will continue to rise [12].

Bone grafts are typically characterized into four groups, including autografts, allografts, xenografts, and alloplasts. While autogenous bone is considered the gold standard for a wide variety of grafting procedures [13], its main drawback includes its fast turnover rate, which prevents its effectiveness for intrabony defect regeneration. Furthermore, a limited supply is another drawback. Therefore, bone allografts harvested from another human cadaver has been the most common alternative. Freeze or fresh-frozen bone, freeze-dried bone allograft (FDBA) and demineralized freeze-dried bone allograft (DFDBA) have all been utilized successfully for the regeneration of intrabony/furcation defects [14–17]. Similarly, while certain countries do not allow the use of allografts, xenografts derived from various animal sources have also been widely used [18–22]. Lastly, alloplasts are synthetically developed bone replacement grafts fabricated from various laboratory materials including hydroxyapatite and beta-tricalcium phosphate. Although they demonstrate some advantages when compared to open flap debridement (OFD) alone [23–29], the majority of clinicians do not fully support their use when compared to allografts or xenografts.

9.4 Biologic agents/growth factors for periodontal regeneration

The use of biologic agents such as growth factors to promote periodontal regeneration has increased tremendously during the last decade in periodontology. A variety of novel research in the mid-1990s focused on developing delivery systems for growth factors accordingly to support periodontal regeneration. Since the regeneration of periodontal tissues is much more complex than most tissues due mainly to the fact it comprises many tissues/cell types from different embryonic origins, a variety of biological agents including enamel matrix derivate (EMD), platelet-derived growth factor-BB (rhPDGF-BB), recombinant human fibroblast growth factor-2 (rhFGF-2), bone morphogenetic proteins BMPs (BMP-2 and BMP-7), teriparatide PTH, and growth differential factor-5 (GDF-5). PRP and PRF have been investigated for periodontal regeneration. The understanding of root cementum development and formation led to the development of EMD where the proteins comprised within EMD, mainly amelogenins, were aimed at mimicking normal tissue development [30–34]. Similarly, rhPDGF was granted FDA approval for both medical and dental purposes and has been the first such growth factor of its kind [35,36]. Its main action is to promote rapid cell migration, proliferation, and angiogenesis to wound sites, and research has further shown it supports intrabony defect regeneration in human randomized clinical trials [37–48].

Derived from megakaryocytes, platelets are small irregular cells with a diameter of 2 to 4 micrometers. Platelets have an average life span of 8 to 12 days, with normal platelets count between 150,000 and 400,000 platelets/microliter. Their key role in hemostasis and being a natural source of growth factor, make platelets a component of paramount importance during wound healing. Depending on the processing technique, different types of platelet concentrates have been described, including but not limited to platelet rich plasma (PRP), pure platelet rich plasma (P-PRP), leukocyte- and platelet rich plasma (L-PRP), and platelet rich fibrin (PRF). The potential of this substances as a biologic agent in periodontology relies on the growth factors stored within platelet alpha granules including platelet-derived growth factor (PDGF), vascular endothelial growth factor (VEGF), insulin-like growth factor (IGF), platelet-derived angiogenic factor, and transforming growth factor-beta (TGF-B) [49]. An alternative method to obtain natural autologous PDGF was first introduced by using PRP, an autologous concentration of growth factors derived from typical platelets following centrifugation. PRP was first utilized extensively by many clinicians in the oral maxillofacial surgery field [50–52] and has since been extensively utilized for intrabony defect regeneration mainly in combination with bone grafts [18,53–67]. While the results from these studies are somewhat controversial, one of the potential reasons for these findings was hypothesized to be due to the use of anti-coagulants in preparation of the PRP.

9.5 Platelet rich fibrin (PRF) as a potential autologous biological agent for periodontal regeneration

Following the regenerative outcomes with PRP, several authors began to hypothesize whether PRF, a natural platelet concentrate without the use of anti-coagulants, could further improve the outcomes observed with PRP. PRF not only differs from its predecessor by its lack of anticoagulant use during preparation, but more importantly it is easier to fabricate (requires one centrifugation cycle with less time, as opposed to two centrifugation cycles with PRP) [68]. There are three main added advantages that further support its use. First, PRF contains a fibrin network that facilitates blood clot formation and tissue repair [69]. Secondly, its growth factor release kinetics have been shown to occur more slowly when compared to PRP, and therefore regeneration may take place over a more extended period of time [70]. Moreover, PRF contains leukocytes and macrophages, known cell types implicated in immunity and host defense [71,72]. Since periodontal defects are the result of invading bacterial pathogens, the inclusion of white blood cells contained within PRF is hypothesized to further act as a bacterial resistant matrix capable of fighting bacterial pathogens.

9.6 Intrabony defect regeneration with PRF: results from controlled clinical trials

To date, 17 randomized clinical trials (RCTs) have investigated the use of PRF for the repair/regeneration of periodontal intrabony defects [73–89]. The various RCTs have compared the additional use of PRF to OFD versus OFD alone and have further investigated its use with various biomaterials and/or antibiotics (Table 9.1). The clinical parameters in Table 9.1 are reported in periodontal pocket depth (PPD) reductions and clinical attachment level (CAL) gains following therapy with PRF. All 17 studies found that the additional use of PRF increased PPD reductions and CAL gains when compared to OFD alone (Table 9.1). Two studies comparing defect healing with PRF versus a bone grafting material (DFDBA) found no significant differences between treatment groups (Figures 9.3–9.11) [80,85]. Three studies found that the use PRF in combination with a bone-grafting material was superior to either PRF alone, or bone-grafting material alone [73,75,86]. It was similarly found that the supplemental use of PRF in combination with a barrier membrane was superior to barrier membrane alone PPD reductions and CAL gains at intrabony defects sites [77]. In a recent study, the additional use of PRF with EMD found no differences between the test and control (EMD alone) groups [84].

In summary, the collected RCTs have all shown that the use of PRF leads to statistically superior CAL gains and PPD reductions when compared to OFD alone and may be combined with either a bone graft or barrier membrane to further enhance results. No differences were reported when EMD was combined with PRF. Despite the large number of RCTs performed to date (17 trials), it remains interesting to point out that no histological study has confirmed whether the results obtained are truly characterized as periodontal "regeneration" versus periodontal

Table 9.1 Effects of PRF on intrabony defect regeneration (PPD = Probing Periodontal Depth; CAL = Clinical Attachment Level; OFD = Open Flap Debridement; PRF = Platelet Rich Fibrin; DFDBA = Demineralized Freeze-Dried Bone Allograft, MF = Metformin; HA = Hydroxyapatite; RSV = Rosuvastatin; DBM = Demineralized Bone Matrix; ALN = Alendronate; ATV = Atorvastatin; EMD = Enamel Matrix Derivative). Data reports significant difference between PRF and control.

Author	Defect #	Healing Time	Groups	ΔPPD (mm)	CAL Gain (mm)	P Value
Thorat (2011)	32	9 months	OFD	3.56	2.13	ΔPPD: <0.01
			OFD + PRF	4.56	3.69	CAL: <0.01
Sharma (2011)	56	9 months	OFD	3.21	2.77	ΔPPD: 0.006
			OFD + PRF	4.55	3.31	CAL: n.s.
Pradeep (2012)	90	9 months	OFD	2.97	2.67	ΔPPD: 0.002
			OFD + PRF	3.90	3.03	GAL: n.s.
Pradeep (2012)	90	9 months	OFD	2.97	2.83	ΔPPD: 0.018
			OFD + PRF	3.77	3.17	GAL: n.s.
Shah (2015)	40	6 months	OFD + DFDBA	3.70	2.97	n.s.
			OFD + PRF	3.67	2.97	
Pradeep (2015)	120	9 months	OFD	3.01	2.96	ΔPPD: <0.001
			OFD + PRF	4.01	4.03	CAL: <0.001 both
			ORF + 1% MF	3.93	3.93	treatment groups
			OFD + 1% MF + PRF	4.90	4.90	
Ajwani (2015)	40	9 months	OFD	1.60	1.30	PPD: <0.001
			OFD + PRF	1.90	1.80	CAL: <0.001
Elgendy (2015)	40	6 months	OFD + HA	3.42	3.55	PPD: <0.02
			OFD + + HA + PRF	3.82	3.90	CAL: <0.027
Agarwal (2016)	60	12 months	OFD +DFDBA	3.60	2.61	PPD: <0.05
			OFD + DFDBA + PRF	4.15	3.73	CAL: <0.05
Panda (2016)	32	9 months	barrier membrane	3.19	3.38	PPD: 0.002
			membrane + PRF	3.88	4.44	CAL = 0.001
Pradeep (2016)	90	9 months	OFD	3.10	2.47	PPD: <0.001
			OFD + PRF	4.03	3.30	CAL: <0.001
			OFD + PRF + 1.2% RSV	4.90	3.93	
Chatterjee (2016)	90	9 months	OFD	3.68	4.14	PPD and CAL: <0.001
			PRF	5.46	6.57	between groups 1 and 2/3
			titanium PRF	6.25	6.74	N.S. btw groups 2 and 3
Chandradas (2016)	36	9 months	OFD	3.00	2.25	PPD: <0.001
			OFD + PRF	3.82	3.27	CAL: <0.001
			OFD + PRF + DBM	4.25	3.92	
Pradeep (2016)	90	9 months	OFD	2.86	3.03	PPD: <0.001
			PRF	3.70	4.20	CAL: <0.001
			PRF + ALN	4.53	5.16	
Martande (2016)	96	9 months	OFD	2.76	2.50	PPD and CAL: <0.001
			OFD + PRF	3.76	3.40	between groups 1 and 2/3
			OFD + PRF + 1.2% ATV	4.06	3.66	N.S. btw groups 2 and 3
Chadwick (2016)	36	6 months	PRF	2.12	1.03	PPD: N.S. CAL: N.S.
			DFDBA	2.00	1.16	
Aydemir Turkal (2016)	28	6 months	EMD	3.88	3.29	PPD: N.S.
			EMD + PRF	4.00	3.42	CAL: N.S.

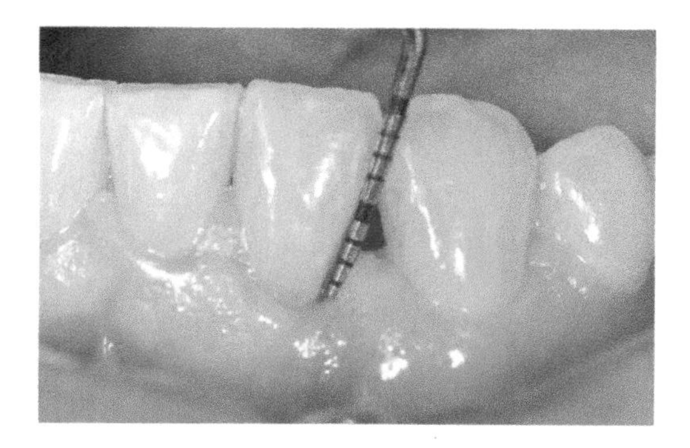

Figure 9.3 Pre-op Probing Depth of a left lower lateral incisor (23D) (Case performed by resident Dr. Jane Chadwick under supervision from Dr. Brian Mealey for Figures 9.3–9.11).

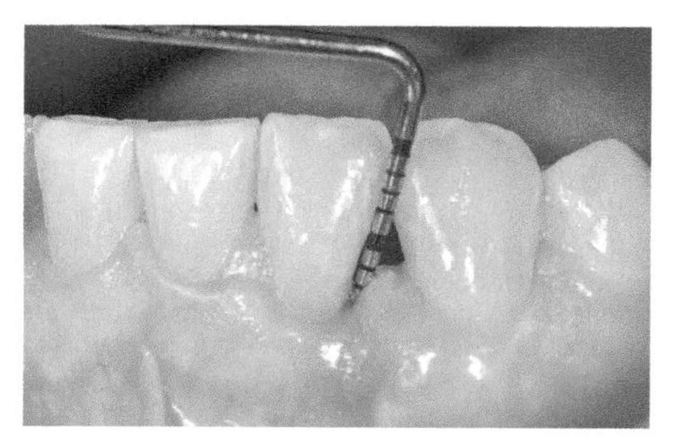

Figure 9.4 Preop bone sounding.

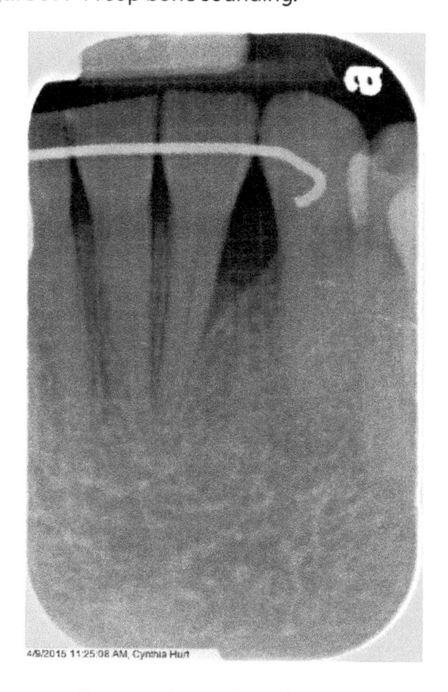

Figure 9.5 Preop radiograph with Fixott-Everett grid.

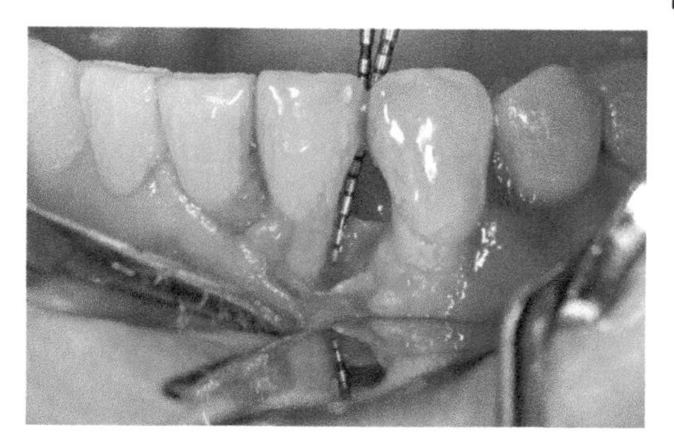

Figure 9.6 Flap reflected, defect debrided, perio probe in defect for measurement.

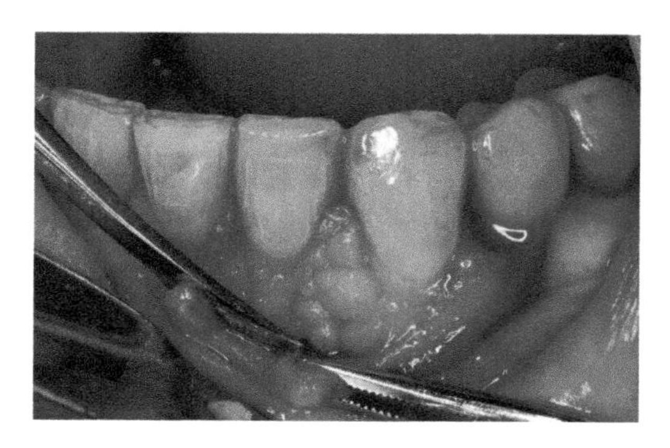

Figure 9.7 PRF place into defect and overfilled (PRF was then compressed with a moist gauze).

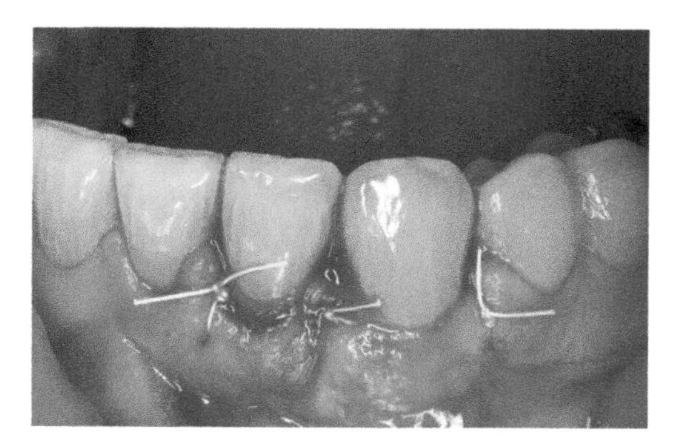

Figure 9.8 Flaps sutured.

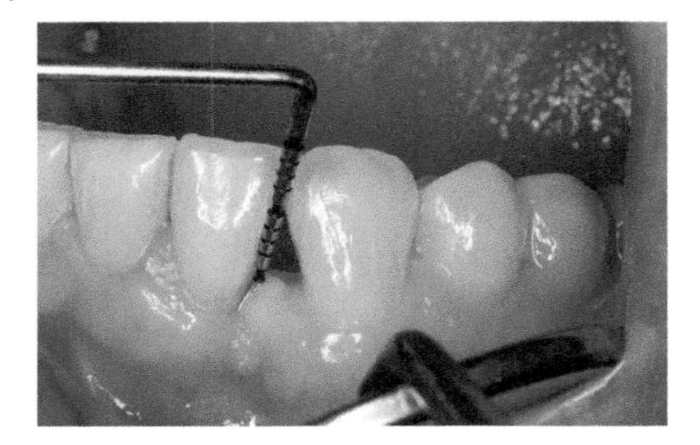

Figure 9.9 Six-month postop probing depth.

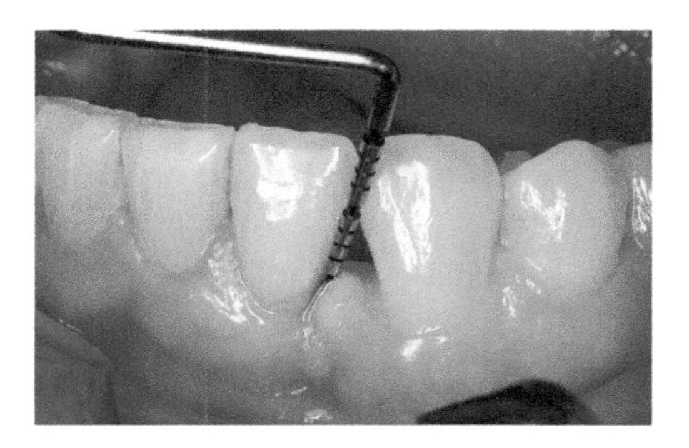

Figure 9.10 Six-month postop bone sounding.

"repair" (Figure 9.12). Future research is therefore needed.

9.7 Furcation defect regeneration with PRF

Similarly, PRF has also been utilized in four RCTs investigating class II furcation defects (Table 9.2). In all studies, PRF was shown to be statistically superior to controls (OFD alone) and resulted in higher CAL gains [90–93]. While these studies reveal the potential for PRF to improve clinical parameters, once again no data exist to date confirming periodontal regeneration via histological evaluation. Furthermore, while a number of studies investigating intrabony defect regeneration have compared PRF to common regenerative modalities including bone grafts, barrier membranes or bioactive factors, no study to date exists for furcation defect regeneration. Therefore, future RCTs remain needed.

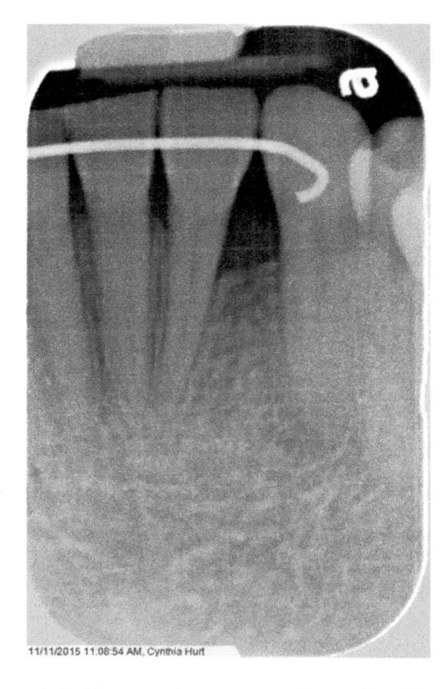

Figure 9.11 Six-month postop radiograph with Fixott-Everett grid—notice the defect fill when compared to Figure 9.5 (Case performed by resident Dr. Jane Chadwick under supervision from Dr. Brian Mealey).

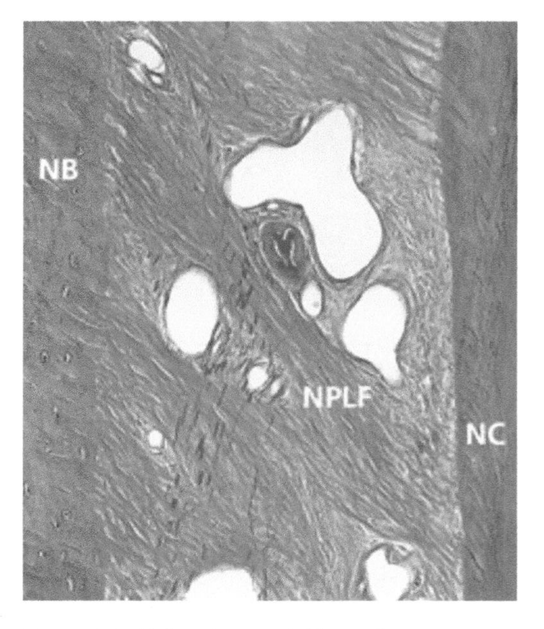

Figure 9.12 Light micrograph illustrating periodontal regeneration as demonstrated by new periodontal ligament fibers (NPLF) inserting into new bone (NB) and new cementum (NC). Source: Bosshardt *et al.* 2015 [2]. Reproduced with permission of John Wiley & Sons.

Table 9.2 Effects of PRF on furcation defect regeneration (OFD = Open Flap Debridement; PRF = Platelet Rich Fibrin; HA = Hydroxyapatite, ALN = Alendronate).

Author	Defect #	Number of Cases	Healing Period	Treatment	Gain in CAL (mm)	P value
Sharma (2011)	Class II Furcations	36	9 months	OFD OFD + PRF	1.28 2.33	<0.001
Bajaj (2013)	Class II Furcations	72	9 months	OFD OFD + PRF	1.37 2.87	<0.05
Pradeep (2016)	Class II Furcations	105	9 months	1. OFD + placebo gel 2. OFD + HA + PRF 3. Rosuvastatin + HA + PRF	1.82 3.31 4.17	<0.05 between all groups
Kanoriya (2016)	Class II Furcations	72	9 months	OFD OFD+ PRF ORF + PRF + ALN	2.41 3.69 4.40	<0.05 between all groups

9.8 Discussion and future research

Despite the fact that PRF is not commonly utilized in routine clinical practice by many clinicians for the regeneration of intrabony defects, it remains interesting to note that 21 RCTs have thus far evaluated its potential for periodontal regeneration either for intrabony or furcation defects. While periodontal regeneration remains complex due to the number of tissues needed to be regenerated (new cementum, periodontal ligament and alveolar bone), as well as the fact Sharpey's fibers need to be oriented functionally to support the tooth apparatus, it remains difficult to assess PRF for periodontal regeneration without histological evidence. Nevertheless, it is known that periodontal disease is caused by bacterial pathogens and an increase in leukocyte number will certainly speed tissue resolution. Furthermore, angiogenesis is an important factor for tissue regeneration, and PRF releases a number of pro-angiogenic and pro-fibrotic agents capable of speeding periodontal tissue repopulation [7,94].

The biological advantages of PRF have been shown to act locally by quickly stimulating a large number of cell types by influencing their recruitment, proliferation, and/or differentiation. These include endothelial cells, gingival fibroblasts, chondrocytes, and osteoblasts, thereby having a potential effect on either soft- or hard-tissue repair [95,96]. While it is known that beneficial effects of PRF may partially be due to the large number of secreted autologous blood-derived growth factors, it remains of interest to determine how these may compare to the food and drug administration (FDA)–approved recombinant proteins PDGF and BMP2 [35,36,97,98]. Interestingly, although recombinant proteins have a regenerative potential well documented in the literature [99–101], their associated costs and other secondary adverse effects including biocompatibility, lower stability and potential swelling, may favor the use of autogenous PRF [102,103]. Future cost-benefit research remains necessary.

Another aspect requiring future research is to investigate histologically whether PRF has the same stimulatory effect on soft and hard tissues as other well-researched recombinant proteins. The literature to date seems to indicate that PRF favors soft-tissue regeneration when compared to hard tissues [104]. Since periodontitis is characterized by not only periodontal ligament breakdown

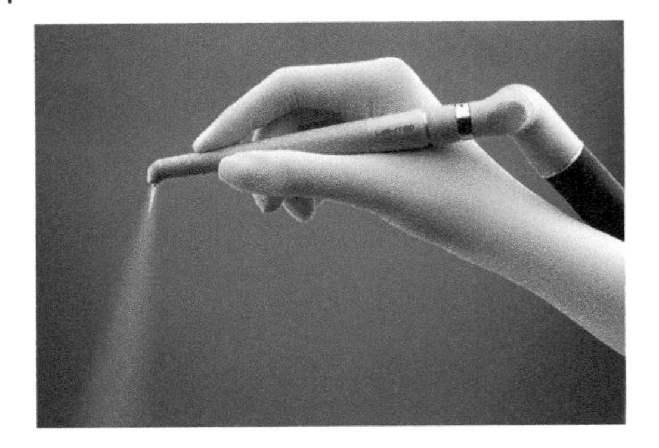

Figure 9.13 Photo of an Erbium:YAG laser. (Image supplied by Dr. Fabrice Baudot).

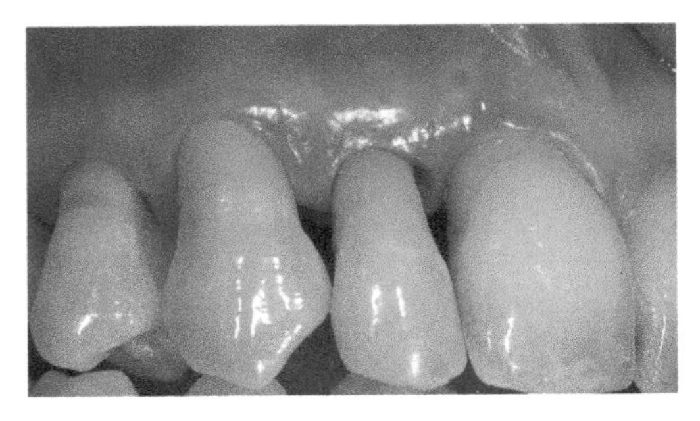

Figure 9.15 Intra-operative view with microsurgical access to the deep periodontium: aggressive periodontitis. Note the tissue stability. (Case performed by Dr. Fabrice Baudot).

but also that of alveolar bone and cementum, the regenerative potential of each of these tissues needs to be further characterized via histological investigations, at least in animal studies.

It remains interesting to point out that blood clot formation alone has been shown to be one of the key necessary features in order for periodontal regeneration to take place, as long as bacterial pathogens have been completely eliminated. Evidence from the literature suggests that blood clot formation alone is enough to treat a number of intrabony defects where space maintenance is not an issue [94]. For such procedures, the additional use of PRF acts primarily in a similar fashion whereby the PRF scaffold can be inserted into the periodontal pocket acting as a clot, favoring tissue regeneration. Future research is therefore needed to determine what factors in the PRF clots (cells/leukocytes, growth factors, or fibrin matrix) are most necessary to help regenerate periodontal tissues.

Interestingly, the use of PRF has been shown to decrease the rate of localized alveolar osteitis 9.5-fold following third molar extractions, suggesting a beneficial wound healing effect of PRF in extraction sites [105].

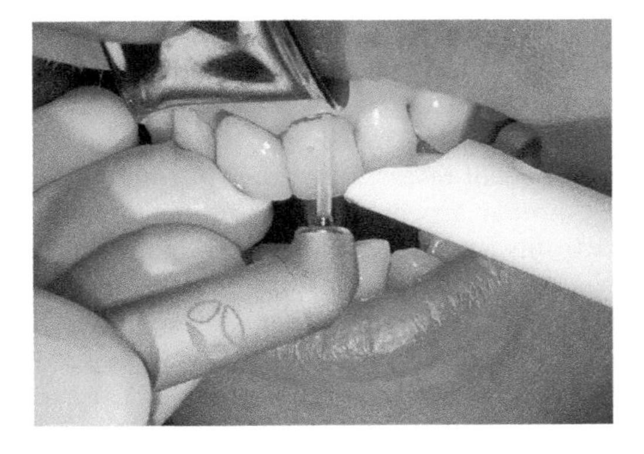

Figure 9.14 The Erbium:YAG laser allows optimal precision required for minimally invasive surgery. (Case performed by Dr. Fabrice Baudot).

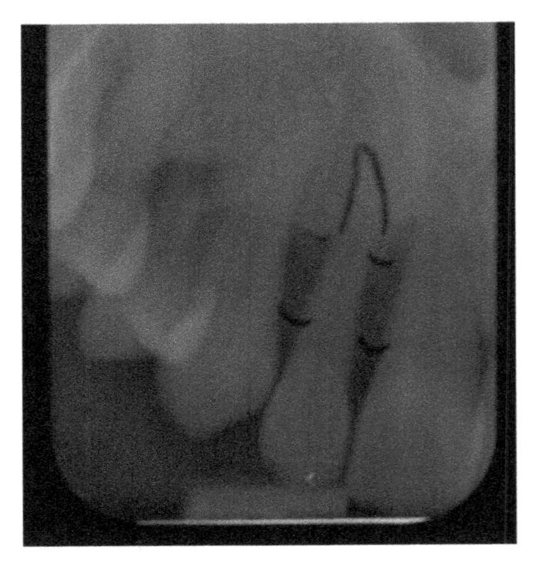

Figure 9.16 Pre-operative x-ray of an aggressive periodontitis, in smoker patient, 45 years old with Vitamin D deficiency. (Case performed by Dr. Fabrice Baudot).

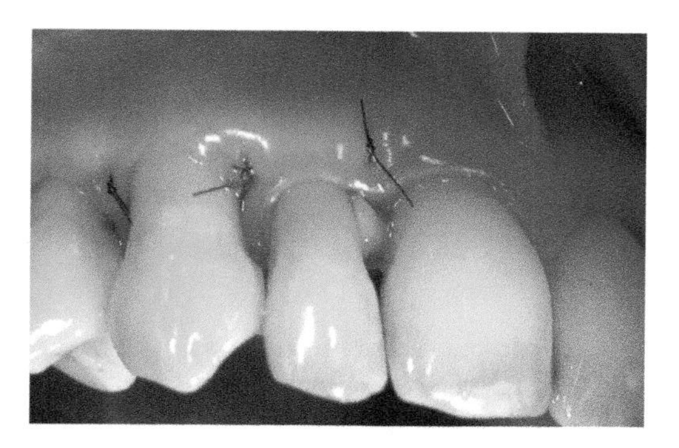

Figure 9.17 Completion of the micro-surgical approach utilizing the Erbium:YAG laser in combination with PRF. The PRF membranes are packed within the intrabony defects and sutured for stability. (Case performed by Dr. Fabrice Baudot).

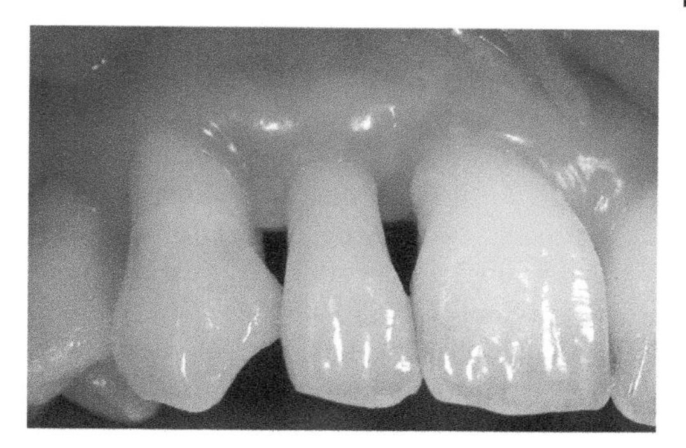

Figure 9.18 Post-operative view after two months of an aggressive periodontitis treated by microsurgical protocol and flapless PRF. Note the access to oral hygiene and the tissue stability after a two-month healing period. (Case performed by Dr. Fabrice Baudot).

This may be due to the presence of leukocytes in PRF. For intrabony periodontal defects, the presence of leukocytes in PRF may improve anti-bacterial host defense, however no basic science experiments have investigated this phenomenon. Furthermore, much research looking into photodynamic therapy (Er:YAG lasers) for periodontal decontamination has been investigated utilizing micro-surgical debridement of pockets (Figures 9.13 and 9.14) [106]. From this perspective, such treatments have been combined with PRF and demonstrated quite favorable results (Figures 9.15–9.18). While this area of research remains preliminary, future investigation aims to reveal this combination approach as a potential source for regeneration of periodontal and peri-implant defects.

In conclusion, the literature shows that the use of PRF is able to significantly improve PPD reductions and CAL gains in a large number of RCTs. Nevertheless, future research is necessary to further characterize histologically periodontal regeneration utilizing PRF.

References

1 Bosshardt DD, Sculean A. Does periodontal tissue regeneration really work? Periodontol 2000. 2009;51:208–19.
2 Bosshardt DD, Stadlinger B, Terheyden H. Cell-to-cell communication–periodontal regeneration. Clinical oral implants research. 2015;26(3):229–39.
3 Eke PI, Dye BA, Wei L, Thornton-Evans GO, Genco RJ, Cdc Periodontal Disease Surveillance workgroup: James Beck GDRP. Prevalence of periodontitis in adults in the United States: 2009 and 2010. J Dent Res. 2012;91(10):914–20.
4 Cullinan MP, Seymour GJ. Periodontal disease and systemic illness: will the evidence ever be enough? Periodontol 2000. 2013;62(1):271–86.
5 Grzesik WJ, Narayanan AS. Cementum and periodontal wound healing and regeneration. Crit Rev Oral Biol Med. 2002;13(6):474–84.
6 Wikesjo UM, Selvig KA. Periodontal wound healing and regeneration. Periodontol 2000. 1999;19:21–39.
7 Wang HL, Greenwell H, Fiorellini J, Giannobile W, Offenbacher S, Salkin L, et al. Periodontal regeneration. Journal of periodontology. 2005;76(9):1601–22.
8 Nyman S, Lindhe J, Karring T, Rylander H. New attachment following surgical

treatment of human periodontal disease. J Clin Periodontol. 1982;9(4):290–6.

9 Pihlstrom BL, McHugh RB, Oliphant TH, Ortiz-Campos C. Comparison of surgical and nonsurgical treatment of periodontal disease. A review of current studies and additional results after 61/2 years. J Clin Periodontol. 1983;10(5):524–41.

10 AlGhamdi AS, Ciancio SG. Guided tissue regeneration membranes for periodontal regeneration–a literature review. Journal of the International Academy of Periodontology. 2009;11(3):226–31.

11 Zhang Y, Zhang X, Shi B, Miron. R. Membranes for guided tissue and bone regeneration. Annals of Oral & Maxillofacial Surgery. 2013;Feb 01;1(1): 10.

12 Place ES, Evans ND, Stevens MM. Complexity in biomaterials for tissue engineering. Nature materials. 2009;8(6): 457–70.

13 Miron RJ, Sculean A, Shuang Y, Bosshardt DD, Gruber R, Buser D, et al. Osteoinductive potential of a novel biphasic calcium phosphate bone graft in comparison with autographs, xenografts, and DFDBA. Clinical oral implants research. 2015.

14 Fucini SE, Quintero G, Gher ME, Black BS, Richardson AC. Small versus large particles of demineralized freeze-dried bone allografts in human intrabony periodontal defects. Journal of periodontology. 1993;64(9):844–7.

15 Harasty LA, Brownstein CN, Deasy MJ. Regeneration of intrabony defects: comparing e-PTFE membrane vs. decalcified freeze dried bone allograft–a pilot study. Periodontal clinical investigations: official publication of the Northeastern Society of Periodontists. 1999;21(1):10–7.

16 Parashis A, Andronikaki-Faldami A, Tsiklakis K. Comparison of 2 regenerative procedures–guided tissue regeneration and demineralized freeze-dried bone allograft–in the treatment of intrabony defects: a clinical and radiographic study. Journal of periodontology. 1998;69(7): 751–8.

17 Reynolds MA, Bowers GM. Fate of demineralized freeze-dried bone allografts in human intrabony defects. Journal of periodontology. 1996;67(2): 150–7.

18 Hanna R, Trejo PM, Weltman RL. Treatment of intrabony defects with bovine-derived xenograft alone and in combination with platelet-rich plasma: a randomized clinical trial. Journal of periodontology. 2004;75(12):1668–77.

19 Hutchens LH, Jr. The use of a bovine bone mineral in periodontal osseous defects: case reports. Compendium of continuing education in dentistry (Jamesburg, NJ: 1995). 1999;20(4):365-8, 70, 72–4 passim; quiz 78.

20 Nevins ML, Camelo M, Rebaudi A, Lynch SE, Nevins M. Three-dimensional micro-computed tomographic evaluation of periodontal regeneration: a human report of intrabony defects treated with Bio-Oss collagen. The International journal of periodontics & restorative dentistry. 2005;25(4):365–73.

21 Richardson CR, Mellonig JT, Brunsvold MA, McDonnell HT, Cochran DL. Clinical evaluation of Bio-Oss: a bovine-derived xenograft for the treatment of periodontal osseous defects in humans. J Clin Periodontol. 1999;26(7): 421–8.

22 Scheyer ET, Velasquez-Plata D, Brunsvold MA, Lasho DJ, Mellonig JT. A clinical comparison of a bovine-derived xenograft used alone and in combination with enamel matrix derivative for the treatment of periodontal osseous defects in humans. Journal of periodontology. 2002;73(4):423–32.

23 Kumar PG, Kumar JA, Anumala N, Reddy KP, Avula H, Hussain SN. Volumetric analysis of intrabony defects in aggressive periodontitis patients following use of a novel composite alloplast: a pilot study. Quintessence international (Berlin, Germany: 1985). 2011;42(5):375–84.

24 Ong MM, Eber RM, Korsnes MI, MacNeil RL, Glickman GN, Shyr Y, et al. Evaluation of a bioactive glass alloplast in treating periodontal intrabony defects. Journal of periodontology. 1998;69(12): 1346–54.

25 Subbaiah R, Thomas B. Efficacy of a bioactive alloplast, in the treatment of human periodontal osseous defects-a clinical study. Medicina oral, patologia oral y cirugia bucal. 2011;16(2):e239–e44.

26 Gera I, Dori F, Keglevich T, Anton S, Szilagyi E, Windisch P. [Experience with the clinical use of beta-tri-calcium phosphate (Cerasorb) as a bone replacement graft material in human periodontal osseous defects]. Fogorvosi szemle. 2002;95(4):143–7.

27 Grover V, Kapoor A, Malhotra R, Uppal RS. Evaluation of the efficacy of a bioactive synthetic graft material in the treatment of intrabony periodontal defects. Journal of Indian Society of Periodontology. 2013;17(1):104–10.

28 Saffar JL, Colombier ML, Detienville R. Bone formation in tricalcium phosphate-filled periodontal intrabony lesions. Histological observations in humans. Journal of periodontology. 1990;61(4):209–16.

29 Singh VP, Nayak DG, Uppoor AS, Shah D. Clinical and radiographic evaluation of Nano-crystalline hydroxyapatite bone graft (Sybograf) in combination with bioresorbable collagen membrane (Periocol) in periodontal intrabony defects. Dental research journal. 2012; 9(1):60–7.

30 Gestrelius S, Andersson C, Johansson AC, Persson E, Brodin A, Rydhag L, et al. Formulation of enamel matrix derivative for surface coating. Kinetics and cell colonization. J Clin Periodontol. 1997; 24(9 Pt 2):678–84.

31 Gestrelius S, Andersson C, Lidstrom D, Hammarstrom L, Somerman M. In vitro studies on periodontal ligament cells and enamel matrix derivative. J Clin Periodontol. 1997;24(9 Pt 2):685–92.

32 Heijl L. Periodontal regeneration with enamel matrix derivative in one human experimental defect. A case report. J Clin Periodontol. 1997;24(9 Pt 2):693–6.

33 Heijl L, Heden G, Svardstrom G, Ostgren A. Enamel matrix derivative (EMDOGAIN) in the treatment of intrabony periodontal defects. J Clin Periodontol. 1997;24(9 Pt 2):705–14.

34 Zetterstrom O, Andersson C, Eriksson L, Fredriksson A, Friskopp J, Heden G, et al. Clinical safety of enamel matrix derivative (EMDOGAIN) in the treatment of periodontal defects. J Clin Periodontol. 1997;24(9 Pt 2):697–704.

35 Steed DL, Donohoe D, Webster MW, Lindsley L. Effect of extensive debridement and treatment on the healing of diabetic foot ulcers. Diabetic Ulcer Study Group. J Am Coll Surg. 1996; 183(1):61–4.

36 Wieman TJ, Smiell JM, Su Y. Efficacy and safety of a topical gel formulation of recombinant human platelet-derived growth factor-BB (becaplermin) in patients with chronic neuropathic diabetic ulcers. A phase III randomized placebo-controlled double-blind study. Diabetes Care. 1998;21(5):822–7.

37 Ronnstrand L, Heldin CH. Mechanisms of platelet-derived growth factor-induced chemotaxis. Int J Cancer. 2001;91(6): 757–62.

38 Nevins M, Camelo M, Nevins ML, Schenk RK, Lynch SE. Periodontal regeneration in humans using recombinant human platelet-derived growth factor-BB (rhPDGF-BB) and allogenic bone. Journal of periodontology. 2003;74(9):1282–92.

39 Camelo M, Nevins ML, Schenk RK, Lynch SE, Nevins M. Periodontal regeneration in human Class II furcations using purified recombinant human platelet-derived growth factor-BB (rhPDGF-BB) with bone allograft. Int J Periodontics Restorative Dent. 2003;23(3):213–25.

40 Rosen PS, Toscano N, Holzclaw D, Reynolds MA. A retrospective consecutive case series using mineralized

allograft combined with recombinant human platelet-derived growth factor BB to treat moderate to severe osseous lesions. The International journal of periodontics & restorative dentistry. 2011; 31(4):335–42.

41 Khoshkam V, Chan HL, Lin GH, Mailoa J, Giannobile WV, Wang HL, et al. Outcomes of Regenerative Treatment with rhPDGF-BB and rhFGF-2 for Periodontal Intrabony Defects: A Systematic Review and Meta-analysis. J Clin Periodontol. 2015.

42 Nevins M, Hanratty J, Lynch SE. Clinical results using recombinant human platelet-derived growth factor and mineralized freeze-dried bone allograft in periodontal defects. The International journal of periodontics & restorative dentistry. 2007;27(5):421–7.

43 Nevins M, Nevins ML, Karimbux N, Kim SW, Schupbach P, Kim DM. The combination of purified recombinant human platelet-derived growth factor-BB and equine particulate bone graft for periodontal regeneration. Journal of periodontology. 2012;83(5):565–73.

44 McGuire MK, Kao RT, Nevins M, Lynch SE. rhPDGF-BB promotes healing of periodontal defects: 24-month clinical and radiographic observations. The International journal of periodontics & restorative dentistry. 2006;26(3):223–31.

45 McGuire MK, Scheyer ET, Schupbach P. Growth factor-mediated treatment of recession defects: a randomized controlled trial and histologic and microcomputed tomography examination. Journal of periodontology. 2009;80(4):550–64.

46 McGuire MK, Scheyer T, Nevins M, Schupbach P. Evaluation of human recession defects treated with coronally advanced flaps and either purified recombinant human platelet-derived growth factor-BB with beta tricalcium phosphate or connective tissue: a histologic and microcomputed tomographic examination. The International journal of periodontics & restorative dentistry. 2009;29(1):7–21.

47 Nevins M, Kao RT, McGuire MK, McClain PK, Hinrichs JE, McAllister BS, et al. Platelet-derived growth factor promotes periodontal regeneration in localized osseous defects: 36-month extension results from a randomized, controlled, double-masked clinical trial. Journal of periodontology. 2013;84(4): 456–64.

48 Rosen PS. Using recombinant platelet-derived growth factor to facilitate wound healing. Compendium of continuing education in dentistry (Jamesburg, NJ: 1995). 2006;27(9): 520–5.

49 Boyapati L, Wang H-L. The role of platelet-rich plasma in sinus augmentation: a critical review. Implant dentistry. 2006;15(2):160–70.

50 Marx RE. Platelet-rich plasma (PRP): what is PRP and what is not PRP? Implant dentistry. 2001;10(4):225–8.

51 Marx RE. Platelet-rich plasma: evidence to support its use. Journal of oral and maxillofacial surgery: official journal of the American Association of Oral and Maxillofacial Surgeons. 2004;62(4): 489–96.

52 Marx RE, Carlson ER, Eichstaedt RM, Schimmele SR, Strauss JE, Georgeff KR. Platelet-rich plasma: Growth factor enhancement for bone grafts. Oral surgery, oral medicine, oral pathology, oral radiology, and endodontics. 1998; 85(6):638–46.

53 Gupta G. Clinical and radiographic evaluation of intra-bony defects in localized aggressive periodontitis patients with platelet rich plasma/hydroxyapatite graft: A comparative controlled clinical trial. Contemporary clinical dentistry. 2014;5(4):445–51.

54 Agarwal A, Gupta ND. Platelet-rich plasma combined with decalcified freeze-dried bone allograft for the treatment of noncontained human intrabony periodontal defects: a

randomized controlled split-mouth study. The International journal of periodontics & restorative dentistry. 2014;34(5): 705–11.

55 Ozdemir B, Okte E. Treatment of intrabony defects with beta-tricalciumphosphate alone and in combination with platelet-rich plasma. Journal of biomedical materials research Part B, Applied biomaterials. 2012;100(4): 976–83.

56 Hassan KS, Alagl AS, Abdel-Hady A. Torus mandibularis bone chips combined with platelet rich plasma gel for treatment of intrabony osseous defects: clinical and radiographic evaluation. International journal of oral and maxillofacial surgery. 2012;41(12):1519–26.

57 Kaushick BT, Jayakumar ND, Padmalatha O, Varghese S. Treatment of human periodontal infrabony defects with hydroxyapatite + beta tricalcium phosphate bone graft alone and in combination with platelet rich plasma: a randomized clinical trial. Indian journal of dental research: official publication of Indian Society for Dental Research. 2011;22(4):505–10.

58 Saini N, Sikri P, Gupta H. Evaluation of the relative efficacy of autologous platelet-rich plasma in combination with beta-tricalcium phosphate alloplast versus an alloplast alone in the treatment of human periodontal infrabony defects: a clinical and radiological study. Indian journal of dental research: official publication of Indian Society for Dental Research. 2011;22(1):107–15.

59 Parimala M, Mehta DS. Comparative evaluation of bovine porous bone mineral. Journal of Indian Society of Periodontology. 2010;14(2):126–31.

60 Dori F, Kovacs V, Arweiler NB, Huszar T, Gera I, Nikolidakis D, et al. Effect of platelet-rich plasma on the healing of intrabony defects treated with an anorganic bovine bone mineral: a pilot study. Journal of periodontology. 2009; 80(10):1599–605.

61 Harnack L, Boedeker RH, Kurtulus I, Boehm S, Gonzales J, Meyle J. Use of platelet-rich plasma in periodontal surgery–a prospective randomised double blind clinical trial. Clinical oral investigations. 2009;13(2):179–87.

62 Dori F, Nikolidakis D, Huszar T, Arweiler NB, Gera I, Sculean A. Effect of platelet-rich plasma on the healing of intrabony defects treated with an enamel matrix protein derivative and a natural bone mineral. J Clin Periodontol. 2008; 35(1):44–50.

63 Piemontese M, Aspriello SD, Rubini C, Ferrante L, Procaccini M. Treatment of periodontal intrabony defects with demineralized freeze-dried bone allograft in combination with platelet-rich plasma: a comparative clinical trial. Journal of periodontology. 2008;79(5):802–10.

64 Yassibag-Berkman Z, Tuncer O, Subasioglu T, Kantarci A. Combined use of platelet-rich plasma and bone grafting with or without guided tissue regeneration in the treatment of anterior interproximal defects. Journal of periodontology. 2007;78(5):801–9.

65 Demir B, Sengun D, Berberoglu A. Clinical evaluation of platelet-rich plasma and bioactive glass in the treatment of intra-bony defects. J Clin Periodontol. 2007;34(8):709–15.

66 Ouyang XY, Qiao J. Effect of platelet-rich plasma in the treatment of periodontal intrabony defects in humans. Chinese medical journal. 2006;119(18): 1511–21.

67 Okuda K, Tai H, Tanabe K, Suzuki H, Sato T, Kawase T, et al. Platelet-rich plasma combined with a porous hydroxyapatite graft for the treatment of intrabony periodontal defects in humans: a comparative controlled clinical study. Journal of periodontology. 2005;76(6): 890–8.

68 Choukroun J, Adda F, Schoeffler C, Vervelle A. Une opportunité en paro-implantologie: le PRF. Implantodontie. 2001;42(55):e62.

69 Toffler M, Toscano N, Holtzclaw D, Corso M, Dohan D. Introducing Choukroun's platelet rich fibrin (PRF) to the reconstructive surgery milieu. J Implant Adv Clin Dent. 2009;1:22–31.
70 Kobayashi E, Fluckiger L, Fujioka-Kobayashi M, Sawada K, Sculean A, Schaller B, et al. Comparative release of growth factors from PRP, PRF, and advanced-PRF. Clinical oral investigations. 2016.
71 Clark RA. Fibrin and wound healing. Annals of the New York Academy of Sciences. 2001;936:355–67.
72 Choukroun J, Diss A, Simonpieri A, Girard MO, Schoeffler C, Dohan SL, et al. Platelet-rich fibrin (PRF): a second-generation platelet concentrate. Part IV: clinical effects on tissue healing. Oral surgery, oral medicine, oral pathology, oral radiology, and endodontics. 2006;101(3):e56–e60.
73 Agarwal A, Gupta ND, Jain A. Platelet rich fibrin combined with decalcified freeze-dried bone allograft for the treatment of human intrabony periodontal defects: a randomized split mouth clinical trail. Acta odontologica Scandinavica. 2016;74(1):36–43.
74 Ajwani H, Shetty S, Gopalakrishnan D, Kathariya R, Kulloli A, Dolas RS, et al. Comparative evaluation of platelet-rich fibrin biomaterial and open flap debridement in the treatment of two and three wall intrabony defects. Journal of international oral health: JIOH. 2015;7(4): 32–7.
75 Elgendy EA, Abo Shady TE. Clinical and radiographic evaluation of nanocrystalline hydroxyapatite with or without platelet-rich fibrin membrane in the treatment of periodontal intrabony defects. Journal of Indian Society of Periodontology. 2015;19(1):61–5.
76 Joseph VR, Sam G, Amol NV. Clinical evaluation of autologous platelet rich fibrin in horizontal alveolar bony defects. Journal of clinical and diagnostic research: JCDR. 2014;8(11):Zc43–7.
77 Panda S, Sankari M, Satpathy A, Jayakumar D, Mozzati M, Mortellaro C, et al. Adjunctive Effect of Autologus Platelet-Rich Fibrin to Barrier Membrane in the Treatment of Periodontal Intrabony Defects. The Journal of craniofacial surgery. 2016;27(3):691–6.
78 Pradeep AR, Nagpal K, Karvekar S, Patnaik K, Naik SB, Guruprasad CN. Platelet-rich fibrin with 1% metformin for the treatment of intrabony defects in chronic periodontitis: a randomized controlled clinical trial. Journal of periodontology. 2015;86(6):729–37.
79 Pradeep AR, Rao NS, Agarwal E, Bajaj P, Kumari M, Naik SB. Comparative evaluation of autologous platelet-rich fibrin and platelet-rich plasma in the treatment of 3-wall intrabony defects in chronic periodontitis: a randomized controlled clinical trial. J Periodontol. 2012;83(12):1499–507.
80 Shah M, Patel J, Dave D, Shah S. Comparative evaluation of platelet-rich fibrin with demineralized freeze-dried bone allograft in periodontal infrabony defects: A randomized controlled clinical study. Journal of Indian Society of Periodontology. 2015;19(1):56–60.
81 Thorat M, Pradeep AR, Pallavi B. Clinical effect of autologous platelet-rich fibrin in the treatment of intra-bony defects: a controlled clinical trial. J Clin Periodontol. 2011;38(10):925–32.
82 Pradeep AR, Bajaj P, Rao NS, Agarwal E, Naik SB. Platelet-Rich Fibrin Combined With a Porous Hydroxyapatite Graft for the Treatment of Three-Wall Intrabony Defects in Chronic Periodontitis: A Randomized Controlled Clinical Trial. J Periodontol. 2012.
83 Sharma A, Pradeep AR. Treatment of 3-wall intrabony defects in patients with chronic periodontitis with autologous platelet-rich fibrin: a randomized controlled clinical trial. Journal of periodontology. 2011;82(12):1705–12.
84 Aydemir Turkal H, Demirer S, Dolgun A, Keceli HG. Evaluation of the adjunctive

effect of platelet-rich fibrin to enamel matrix derivative in the treatment of intrabony defects. Six-month results of a randomized, split-mouth, controlled clinical study. Journal of clinical periodontology. 2016;43(11):955–64.

85 Chadwick JK, Mills MP, Mealey BL. Clinical and Radiographic Evaluation of Demineralized Freeze-Dried Bone Allograft Versus Platelet-Rich Fibrin for the Treatment of Periodontal Intrabony Defects in Humans. Journal of periodontology. 2016;87(11):1253–60.

86 Chandradas ND, Ravindra S, Rangaraju VM, Jain S, Dasappa S. Efficacy of platelet rich fibrin in the treatment of human intrabony defects with or without bone graft: A randomized controlled trial. Journal of International Society of Preventive & Community Dentistry. 2016;6(Suppl 2):S153–S9.

87 Chatterjee A, Pradeep AR, Garg V, Yajamanya S, Ali MM, Priya VS. Treatment of periodontal intrabony defects using autologous platelet-rich fibrin and titanium platelet-rich fibrin: a randomized, clinical, comparative study. Journal of investigative and clinical dentistry. 2016.

88 Martande SS, Kumari M, Pradeep AR, Singh SP, Suke DK, Guruprasad CN. Platelet-Rich Fibrin Combined With 1.2% Atorvastatin for Treatment of Intrabony Defects in Chronic Periodontitis: A Randomized Controlled Clinical Trial. Journal of periodontology. 2016;87(9): 1039–46.

89 Pradeep AR, Garg V, Kanoriya D, Singhal S. Platelet-Rich Fibrin With 1.2% Rosuvastatin for Treatment of Intrabony Defects in Chronic Periodontitis: A Randomized Controlled Clinical Trial. Journal of periodontology. 2016;87(12): 1468–73.

90 Sharma A, Pradeep AR. Autologous platelet-rich fibrin in the treatment of mandibular degree II furcation defects: a randomized clinical trial. Journal of periodontology. 2011;82(10):1396–403.

91 Bajaj P, Pradeep AR, Agarwal E, Rao NS, Naik SB, Priyanka N, et al. Comparative evaluation of autologous platelet-rich fibrin and platelet-rich plasma in the treatment of mandibular degree II furcation defects: a randomized controlled clinical trial. Journal of periodontal research. 2013.

92 Pradeep AR, Karvekar S, Nagpal K, Patnaik K, Raju A, Singh P. Rosuvastatin 1.2 mg In Situ Gel Combined With 1:1 Mixture of Autologous Platelet-Rich Fibrin and Porous Hydroxyapatite Bone Graft in Surgical Treatment of Mandibular Class II Furcation Defects: A Randomized Clinical Control Trial. Journal of periodontology. 2016;87(1): 5–13.

93 Kanoriya DD, Pradeep DA, Garg DV, Singhal DS. Mandibular Degree II Furcation Defects Treatment With Platelet Rich Fibrin and 1% Alendronate Gel Combination: A Randomized Controlled Clinical Trial. Journal of periodontology. 2016:1–13.

94 Wang HL, Boyapati L. “PASS” principles for predictable bone regeneration. Implant dentistry. 2006;15(1):8–17.

95 Roy S, Driggs J, Elgharably H, Biswas S, Findley M, Khanna S, et al. Platelet-rich fibrin matrix improves wound angiogenesis via inducing endothelial cell proliferation. Wound repair and regeneration: official publication of the Wound Healing Society [and] the European Tissue Repair Society. 2011; 19(6):753–66.

96 Chen FM, Wu LA, Zhang M, Zhang R, Sun HH. Homing of endogenous stem/progenitor cells for in situ tissue regeneration: Promises, strategies, and translational perspectives. Biomaterials. 2011;32(12):3189–209.

97 White AP, Vaccaro AR, Hall JA, Whang PG, Friel BC, McKee MD. Clinical applications of BMP-7/OP-1 in fractures, nonunions and spinal fusion. International orthopaedics. 2007;31(6): 735–41.

98 Miron RJ, Zhang YF. Osteoinduction: a review of old concepts with new standards. Journal of dental research. 2012;91(8):736–44.

99 Young CS, Ladd PA, Browning CF, Thompson A, Bonomo J, Shockley K, et al. Release, biological potency, and biochemical integrity of recombinant human platelet-derived growth factor-BB (rhPDGF-BB) combined with Augment(TM) Bone Graft or GEM 21S beta-tricalcium phosphate (beta-TCP). Journal of controlled release: official journal of the Controlled Release Society. 2009;140(3):250–5.

100 Park YJ, Lee YM, Lee JY, Seol YJ, Chung CP, Lee SJ. Controlled release of platelet-derived growth factor-BB from chondroitin sulfate-chitosan sponge for guided bone regeneration. J Control Release. 2000;67(2-3):385–94.

101 Wissink MJ, Beernink R, Poot AA, Engbers GH, Beugeling T, van Aken WG, et al. Improved endothelialization of vascular grafts by local release of growth factor from heparinized collagen matrices. J Control Release. 2000;64(1-3):103–14.

102 Delgado JJ, Evora C, Sanchez E, Baro M, Delgado A. Validation of a method for non-invasive in vivo measurement of growth factor release from a local delivery system in bone. J Control Release. 2006; 114(2):223–9.

103 Oe S, Fukunaka Y, Hirose T, Yamaoka Y, Tabata Y. A trial on regeneration therapy of rat liver cirrhosis by controlled release of hepatocyte growth factor. J Control Release. 2003;88(2):193–200.

104 Miron RJ, Fujioka-Kobayashi M, Bishara M, Zhang Y, Hernandez M, Choukroun J. Platelet-Rich Fibrin and Soft Tissue Wound Healing: A Systematic Review. Tissue engineering Part B, Reviews. 2016.

105 Hoaglin DR, Lines GK. Prevention of localized osteitis in mandibular third-molar sites using platelet-rich fibrin. International journal of dentistry. 2013; 2013:875380.

106 Sculean A, Aoki A, Romanos G, Schwarz F, Miron RJ, Cosgarea R. Is Photodynamic Therapy an Effective Treatment for Periodontal and Peri-Implant Infections? Dental clinics of North America. 2015; 59(4):831–58.

10

Platelet Rich Fibrin as an Adjunct to Implant Dentistry

Howard Gluckman

Abstract

Dental implants have gradually become the standard of care for the treatment of missing teeth. Today the potential for osseointegration is no longer considered a question, but rather a certainty in implant dentistry. As with all successful techniques, the focus has now shifted to the finer details of treatment protocols and techniques. In recent years, the speed and quality of osseointegration and interventions to improve the bone type to enhance primary stability has received much attention. This, in turn, has shortened the time to implant loading as well as the ability to achieve desired treatment goals. Other critical issues now include the long-term aesthetic stability, which is affected by the periodontal biotype, the quantity and quality of bone supporting the implant, the soft tissue surrounding the implant, and its restoration among others. Consequently, the issue of maintenance of these supporting tissues is now known to be critical for the long-term health and stability of the implant.

Implant placement has, therefore, many factors to consider, as has been highlighted throughout this textbook. However, this chapter on implant dentistry would be remiss without mentioning the importance of bone and soft tissues surrounding the implant for long-term success. Today, the symbiotic relationship between bone and soft tissue to maintain the integrity of the implant is increasingly being understood. Past and current trends have focused on bone and its augmentation as keys to implant success, however, it is the symbiotic relationship between the bone and soft tissue that maintains long-term health and aesthetics. The bone supports the soft tissue and in return the soft tissue reinforces bone stability. For this reason, it is essential to ensure that implant sites are developed appropriately to ensure optimum bone and soft tissues. The focus of this chapter, therefore, deals with the issues of tissue healing around implants, with a focus on bone healing during osseointegration as well as soft-tissue enhancement around implants with PRF to favor faster treatment protocols and contribute to their long-term maintenance.

Highlights

- An overview of the reported clinical scenarios that apply PRF during implant placement
- Maintainenance of peri-implant crestal bone following integration and loading: PRF and soft tissue
- Osseointegration with emphasis on how growth factors affect the integration process
- Techniques to increase primary stability in poor bone quality
- The future of PRF at implant sites

Platelet Rich Fibrin in Regenerative Dentistry: Biological Background and Clinical Indications, First Edition.
Edited by Richard J. Miron and Joseph Choukroun.

10.1 Introduction

It is well understood that tooth loss leads to a reduction in ridge tissue and the most obvious benefit of PRF as a biomaterial is that it may accelerate growth and healing during the augmentation and reconstruction of those sites [1]. One of the first instances where the clinician may use PRF is within extraction sockets to limit dimensional changes post-extraction, presumably with the intention of later placing implants. The chapter by Miron and Du Toit addresses the topic of socket management with PRF in detail. To follow thereon, the topic of utilizing PRF at placed implants is covered within this chapter. As such, the clinician may have numerous questions in this regard: can I or should I use PRF when I place implants? What are the benefits? When or how should I use PRF? Unfortunately to date the literature can only in part contribute to answering these. What is certain is that the loss of ridge architecture following tooth extraction often demands augmentation to provide adequate, healthy hard and soft tissue to accommodate the future implant [2,3]. The literature is abundant with sound data that prescribes to the clinician the parameters needed—the quantity of healthy bone and soft tissue [4,5]. Indeed, numerous authors have reported on combining PRF with augmentation materials at implant sites [6,7]. The distinction is again made that pre-implant site development is not addressed in this chapter and rather its use with implants is the focus.

A second distinction can also be made between PRF's contribution to hard-tissue healing and soft-tissue healing. To address the latter, it may be noted that the critical importance of soft-tissue quality and volume at implants is a more recent focus of attention [4,8,9]. Sufficient, stable bone is key to the long-term success of implants and the difficulty in predictably regenerating this bone when lost remains a major challenge [2]. It has been shown that a minimum of 2 to 4 mm of bone around the implant is essential to maintain stability of the soft tissue. Vice versa, it is essential that a minimum of 2 to 3 mm of attached soft-tissue thickness in both the vertical and horizontal dimension be present to protect bone from resorption [4,5]. Far too often, one or the other of these components is neglected which leads to potential long-term breakdown [10–12]. As such, the clinician may seek to better understand what effects PRF may provide, not only during osseointegration but also for the healing of soft and hard tissues during implant placement.

Hereafter the topic of PRF's use with dental implants is explored, describing the contributions of this material's growth promoting factors that may contribute to the success and performance of these biomedical devices. Its use during implant placement may include the treatment of peri-implant defects, osseointegration, and soft-tissue healing at implant sites.

10.2 PRF treatment of peri-implant defects

The two peri-implant defect types receiving the most attention is coronal bone loss seen in peri-implantitis and the buccal gap at immediate implant placement. It is widely known that immediate implant placement dictates a more palatal or lingual approach and a deeper placement to establish primary stability. The so-called buccal gap is observed as the implant is placed away from the buccal plate (Figure 10.1) [5]. The literature reports on a variety of approaches to manage this gap; although no intervention other than allowing a whole blood clot to organize into bone, or grafting this space with an assortment of materials [5,13,14]. It is apparent that PRF may contribute its leukocyte cytokines and growth factors to this process that may have a positive influence on the healing of this bony defect (Figure 10.2). Lee and coworkers created buccal gap defects during implant placement to experimentally simulate this in an animal model [15]. Positive results were demonstrated with an increase

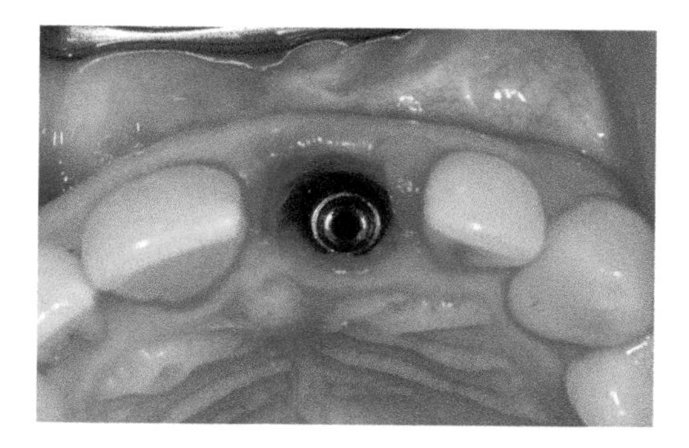

Figure 10.1 Implant placement slightly lingually; a buccal gap is created between the implant surface and the buccal bone wall.

in bone volume in the defect area and in the interthread spaces when augmented with PRF. Additional studies have also shown that PRF alone or with particulate bone material in non-infective peri-implant defects showed high bone to implant contact (BIC) of 61% and 73% respectively [16,17]. As such the literature seems to support the use of PRF as beneficial during the filling within this buccal gap during immediate placement, or in combination with a bone biomaterial.

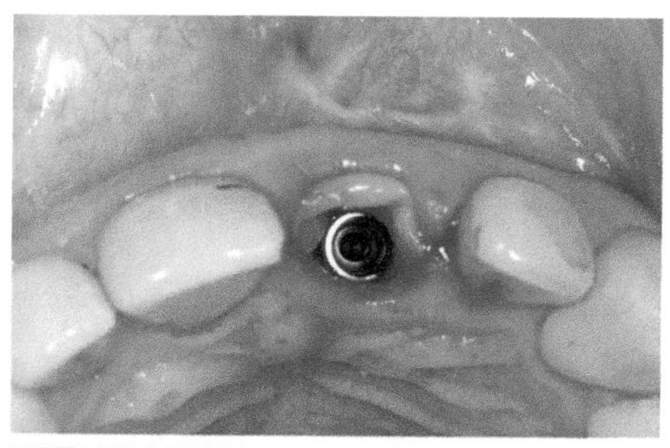

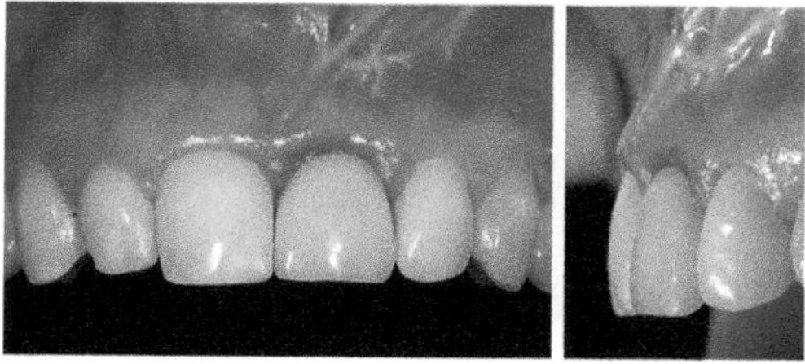

Figure 10.2 The buccal gap filled with PRF.

Contrary to the augmentation of the buccal gap, treating peri-implant defects as a result of peri-implantitis is far more complex [18]. This topic remains largely unresolved and its exact etiology with reliable treatment options is poorly understood [19]. That said, various reports have now investigated the use of PRF in human studies [20]. In such a study, the implants had full thickness flaps raised and decontaminated. The experimental group additionally utilized PRF placed within the bone defect before the flap was closed. When healing occurred with PRF, a minor difference in probing depth reduction was seen [20]. Furthermore, clinical attachment levels seemed to benefit and an increase in keratinized mucosa was reported. These results suggest that PRF may be beneficial for the treatment of peri-implantitis defects; however, much further research remains necessary to validate these preliminary findings. Again, the clinician should be aware that the treatment of peri-implantitis is at present unpredictable, with great variations in bone defects and diverse responses to treatment [21].

10.3 PRF and soft-tissue healing at implants

It has been shown that thick soft tissue favors coronal peri-implant bone stability [4,5,8]. As mentioned previously, a symbiosis relationship between bone and soft tissue is necessary to maintain the stability and integrity of the implant. Bone and its augmentation in numerous reconstruction techniques traditionally has been a keen topic in implant dentistry [2]. Current understanding now stresses the importance of bone to maintain the soft tissue and the soft tissue to reinforce bone stability. The lack of adequate soft- and hard-tissue development could be one of the reasons why high levels of peri-implantitis is observed in the current literature [22]. This raises the question, "could PRF contribute to soft-tissue healing and augmentation when placed within soft-tissue flaps raised during

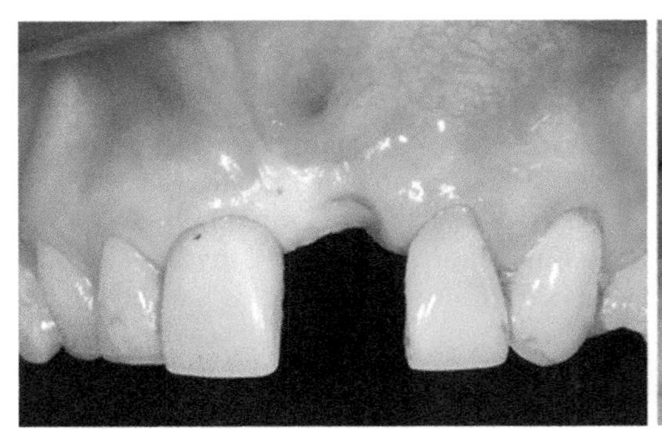

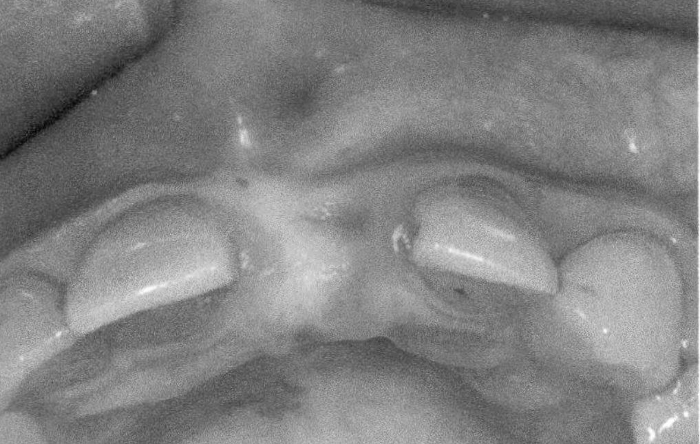

Figure 10.3 Case presentation with a missing central incisor. Lack of facial-lingual thickness.

implant placement?" The concept certainly seems biologically plausible by locally applying an autogenous biomaterial rich in growth factors that stimulate neoangiogenesis and collagen formation within the soft-tissue flap atop an implant (Figures 10.3–10.9). Moreover, PRF when compressed into membranes can maintain the integrity of an augmentation procedure, enhancing site protection when used in conjunction with other barrier membranes, and contributing to the healing of the overlying flap [23,24].

While to date, approximately 164 publications across the health sciences have reported on PRF and its effect on soft-tissue regeneration and healing, only one study has reported on PRF and soft-tissue healing at placed implants [24]. Hehn and coworkers had experimented with the insertion of PRF within a split flap at implant placement and reported this to reduce soft-tissue thickness [25]. These findings here suggest that splitting the flap may unnecessarily strains the soft-tissue healing in addition to a full mucoperiosteal flap raised for implant insertion. An ideal procedure would be to place the PRF beneath the flap without additionally dividing the tissue. Chapter 2 on the biological background of PRF may further

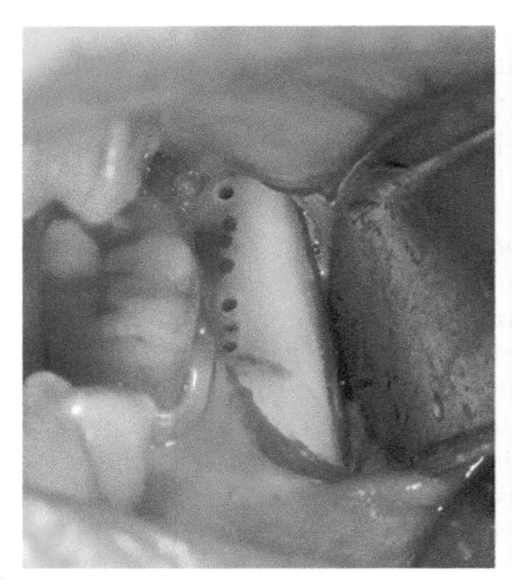

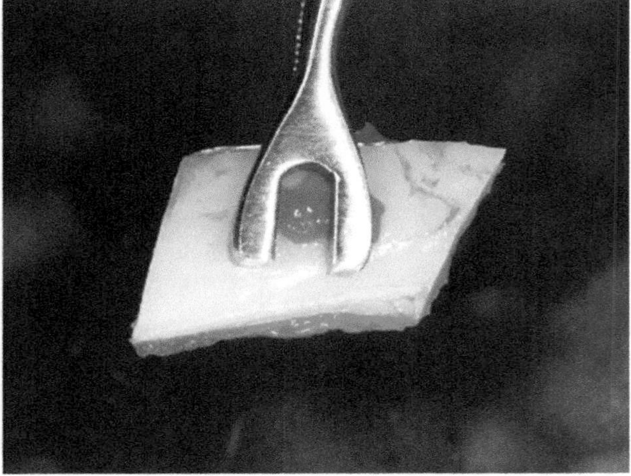

Figure 10.4 Autogenous bone block harvested from the lower ramus to be utilized in the case presented in Figure 10.3.

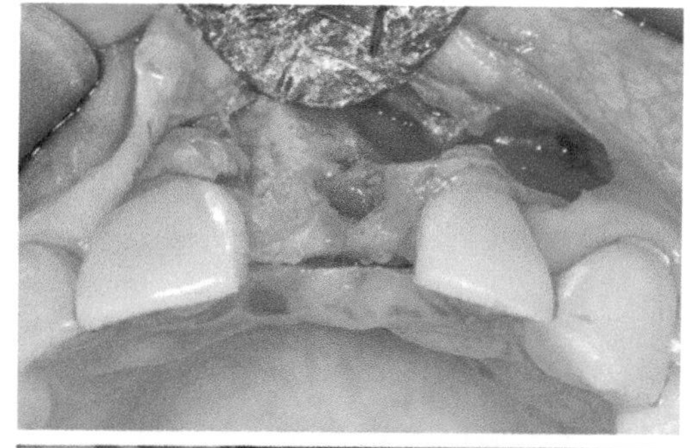

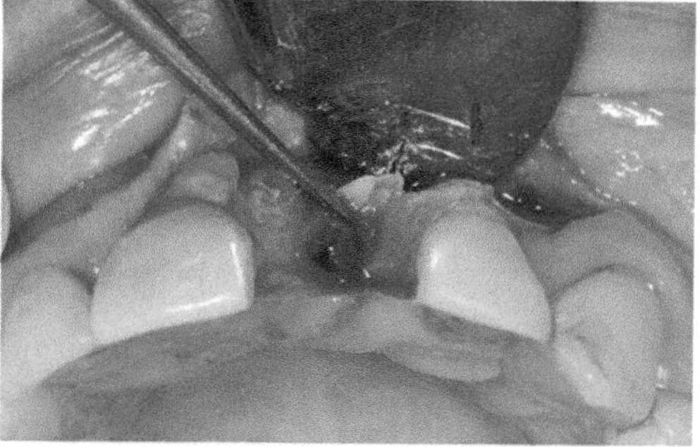

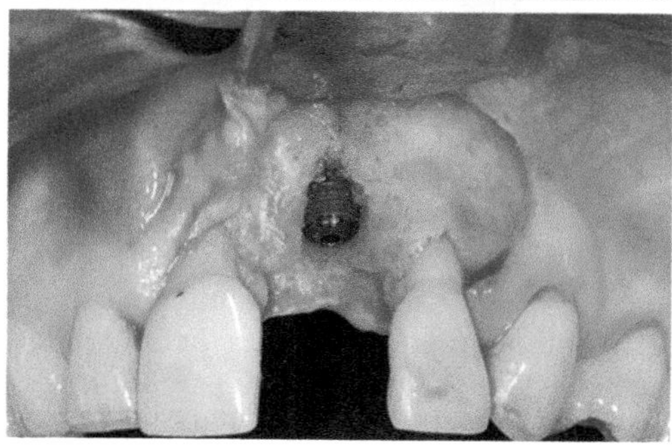

Figure 10.5 Implant placement in the esthetic zone utilizing a bone-level implant.

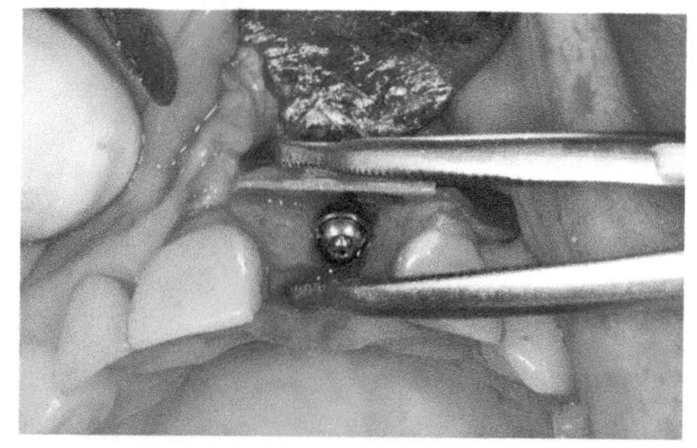

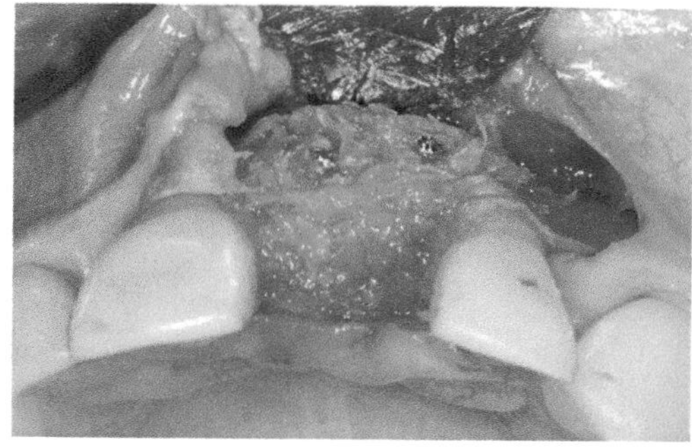

Figure 10.6 Contour augmentation in the esthetic zone utilizing an autogenous bone block filled with particulate bone graft.

shed light on the topic of soft-tissue healing with PRF.

10.4 Osseointegration

The term osseointegration was introduced by Brånemark following his work in the early 1950s, and at first was considered a "functional ankylosis," but was further revised as "a direct structural and functional connection between ordered, living bone and the surface of a load-bearing implant"[26]. In essence, the placement of a biologically inert material such as titanium or zirconium will lead to the apposition of bone around the implant, which is strong enough to withstand the forces of occlusion. This demonstrates the normal physiology of bone in function with both deposition and resorption with respect to the load of the implant following integration. The phases of osseointegration are synonymous with routine inflammation and wound healing seen in traumatic bone injury [27]. Trauma by the osteotomy drill cuts and orderly fractures bone, and ruptures its supplying blood vessels in the process. This surgical intervention initiates a cascade of complex but orderly wound healing events, highlighted by hemostasis, inflammation, proliferation, and tissue maturation [28].

The implant osteotomy fills with blood that coats the implant as it is inserted [29]. Initially, its support is derived entirely from friction with the bone, and is defined as primary stability. Later, secondary stability is derived

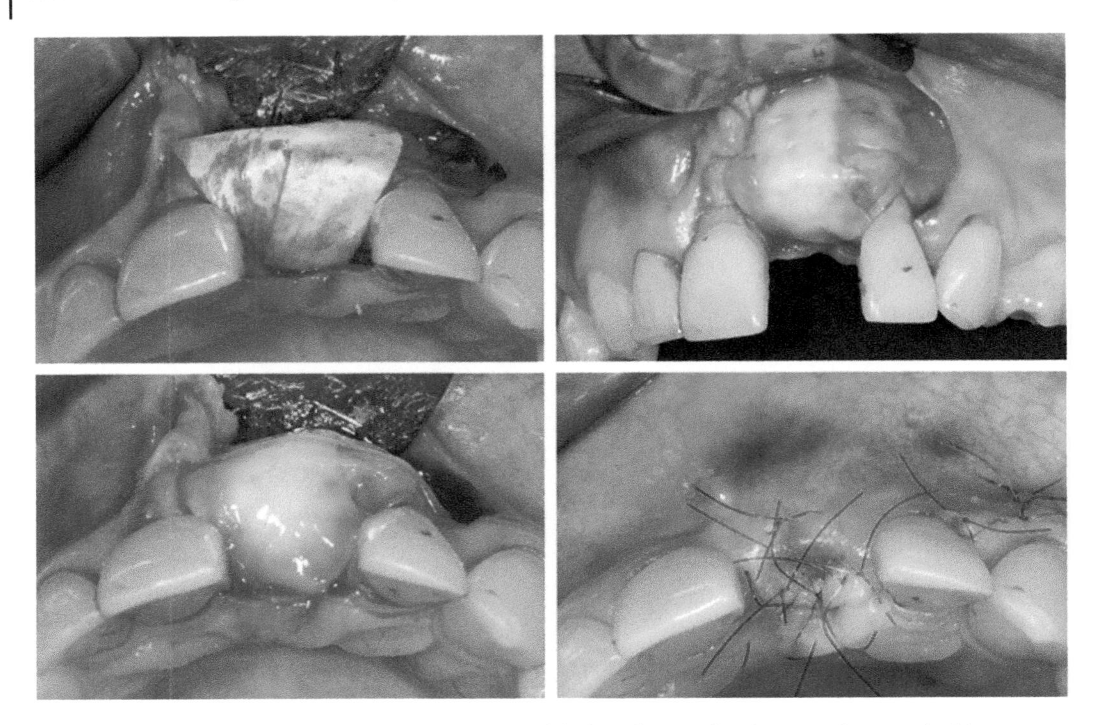

Figure 10.7 Defect augmented with autogenous bone block and particulate bone graft covered with a collagen barrier membrane and several layers of PRF membranes.

as the blood and cellular products produce healing that apposes newly formed bone on the implant surface. Following insertion, platelets are activated and aggregate, forming a clot that seals the ruptured vessels at the osteotomy [29,30]. The platelets degranulate and release a variety of growth factors and cytokines that stimulate perivascular cells during neoangiogenesis [30]. Thereafter, activated fibrin within the forming clot provides a provisional matrix within the wound microspaces surrounding the implant surface [29,30]. Inflammatory cells are then recruited from the vessels and into the wound to participate in clearing debris. This ingress of leukocytes also contributes to the overall increase in release of inflammatory cytokines that recruit future cells, kill bacteria, clean the wound, and promote healing. The inflammatory cytokines recruit macrophages that migrate to the area to remove tissue debris and mediate the inflammatory process [30]. Macrophages also secrete growth factors that recruit fibroblasts to synthesize collagen to reinforce the wound matrix [30]. Osteoclasts initially resorb the microscopic fractured bone, and in turn release growth factors from bone that stimulate osteoblasts. The perivascular cells also migrate to the healing bone and implant surface and differentiate into osteoblasts [29,30]. These cells then produce a matrix that mineralizes, producing

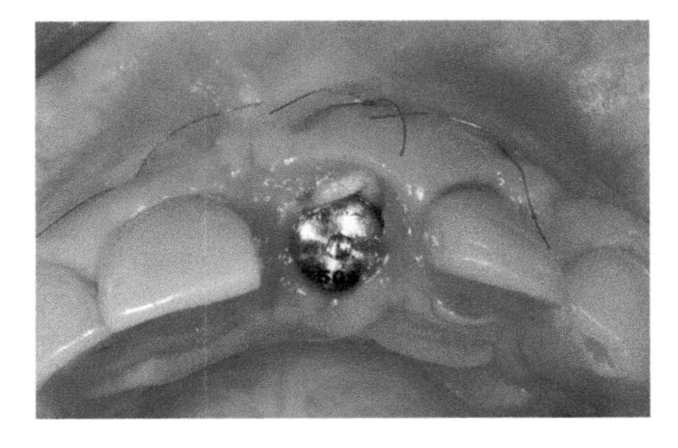

Figure 10.8 PRF membrane utilized on the buccal surface of the abutment.

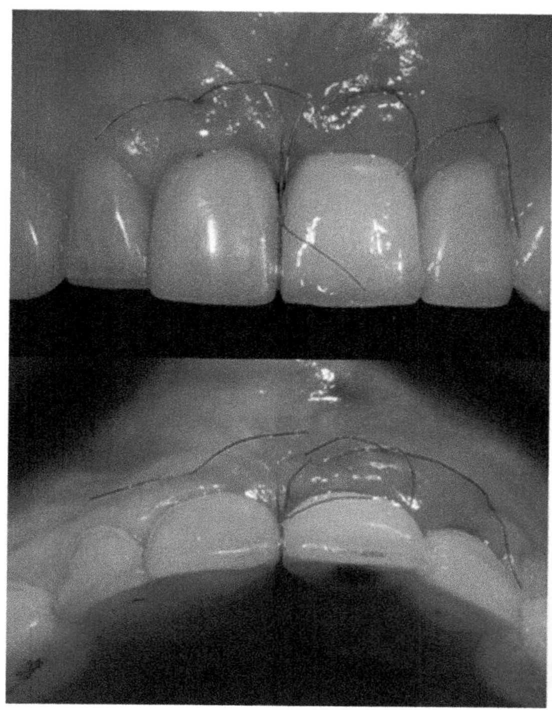

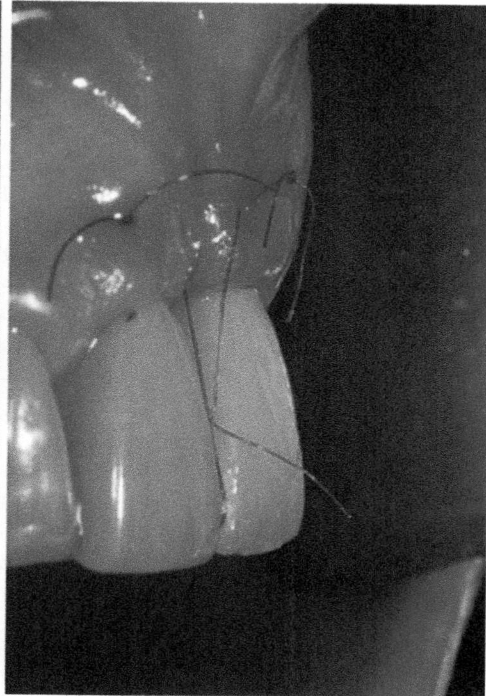

Figure 10.9 Provisionalization of the left maxillary central incisor.

woven bone within the first and second weeks. With time the bone is remodeled and ordered into trabeculae via osteoblast and osteoclast interactions [29,30].

Since these highly complex interactions between cells and their products of inflammation is the basis of osseointegration, it is therefore biologically feasible to apply PRF in the osteotomy to promote these processes (Figure 10.10). Although the scientific data is sparse with respect to PRF and implants, there is an enormous amount of data that can be extrapolated to contribute to educated clinical decision making.

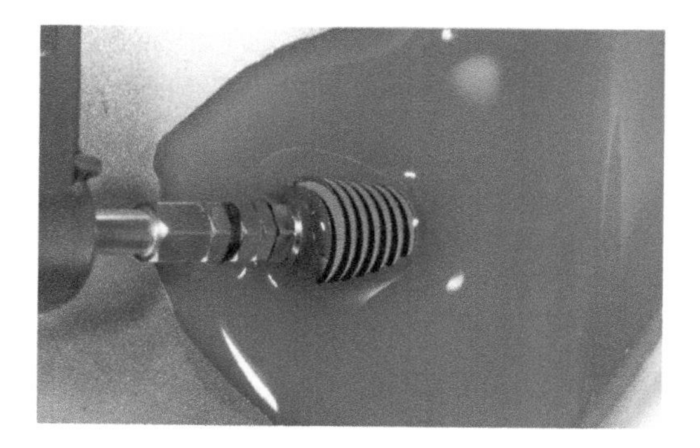

Figure 10.10 Implant surface coated with blood-derived growth factors prior to implant placement.

10.5 Techniques to improve primary stability in poor bone quality

Primary stability is key for the success of osseointegration [31]. Fibrous encapsulation of the implant may result when there is no primary stability leading to early failure. It is essential during the first 6 weeks following implant placement until secondary stability is established [27]. Gaining stability during implant placement is easily accomplished in hard bone (types 1 and 2). However, in type 3, 4, and 5 bone, this is not as predictably achieved. As such, various techniques have been proposed with the aim of improving primary stability in such cases.

1. **Under-preparation of the osteotomy site**
   This is an old technique typically omitting the final osteotomy preparation drill from the drilling sequence [32]. The rationale of the technique is that the implant itself will then partially compact the bone as it is inserted and hence improve primary stability. This leads to an improvement in the initial BIC due to the compression of the fine trabeculae. Utilizing this approach depends on the initial bone density, since the softer the bone, the less drills are required, and a wider implant may be placed to increase the compression and thus favors primary stability. This is a very simple concept however very experience-dependent; and inadvertent over-compression of the osteotomy may result in bone loss [33].
2. **Osteotome bone condensation**
   In this technique the osteotomy is not prepared by a drilling sequence but rather sequential compression by sharp osteotomes [34]. These lancing instruments apply force by hand and mallet to advance the osteotomy size correct to the implant. In the lower jaw mobility renders the technique obsolete, and thus it is primarily utilized in the maxilla where bone density is poorer and the head remains immobile. The technique is, however, quite traumatic since the malleting is not well tolerated by most patients and should be avoided when possible. If the technique is to be used, the operator's leg may support the head to dissipate the force. The clinician is to note there have been reports of vestibulocochlear disturbances resulting from malleting force and the patient may suffer from a postoperative vertigo [35].
   Like the "under preparation of the osteotomy drilling" technique, osteotome preparation has been shown to result in bone loss [36]. This is possibly a result of over-compression of the bone beyond its elastic limit.
3. **Osseodensification**
   This technique has been newly introduced and utilizes a specialized set of burs with uniquely designed flutes that when operated in reverse will condense the bone instead of removing it by cutting [37]. This results in bone particles being deposited in the wall of the osteotomy rather than being carried out. Histological confirmation of a greater BIC and denser bone at the implant site with higher implant stability quotient values (ISQ) have been reported [37,38].
4. **Implant design**
   The design of the implant plays a major role in primary stability with two aspects being important. The first is the implant's body design. Parallel walled implants will have poorer primary stability than an implant that has a tapered design. The tapered design itself has the ability to increase the primary stability as a result of a wedging effect [39]. The second factor is its thread design. Implants with very short threads, and threads spaced closely together, tend to have poorer primary stability than implants with wider and more aggressive cutting threads. Logically, better primary stability can be achieved with implants having more aggressive threads in poor bone density [40]. One would usually use this in conjunction with the under-preparation of the osteotomy. It is important to note that wider threads in practicality equate to a wider implant. The operator needs to be aware of the space required to accommodate these.

10.6 The use of PRF at osteotomy preparation

The high predictability of osseointegration has prompted clinicians and researchers to push the boundary to accelerate healing and expedite the completion of treatment. Developments in micro-roughened implant surface technology has largely facilitated this and successfully shown to increase ISQ at shorter time intervals [41]. This means a restoration present in the mouth earlier for the patient and patient functioning earlier than previously possible. The downside, however, is that micro-roughened implant surfaces may be more susceptible to bacterial colonization and peri-implantitis [42].

Numerous studies over the years have investigated implant surfaces enhanced with growth factors with varying results [43]. Some studies utilizing cell adhesion molecules or bone morphogenic proteins (BMPs) can increase osteoblastic differentiation and functional integration and have shown increases in BIC values [44]. PRF delivers platelets and leukocytes to the wound or osteotomy and releases growth factors locally (namely platelet-derived growth factor [PDGF], transforming growth factor-β, insulin-like growth factor (IGF), and vascular endothelial growth factor (VEGF)) that accelerate the healing process by attracting undifferentiated endothelial cells and mesenchymal cells to the injured site [27,28,45]. This theoretically could improve the healing response around implants (Figures 10.11–10.14). A recent study reported increased ISQ values during the early healing

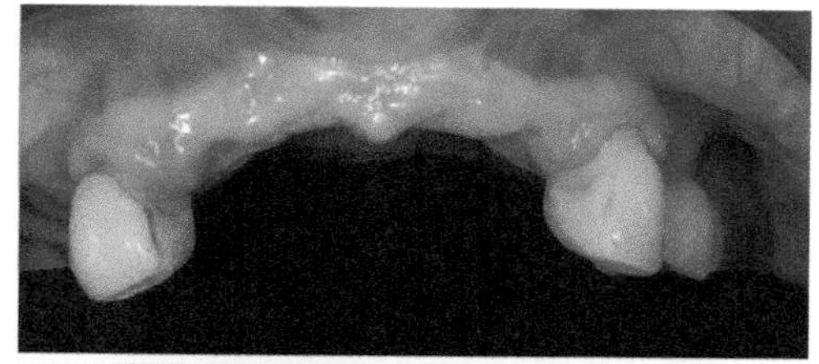
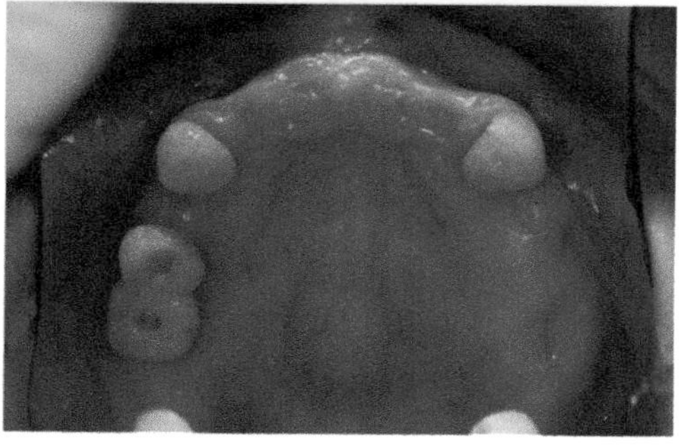

Figure 10.11 Case presentation with four missing maxillary incisors.

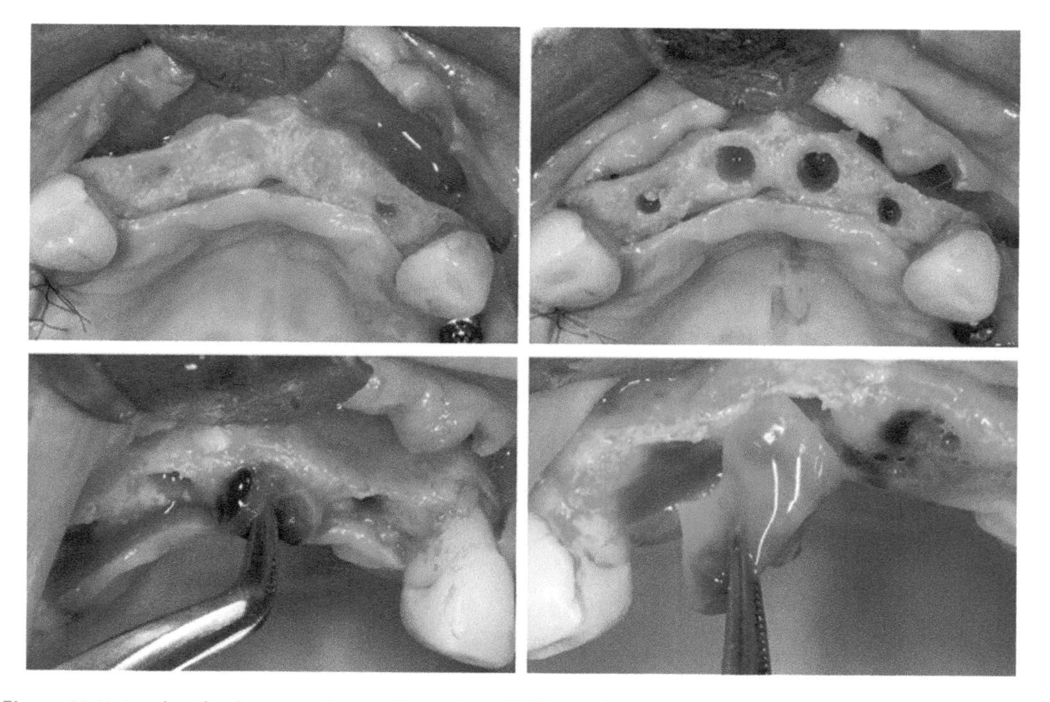

Figure 10.12 Implant bed preparation and insertion of PRF membranes into defect sites.

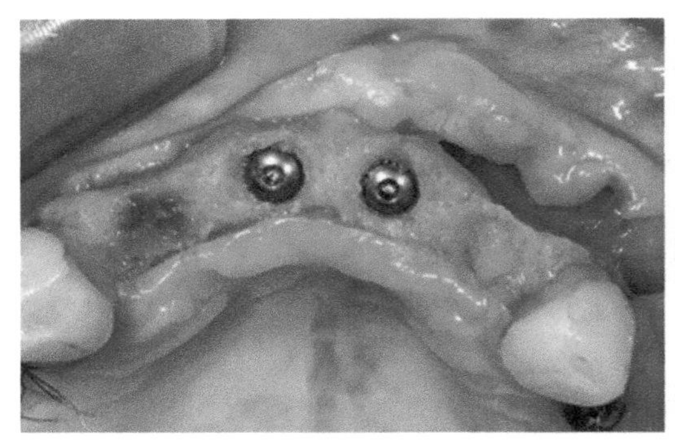
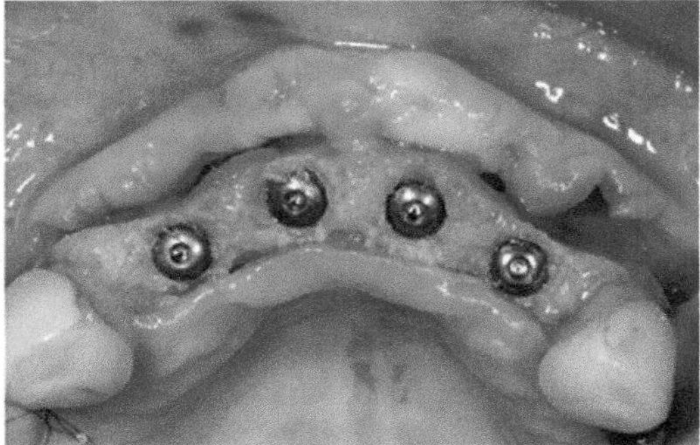

Figure 10.13 Implant placement with PRF membranes utilized on the buccal surface.

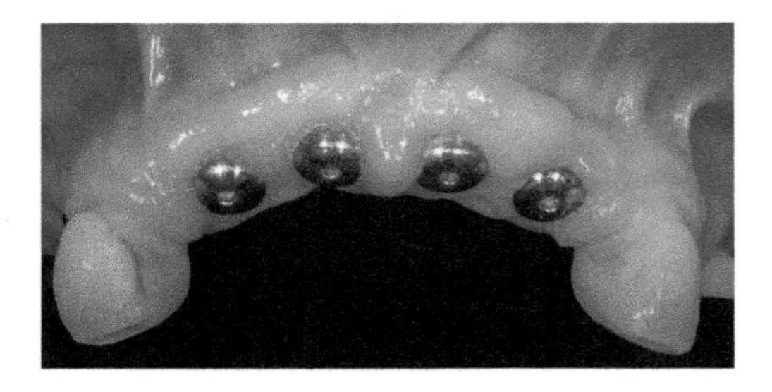

Figure 10.14 Final case presentation with four implants placed in the anterior maxilla.

period when PRF was applied inside the osteotomy during insertion and the implant itself coated in plasma extruded from the PRF [46]. However, these studies have showed statistically significant improvement in type 2 bone, limited data exists supporting other types of bone, and it is typically types 3 and 4 of poorer density that presents clinical challenges. The significance of PRF and implants seems to be limited to the early stages of osseointegration. This is an interesting development in PRF's uses and deserves much further research.

10.7 The future of PRF and implants

A consistent theme in discussions regarding PRF is that experts on the topic are recommending more research to substantiate the exciting possibilities it presents. The potential for PRF in conjunction with implant therapy is limitless. While some studies have investigated PRF's value in accelerating osseointegration, some evidence has been provided and even more will be needed to fully determine its evidence-based validity. Likely a great opportunity presents in inquiring PRF's potential when combined with particulate bone material at guided bone regeneration (GBR) procedures with implants. Similarly, the question whether PRF can augment soft tissue thickness at implants and contribute to coronal bone stability remains unanswered. These are exciting times in implant dentistry and much awaits to be discovered regarding the use of PRF in conjunction with placed dental implants.

References

1 Scala A, Lang NP, Schweikert MT, Oliveira JA, Rangel-Garcia I, Botticelli D. Sequential healing of open extraction sockets. An experimental study in monkeys. Clinical oral implants research. 2014;25(3):288–95.

2 Esposito M, Grusovin MG, Felice P, Karatzopoulos G, Worthington HV, Coulthard P. Interventions for replacing missing teeth: horizontal and vertical bone augmentation techniques for dental implant treatment. The Cochrane Library. 2009.

3 Esposito M, Maghaireh H, Gabriella Grusovin M, Ziounas I, Worthington HV.

Soft tissue management for dental implants: what are the most effective techniques? A Cochrane systematic review. European journal of oral implantology. 2012;5(3).
4 Puisys A, Linkevicius T. The influence of mucosal tissue thickening on crestal bone stability around bone-level implants. A prospective controlled clinical trial. Clinical oral implants research. 2015;26(2): 123–9.
5 Levine RA, Huynh-Ba G, Cochran DL. Soft tissue augmentation procedures for mucogingival defects in esthetic sites. International Journal of Oral & Maxillofacial Implants. 2014;29.
6 Xuan F, Lee C-U, Son J-S, Jeong S-M, Choi B-H. A comparative study of the regenerative effect of sinus bone grafting with platelet-rich fibrin-mixed Bio-Oss® and commercial fibrin-mixed Bio-Oss®: an experimental study. Journal of Cranio-Maxillofacial Surgery. 2014;42(4): e47–e50.
7 Simonpieri A, Del Corso M, Vervelle A, Jimbo R, Inchingolo F, Sammartino G, et al. Current knowledge and perspectives for the use of platelet-rich plasma (PRP) and platelet-rich fibrin (PRF) in oral and maxillofacial surgery part 2: Bone graft, implant and reconstructive surgery. Current pharmaceutical biotechnology. 2012;13(7):1231–56.
8 Linkevicius T, Puisys A, Steigmann M, Vindasiute E, Linkeviciene L. Influence of vertical soft tissue thickness on crestal bone changes around implants with platform switching: a comparative clinical study. Clinical implant dentistry and related research. 2015;17(6):1228–36.
9 Bassetti RG, Stähli A, Bassetti MA, Sculean A. Soft tissue augmentation around osseointegrated and uncovered dental implants: a systematic review. Clinical oral investigations. 2016:1–18.
10 Puisys A, Linkevicius T. The influence of mucosal tissue thickening on crestal bone stability around bone-level implants. A prospective controlled clinical trial. Clinical oral implants research. 2015;26(2): 123–9.
11 Fu JH, Lee A, Wang HL. Influence of tissue biotype on implant esthetics. The International journal of oral & maxillofacial implants. 2011;26(3):499–508.
12 Lee A, Fu JH, Wang HL. Soft tissue biotype affects implant success. Implant dentistry. 2011;20(3):e38–e47.
13 Degidi M, Daprile G, Nardi D, Piattelli A. Buccal bone plate in immediately placed and restored implant with Bio-Oss® collagen graft: a 1-year follow-up study. Clinical oral implants research. 2013; 24(11):1201–5.
14 Maia LP, Reino DM, Muglia VA, Almeida AL, Nanci A, Wazen RM, et al. Influence of periodontal tissue thickness on buccal plate remodelling on immediate implants with xenograft. Journal of clinical periodontology. 2015;42(6):590–8.
15 Lee J-W, Kim S-G, Kim J-Y, Lee Y-C, Choi J-Y, Dragos R, et al. Restoration of a peri-implant defect by platelet-rich fibrin. Oral surgery, oral medicine, oral pathology and oral radiology. 2012;113(4): 459–63.
16 Hao P-J, Wang Z-G, Xu Q-C, Xu S, Li Z-R, Yang P-S, et al. Effect of umbilical cord mesenchymal stem cell in peri-implant bone defect after immediate implant: an experiment study in beagle dogs. International journal of clinical and experimental pathology. 2014;7(11):8271.
17 Şimşek S, Özeç İ, Kürkçü M, Benlidayi E. Histomorphometric evaluation of bone formation in peri-implant defects treated with different regeneration techniques: an experimental study in a rabbit model. Journal of Oral and Maxillofacial Surgery. 2016.
18 Esposito M, Grusovin MG, Worthington HV. Treatment of peri-implantitis: what interventions are effective? A Cochrane systematic review. Eur J Oral Implantol. 2012;5(Suppl 1):21–41.
19 Tomas A, Luigi C, David C, Hugo DB. “Peri-Implantitis”: A Complication of a Foreign Body or a Man-Made “Disease”.

Facts and Fiction. Clinical implant dentistry and related research. 2016.

20 Guler B, Uraz A, Yalım M, Bozkaya S. The Comparison of Porous Titanium Granule and Xenograft in the Surgical Treatment of Peri-Implantitis: A Prospective Clinical Study. Clinical implant dentistry and related research. 2016.

21 Schwarz F, Herten M, Sager M, Bieling K, Sculean A, Becker J. Comparison of naturally occurring and ligature-induced peri-implantitis bone defects in humans and dogs. Clinical oral implants research. 2007;18(2):161–70.

22 Monje A, Aranda L, Diaz K, Alarcón M, Bagramian R, Wang H, et al. Impact of Maintenance Therapy for the Prevention of Peri-implant Diseases: A Systematic Review and Meta-analysis. Journal of dental research. 2016;95(4):372.

23 Panda S, Sankari M, Satpathy A, Jayakumar D, Mozzati M, Mortellaro C, et al. Adjunctive Effect of Autologus Platelet-Rich Fibrin to Barrier Membrane in the Treatment of Periodontal Intrabony Defects. Journal of Craniofacial Surgery. 2016;27(3):691–6.

24 Miron RJ, Fujioka-Kobayashi M, Bishara M, Zhang Y, Hernandez M, Choukroun J. Platelet-Rich Fibrin and Soft Tissue Wound Healing: A Systematic Review. Tissue Engineering Part B: Reviews. 2016.

25 Hehn J, Schwenk T, Striegel M, Schlee M. The effect of PRF (platelet-rich fibrin) inserted with a split-flap technique on soft tissue thickening and initial marginal bone loss around implants: results of a randomized, controlled clinical trial. International Journal of Implant Dentistry. 2016;2(1):1.

26 Branemark P-I. Osseointegration and its experimental background. The Journal of prosthetic dentistry. 1983;50(3):399–410.

27 Terheyden H, Lang NP, Bierbaum S, Stadlinger B. Osseointegration–communication of cells. Clinical oral implants research. 2012;23(10):1127–35.

28 Terheyden H, Stadlinger B, Sanz M, Garbe AI, Meyle J. Inflammatory reaction–communication of cells. Clinical oral implants research. 2014;25(4):399–407.

29 Davies JE. Understanding peri-implant endosseous healing. Journal of dental education. 2003;67(8):932–49.

30 Gruber R, Stadlinger B, Terheyden H. Cell-to-cell communication in guided bone regeneration: molecular and cellular mechanisms. Clinical oral implants research. 2016.

31 Lioubavina-Hack N, Lang NP, Karring T. Significance of primary stability for osseointegration of dental implants. Clinical oral implants research. 2006;17(3): 244–50.

32 Turkyilmaz I, Aksoy U, McGlumphy EA. Two alternative surgical techniques for enhancing primary implant stability in the posterior maxilla: a clinical study including bone density, insertion torque, and resonance frequency analysis data. Clinical implant dentistry and related research. 2008;10(4):231–7.

33 Stavropoulos A, Cochran D, Obrecht M, Pippenger B, Dard M. Effect of osteotomy preparation on osseointegration of immediately loaded, tapered dental implants. Advances in dental research. 2016;28(1):34–41.

34 Nóbrega AR, Norton A, Silva JA, Silva JPD, Branco FM, Anitua E. The Osteotome Versus Conventional Drilling Technique for Implant Site Preparation: A Comparative Study in the Rabbit. International Journal of Periodontics & Restorative Dentistry. 2012;32(3).

35 Sammartino G, Mariniello M, Scaravilli MS. Benign paroxysmal positional vertigo following closed sinus floor elevation procedure: mallet osteotomes vs. screwable osteotomes. A triple blind randomized controlled trial. Clinical oral implants research. 2011;22(6):669–72.

36 Strietzel FP, Nowak M, Küchler I, Friedmann A. Peri-implant alveolar bone loss with respect to bone quality after use of the osteotome technique. Clinical oral implants research. 2002;13(5): 508–13.

37 Huwais S, Meyer EG. A Novel Osseous Densification Approach in Implant Osteotomy Preparation to Increase Biomechanical Primary Stability, Bone Mineral Density, and Bone-to-Implant Contact. The International journal of oral & maxillofacial implants. 2016.

38 Trisi P, Berardini M, Falco A, Vulpiani MP. New Osseodensification Implant Site Preparation Method to Increase Bone Density in Low-Density Bone: In Vivo Evaluation in Sheep. Implant dentistry. 2016;25(1):24.

39 Romanos GE, Delgado-Ruiz RA, Sacks D, Calvo-Guirado JL. Influence of the implant diameter and bone quality on the primary stability of porous tantalum trabecular metal dental implants: an in vitro biomechanical study. Clinical oral implants research. 2016.

40 Lee S-Y, Kim S-J, An H-W, Kim H-S, Ha D-G, Ryo K-H, et al. The effect of the thread depth on the mechanical properties of the dental implant. The journal of advanced prosthodontics. 2015;7(2): 115–21.

41 Smeets R, Stadlinger B, Schwarz F, Beck-Broichsitter B, Jung O, Precht C, et al. Impact of dental implant surface modifications on osseointegration. BioMed research international. 2016;2016.

42 Esposito M, Coulthard P, Thomsen P, Worthington H. The role of implant surface modifications, shape and material on the success of osseointegrated dental implants. A Cochrane systematic review. The European journal of prosthodontics and restorative dentistry. 2005;13(1): 15–31.

43 Scheller EL, Krebsbach PH. Using Soluble Signals to Harness the Power of the Bone Marrow Microenvironment for Implant Therapeutics. The International journal of oral & maxillofacial implants. 2011;26: 70.

44 Liu Y, Enggist L, Kuffer AF, Buser D, Hunziker EB. The influence of BMP-2 and its mode of delivery on the osteoconductivity of implant surfaces during the early phase of osseointegration. Biomaterials. 2007;28(16):2677–86.

45 Miron R, Fujioka-Kobayashi M, Bishara M, Zhang Y, Hernandez M, Choukroun J. Platelet Rich Fibrin and Soft Tissue Wound Healing: A Systematic Review. Tissue engineering Part B, Reviews. 2016.

46 Öncü E, Bayram B, Kantarcı A, Gülsever S, Alaaddinoğlu E-E. Posıtıve effect of platelet rich fibrin on osseointegration. Medicina Oral, Patología Oral y Cirugía Bucal. 2016; 21(5):e601.

11

Guided Bone Regeneration with Platelet Rich Fibrin

Richard J. Miron, Michael A. Pikos, Yufeng Zhang, and Tobias Fretwurst

Abstract

Barrier membranes have played a prominent role in regenerative dentistry since the mid-1980s by preventing infiltration of fast-growing soft tissues from slower-growing bone and mineralized tissues. These concepts were first applied to teeth in what is now known as "guided tissue regeneration" (GTR) and were shortly thereafter utilized in bone as "guided bone regeneration" (GBR). Over the years, much development has been made with respect to the osteoconduction and biocompatibility of bone-grafting materials as well as barrier membranes. While original PTEF non-resorbable membranes were first utilized requiring a second surgical procedure, thereby increasing patient morbidity, more recently various biodegradable collagen membranes, biodegradable polymers, as well as platelet rich fibrin (PRF) have been developed as next-generation membranes for GBR procedures. Similarly, bone-grafting materials were first utilized as passive materials, yet have more recently gained additional advantages by employing biologics to speed new bone formation, including various growth factors and bioactive modifiers. Despite bone morphogenetic proteins being deemed the gold standard to facilitate new bone formation, a concurrent wave of research derived from platelet concentrates (platelet rich plasma (PRP)) have been found to speed angiogenesis, a key component of bone regeneration. While the effects of utilizing PRP has been heavily debated in the literature due to their incorporation of anti-coagulants, a second more autologous platelet concentrate (PRF) has seen more frequent use in dentistry due to its easier preparation protocols and additional handling benefits. This chapter focuses on the history of GBR, currently utilized biomaterials, and discusses the advantages and limitations for combining PRF into routine GBR procedures.

Highlights

- History of guided bone regeneration (GBR)
- Currently utilized biomaterials for GBR
- Documented evidence supporting PRF in GBR
- Clinical cases combining PRF with bone grafting materials for GBR
- Clinical cases using PRF as a barrier membrane
- Discussion over the additional benefit to combining PRF with bone grafts
- Future perspectives

11.1 Introduction

Guided tissue regeneration (GTR) and guided bone regeneration (GBR) have been pivotal techniques utilized by oral surgeons,

Platelet Rich Fibrin in Regenerative Dentistry: Biological Background and Clinical Indications, First Edition.
Edited by Richard J. Miron and Joseph Choukroun.

periodontists, and more frequently general dentists for the successful and predictable regeneration of periodontal and bone tissues. Interestingly, in the mid-1980s, a series of studies occurred based on the hypothesis that in order to optimize tissue regeneration of periodontal and alveolar bony structures, the overlaying fast-growing soft tissues needed to be excluded [1]. Since then, a plethora of research in both the periodontal field as well as the bone regeneration field have exploded in popularity with various methods and biomaterials being utilized to facilitate this task.

Another popular trend in recent years has been related to the development of platelet rich fibrin (PRF), which was initially introduced in 2001 [2]. Since then, a rapid growth in use has been observed due to its 100% naturally derived autologous source of growth factors obtained at relatively low cost. PRF differs significantly from previous platelet formulations including platelet rich plasma (PRP) and platelet rich growth factors (PRGF) in that it does not contain anti-coagulants and thus forms a fibrin clot during the centrifugation process. It is therefore not a liquid and instead acts as a clot containing numerous autologous growth factors. PRF can either be cut into small pieces and combined with various bone biomaterials/grafting materials, or subsequently flattened and utilized as a barrier membrane in GTR/GBR procedures. It offers numerous advantages when compared to traditional collagen membranes in that it contains autologous growth factors as well as living host-immune leukocytes. These cells act to fight against incoming pathogens and therefore the rate of infection may be reduced as much as 10-fold [3]. For these reasons, PRF membranes bear the advantage in that they may be left exposed to the oral cavity without much fear of contamination due to their abundant supply of host-immune cells capable of fighting pathogens from the oral cavity. Nevertheless, while the effects of PRF on angiogenesis have been well documented, the subsequent influence on bone regeneration and GBR procedures has been scarce. The majority of the literature to date has focused solely on its influence on soft-tissue wound healing [4] with limited data available investigating its effect on bone regeneration. This chapter aims to provide an overview of GBR and the most commonly utilized biomaterials, and thereafter highlights the effects of PRF in GBR procedures either utilized in combination with a bone-grafting material, or serving as a barrier membrane.

11.2 Overview of GBR

In order to maintain stable teeth and implants, a sufficient quantity of bone volume in the vertical and horizontal dimensions of the alveolar ridge is mandatory [5]. Interestingly, the concept of GBR and the use of barrier membranes were introduced in the field of periodontology and implant dentistry nearly 30 years ago [6–9]. These concepts were derived from the fact that different rates of cell growth and migration properties were observed between alveolar soft tissues when compared to underlying hard tissues [6]. The concept originally attempted to hamper fast-growing non-functional epithelial cells from infiltrating into bone defects to allow for the unimpaired healing of slower growing bone [10] (Figure 11.1 and 11.2). Over the years, a variety of additional parameters including space maintenance, ability to form a blood clot, mechanical stabilization, cellular infiltration potential, biocompatibility, and resorption properties have been investigated to achieve more favorable bone tissue healing [11].

Although originally synthetic expanded polytetrafluoroethylene (PTFE) membranes were shown to provide successful outcomes [6,7], it was later argued that a second surgical intervention mandatory to remove the barrier membrane provided additional patient morbidity, which could be prevented by utilizing biodegradable materials [12,13]. For these reasons, resorbable collagen and synthetic membranes have become available in

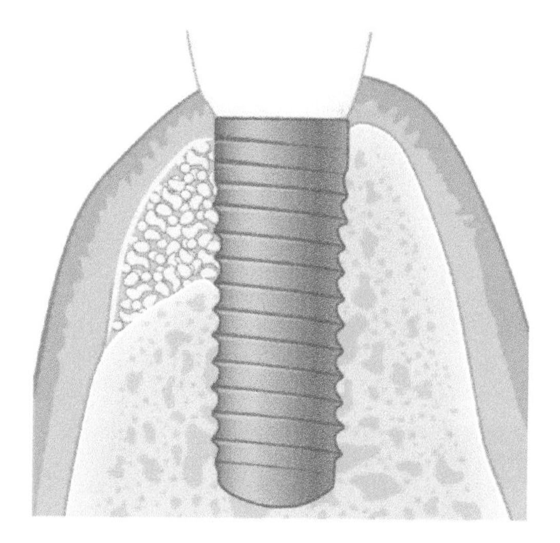

Figure 11.1 Illustration of standard guided bone regeneration procedure around a dental implant. First the bone-grafting material is placed in the bone defect and thereafter a barrier membrane is utilized to prevent soft-tissue infiltration into bone. Regeneration may then take place due to the space maintenance ability of the barrier membrane.

the last decade practically replacing original PTFE membranes.

Overall, GBR has seen extremely high predictable results with well-established and well-documented protocols leading to high implant survival rates ranging from 91.9% to 92.6% during a median follow-up of 12.5 years in current prospective long-term studies [5]. Various animal and clinical studies have further demonstrated the successful applicability of GTR in periodontal defects including intrabony, furcation recession, and supra-alveolar defects [14–17]. Nevertheless, a sufficient primary wound closure is mandatory using standard GBR-techniques to prevent soft-tissue ingrowth, bacterial contamination, early membrane degradation, or soft-tissue dehiscence and graft exposure.

Membranes for GBR have ranged tremendously with hundreds of commercially available products now available. Furthermore, bone grafting and bone substitute materials have reached a multi-billion-dollar per year industry with an exponential growth in commercially available products brought to market on a yearly basis [5,18]. Below we summarize the available options and later present PRF as a low-cost, easily producible membrane derived from 100% autologous sources as its potential use in combination with bone grafting materials as well as acting as a functional living autogenous barrier membrane.

11.3 Available options of GBR

Fundamental requirements for biomaterials utilized in GBR are biocompatibility of the material to prevent an adverse host reaction and certain degradability properties to allow adequate bone regeneration and eventual replacement with native host bone. Ideally, GBR materials must provide proper mechanical strength to guarantee space maintenance for migrating cells from the surrounding bone tissue to facilitate bone regeneration. Therefore, barrier membranes must prevent the infiltration of fibrous tissue (cell-occlusiveness properties) to avoid impaired bone healing, whereas the bone-grafting material must facilitate the migration of osteogenic cells such as osteoblasts to the material surface [19]. A wide range of barrier membranes have been made commercially available for various clinical approaches with distinct advantages and disadvantages of each presented in Table 11.1 and summarized below [19–21].

11.4 Non-resorbable PTFE membranes

Non-resorbable membranes include expanded, high-density and titanium-reinforced expanded polytetrafluoroethylene (e-,d-PTFE and Ti-e-PTFE) membranes [21]. In general, the main disadvantage of synthetic non-resorbable membranes is the requirement for a second surgical intervention to remove the membrane since

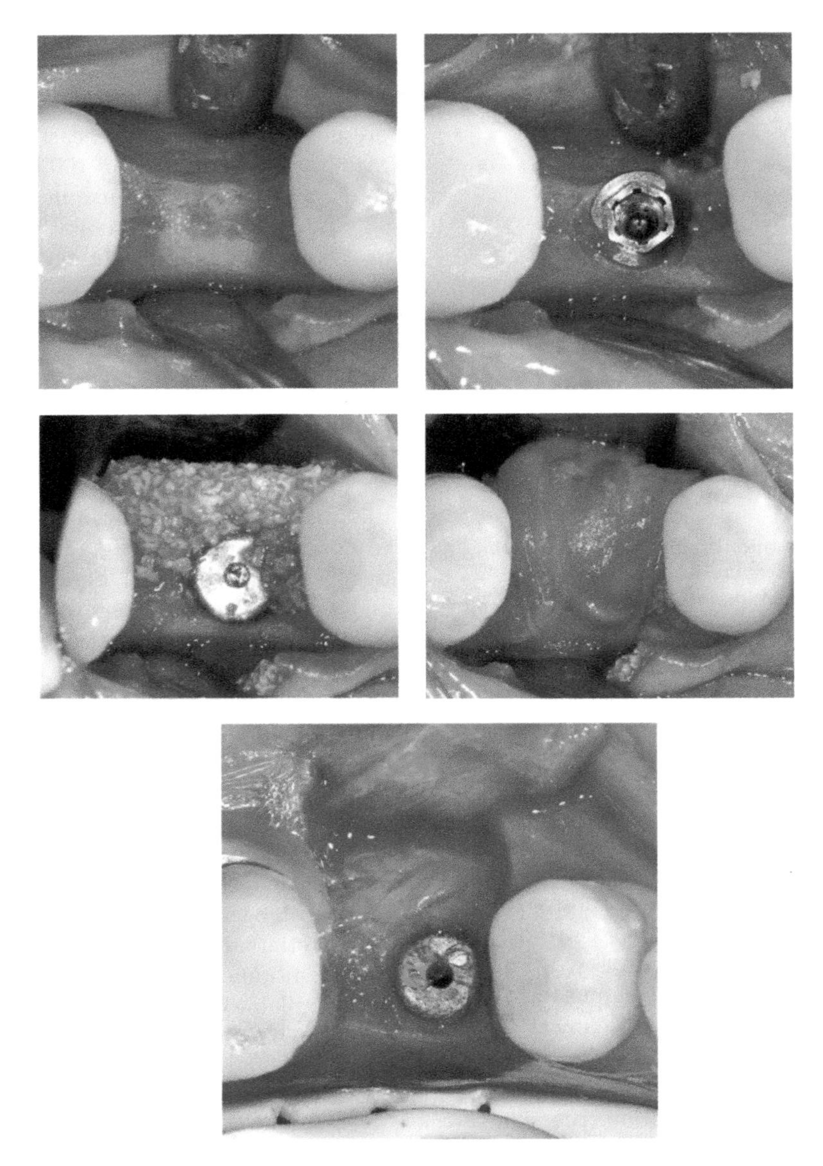

Figure 11.2 Clinical demonstration of a GBR procedure performed in a horizontal deficiency of the alveolar crest around a dental implant. Following implant placement, bone-grafting materials may be packed on the buccal aspect with a barrier membrane utilized to prevent soft-tissue infiltration. Lower image demonstrates re-entry after 5 months with new bone formation.

they are not biodegradable (Figure 11.3) [22]. Although the use of ePTFE membranes have demonstrated higher levels of new bone formation and clinical attachment levels around teeth [23], the requirement of a second surgical intervention to remove the barrier 4 to 6 weeks after implantation is a significant drawback often resulting in re-injury of tissues [19]. Furthermore, the second surgical procedure leads to extra surgical time and therefore incurs additional costs and patient discomfort. For the above-mentioned reasons, PTFE membranes are seldom utilized in modern dentistry.

Table 11.1 List of available membranes for guided tissue regeneration. Source: Zhang *et al.* 2013 [19]. CC-BY.

Membranes		Commercial name	Manufacturer and nation	Material	Properties	Comments
Non-resorbable membranes	e-PTFE	Gore-Tex	W. L. Gore & Associates, Inc., USA	e-PTFE	Good space maintainer Easy to handle	Longest clinical experience
		Gore-Tex-TI	W. L. Gore & Associates, Inc., USA	Ti-e-PTFE	Most stable space maintainer Filler material unnecessary	Titanium should not be exposed Commonly used in ridge augmentation
	d-PTFE	High-density Gore-Tex	W. L. Gore & Associates, Inc., USA	d-PTFE	0.2 μm pores	Avoid a secondary surgery
		Cytoplast	Osteogenics Biomedical., USA		<0.3 μm pores	Primary closure unnecessary
		TefGen FD	Lifecore Biomedical, Inc., USA		0.2–0.3 μm pores	Easy to detach
		Non-resorbable ACE	Surgical supply, Inc., USA		<0.2 μm pores 0.2 mm thick	Limited cell proliferation
	Titanium mesh	Ti-Micromesh ACE	Surgical supply, Inc., USA	Ti	1700mm pores 0.1mm thick	Ideal long term survival rate
		Tocksystem Mesh	Tocksystem, Italy		0.1 to 6.5mm pore 0.1mm thick	Minimal resorption and inflammation
		Frios BoneShields	Dentsply Friadent, Germany		0.03mm pores 0.1mm thick	Sufficient bone to regenerate
		M-TAM			1700mm pores 0.1 to 0.3mm thick	Excellent tissue compatibility

Synthetic resorbable membranes	OsseoQuest	W. L. Gore & Associates, Inc., USA	Hydrolyzable polyester	Resorption: 16–24 weeks	Good tissue integration
	Biofix	Bioscience Oy, USA	Polyglycolic acid	Resorption: 24–48 weeks	Isolate the space from cells from soft tissue and bacteria
	Vicryl	Johnson & Johnson, USA	Polyglactin 910 Polyglicolid/polyl actid 9:1	Well adaptable Resorption: 4–12 weeks	Woven membrane Four prefabricated shapes
	Atrisorb	Tolmar, Inc., USA	Poly-DL-lactide and solvent	Resorption: 36–48 weeks Interesting resorptive characteristics	Custom fabricated membrane "Barrier Kit"
	EpiGuide	Kensey Nash corporation, USA	Poly-DL-lactic acid	Three-layer membrane Resorption: 6–12 weeks	Self-supporting Support developed blood clot
	Resolut	W. L. Gore & Associates, Inc., USA	Poly-DL-lactid/Co-glycolid	Resorption: 10 weeks Good space maintainer	Good tissue integration Separate suture material
	Vivosorb	Polyganics B.V. NL	DL-lactide-ε-caprolactone (PLCL)	Anti-adhesive barrier Up to 8 weeks' mechanical properties	Act as a nerve guide

(continued)

Table 11.1 (*Continued*)

Membranes	Commercial name	Manufacturer and nation	Material	Properties	Comments
Natural biodegradable material	Plasma rich in growth factors(PRGF-Endoret)	BTI Biotechnology Institute, Vitoria, Spain	Patients' own blood	Abundant growth factors and proteins mediate cell behaviors Different formulations for various usages Total resorption	Enhance osseointegration and initial implant stability Promote new bone formation Encourage soft tissue recovery
	Bio-Gide	Osteohealth Company, SUI	Porcine I and III	Resorption: 24 weeks Mechanical strength: 7.5 MPa	Usually used in combination with filler materials
	Bio-mend	Zimmer, USA	Bovine I	Resorption: 8 weeks Mechanical strength: 3.5–22.5 MPa	Fibrous network Modulate cell activities
	Biosorb membrane	3M ESPE, USA	Bovine I	Resorption: 26–38 weeks	Tissue integration
	Neomem	Citagenix, CAN	Bovine I	Double-layer product Resorption: 26–38 weeks	Used in severe cases
	OsseoGuard	BIOMET 3i, USA	Bovine I	Resorption: 24–32 weeks	Improve the aesthetics of the final prosthetics
	Ossix	OraPharma, Inc., USA	Porcine I	Resorption: 16–24 weeks	Increase the woven bone

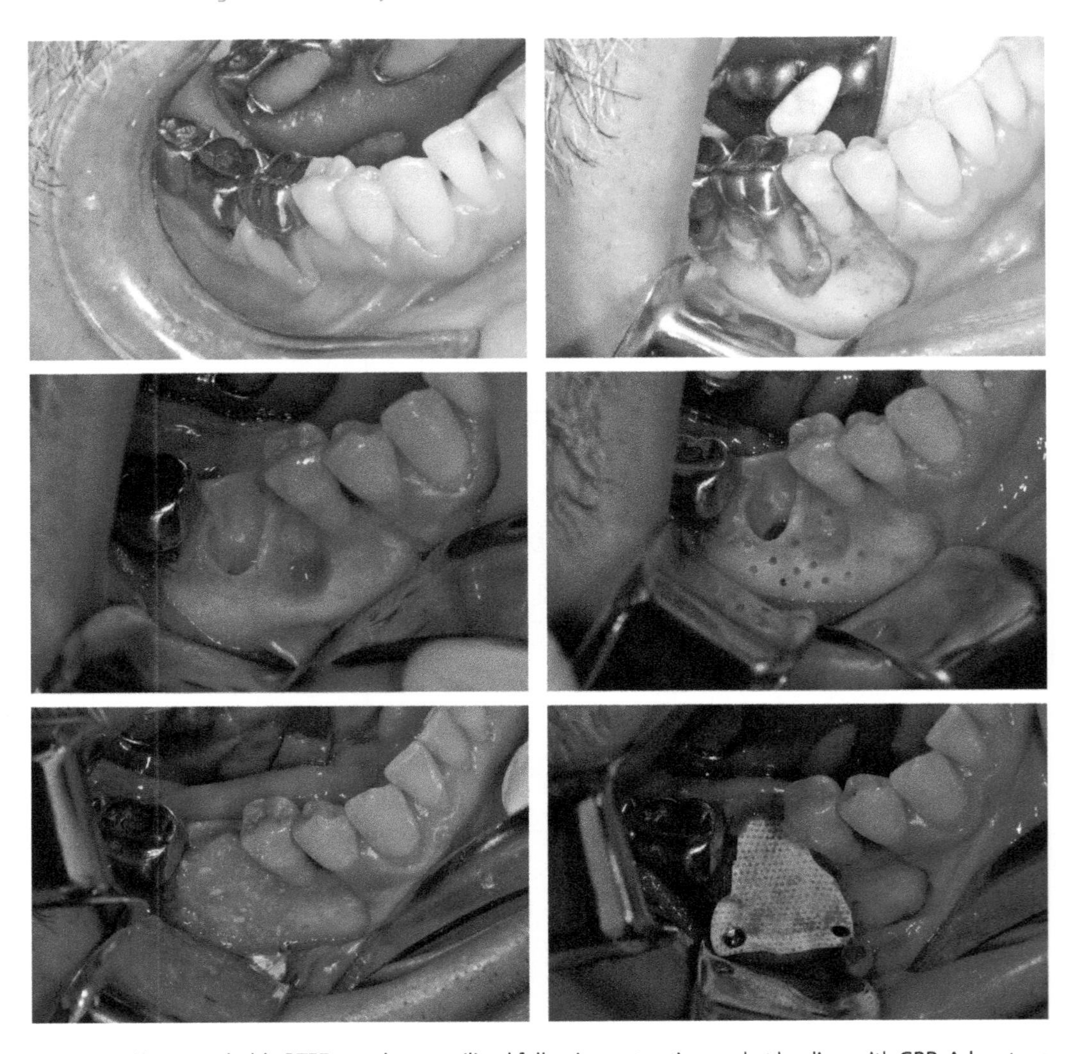

Figure 11.3 Non-resorbable PTFE membrane utilized following extraction socket healing with GBR. Advantages include their ability to prevent soft-tissue infiltration. Their main drawback is, however, the requirement of a second surgical procedure required to remove the non-resorbable membrane (Case performed by Dr. Michael A. Pikos).

11.5 Titanium mesh

Due to the high biocompatibility and strength of titanium, titanium-reinforced barrier membranes were introduced as an option for GBR (Figure 11.4). This allows for superior mechanical support, which favors a larger space for bone and tissue regrowth without compression on the underlying bone. Based on these advantages, titanium meshes have been more frequently utilized as non-resorbable membranes [24].

11.6 Collagen-based resorbable membranes

The main advantage of this second generation resorbable barrier membranes is that

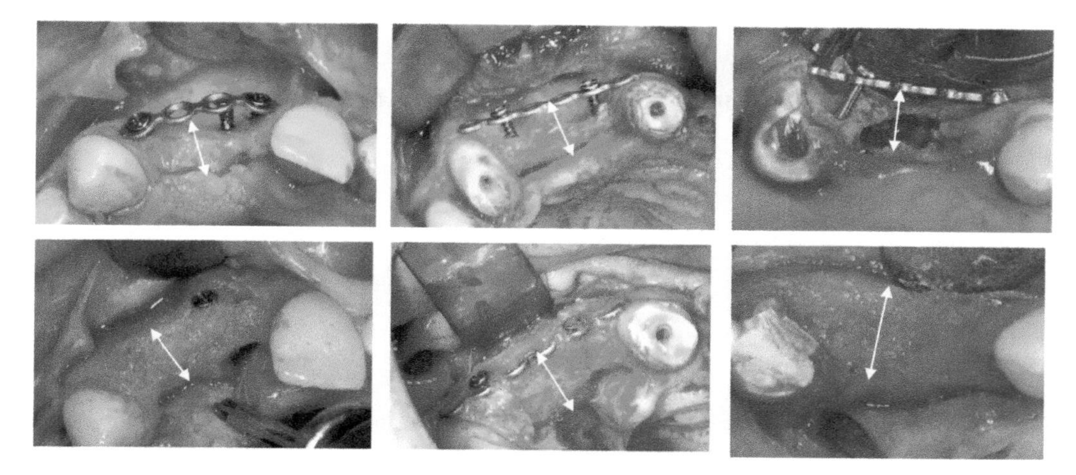

Figure 11.4 Large GBR procedure performed with a titanium grid to protect the graft from pressure. Due to their high mechanical strength, titanium meshes are frequently utilized due to their space-maintenance ability and superior strength (Case performed by Dr. Dominique Caspar).

they permit a single-step procedure, thus alleviating patient discomfort and additional morbidity/tissue damage caused by a second surgery. Initially, one of the main disadvantages of resorbable membranes was the unpredictable resorption time, which directly affects new bone formation [25]. Various barrier membranes each reporting different resorption rates are presented in Table 11.1 (Figure 11.5). These may be derived from human skin, bovine achilles tendon, or porcine skin and have been characterized by their excellent cell affinity and biocompatibility. While they are most frequently utilized, drawbacks include their lack of space-maintenance ability/rigidity, high costs, potential for creating a foreign body reaction, and risk of infection if left exposed to the oral cavity.

11.7 Synthetic resorbable membranes

In addition to collagen resorbable membranes, a series of synthetic resorbable membranes fabricated from polyesters (e.g., poly(glycolic acid) (PGA), poly(lactic acid) (PLA), poly(-caprolactone) (PCL), and their copolymers have been introduced (Table 11.1) [19,26]. Their main advantage is that polyglycolide or polylactide can be made in large quantities at low costs with different physical, chemical, and mechanical properties. Their main disadvantage has been the fact they are more prone to foreign body reactions thereby influencing their wound healing properties. For these reasons, collagen barrier membranes are more frequently utilized.

11.8 Plasma-rich proteins as growth factors for membranes

One area of research that has gained more popularity over the past decade has been the use of platelet concentrates as potential barrier membranes. Since the 1990s, it has been known that platelets are critical during the wound-healing process. PRP was one of the first autologous modifications that could be combined with barrier membranes but its main limiting factor included the use of additional anticoagulants preventing the natural healing process [27–30].

More recently, PRF was developed [31–35]. The PRF preparation is much simpler only

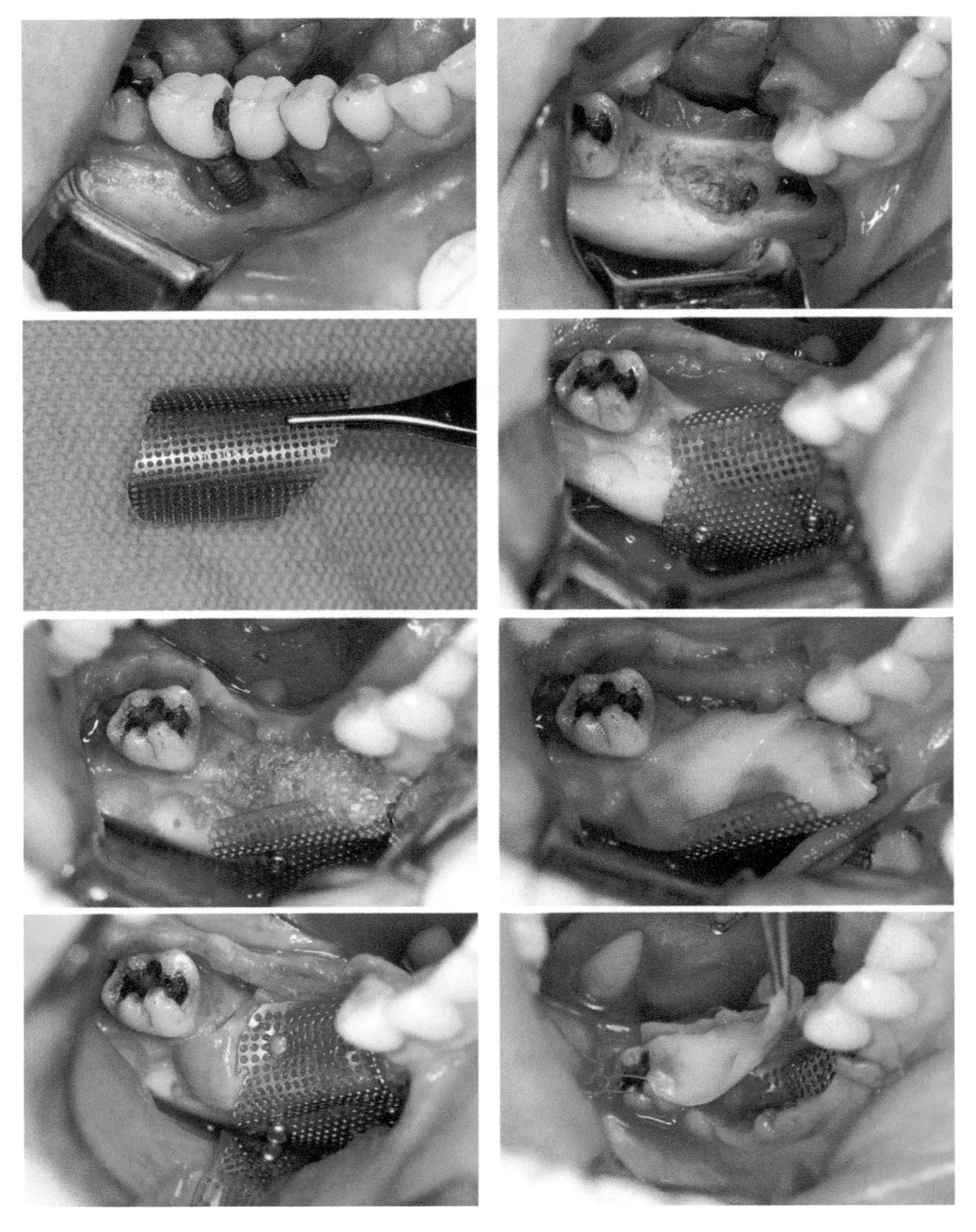

Figure 11.5 Large GBR procedure performed with a titanium mesh to protect the graft from pressure. Due to the high mechanical strength, titanium meshes are frequently utilized due to their space-maintenance ability. Platelet rich fibrin (PRF) is utilized above and below the titanium to improve vascularization to both bone and soft tissues (Case performed by Dr. Michael A. Pikos).

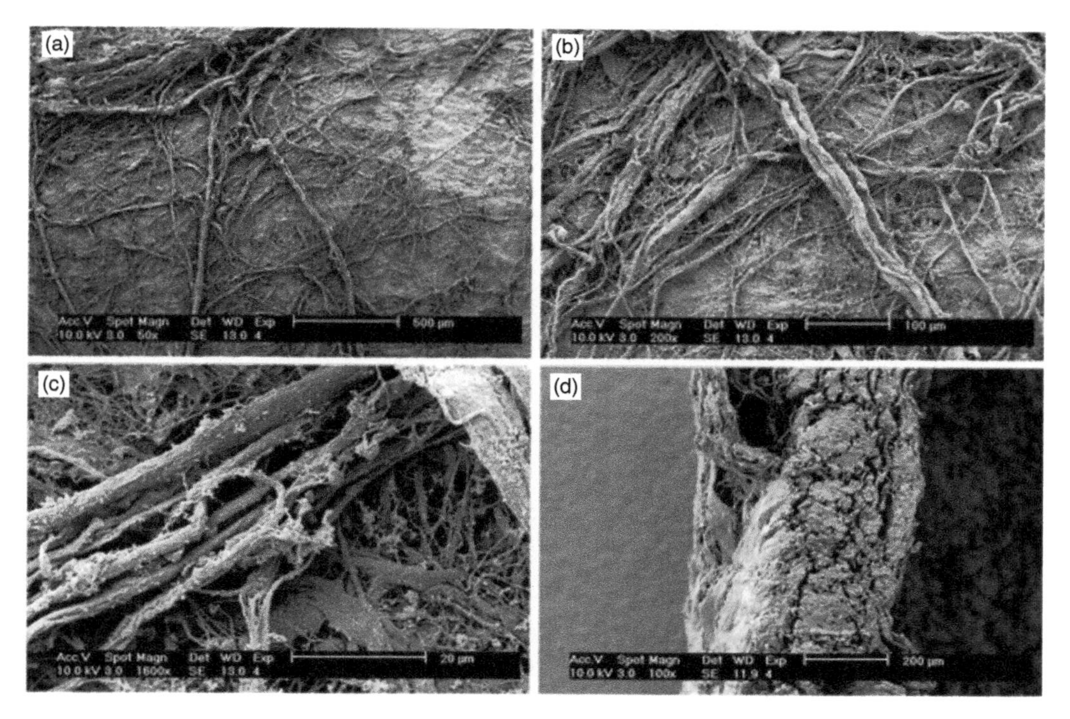

Figure 11.6 Scanning electron microscopy (SEM) analysis of collagen barrier membrane. a,b Membrane surface reveals many collagen fibrils that are intertwined with one another with various diameters and directions (magnification $A = \times 50$, $B = \times 200$). c High-resolution SEM demonstrates collagen fibrils ranging in diameter between 1 and 5 µm (magnification = ×1,600). d Cross-sectional view of collagen barrier membrane of approximately 300 µm (magnification = ×100). Source: Miron *et al.* 2013 [36]. Reproduced with permission of Springer-Verlag.

requiring one centrifugation cycle and is less expensive not requiring any anticoagulant/activator additives. PRF clots may also be compressed into flattened fibrin able to serve as a barrier membrane during GBR procedures (Figure 11.6) [36]. This fibrin scaffold can then be used as a natural barrier membrane alone or subsequently cut and combined with bone grafts discussed later in this chapter.

11.9 Choice of bone-grafting materials during GBR procedures

An extensive array of bone grafts is currently available on the market. While the goal of this chapter is not to go in detail of the available options, it is noteworthy, however, to mention that most GBR procedures are routinely augmented with bone grafts, which may consist of either utilizing autografts, allografts, xenografts, and alloplasts (synthetic bone grafts) (Table 11.2) [37]. Naturally, autogenous bone grafts are still considered the gold standard due to their combined osteoconductive, osteoinductive, and osteogenic properties [38]. However, the availability is limited and the harvesting procedure leads to donor site morbidity [39]. Allografts demonstrate good osteoconductive properties and certain classes are known to be slightly osteoinductive, which is attributed to the release of bone morphogenetic proteins (BMPs) in the demineralized grafts [40]. Xenografts are available from different species (bovine, porcine, equine) and have exclusive osteoconductive properties. Similarly, synthetic materials (hydroxyappatite, tri-calcium phosphate, biphasic calcium phosphate, and bioactive glass) display osteoconductive properties with no

Table 11.2 Classification of bone grafting materials used for the regeneration of periodontal intrabony defects.

Material Characteristic	Ideal	Autograft	Allograft	Xenograft	Alloplast
Biocompatibility	+	+	+	+	+
Safety	+	+	+	+	+
Surface characteristics	+	+	+	+	+
Geometry	+	+	+	+	+
Handling	+	+	+/−	+	+
Mechanical characteristics	+	+	+/−	+	−
Osteogenic	+	+	−	−	−
Osteoinductivity	+	+	+/−	−	−
Osteoconductivity	+	+	+	+	+

osteogenic or osteoinductive potential currently available on the market [37,39,41.]

11.10 Alternative strategies to induce new bone formation during GBR procedures

All bone-grafting materials provide the essential osteoconductive properties in that they facilitate three-dimensional bone regrowth. Nevertheless, the main feature sought by many clinicians is the ability for a bone grafting material to provide osteoinduction [42]. Therefore, two main strategies exist, whereby bone grafting materials may either be combined with 1) osteogenic cells or mesenchymal stem cells or 2) bioactive growth factors [43–45]. This first approach aims to utilize mesenchymal stem cells for regenerative procedures by isolating stem cells and seeding them directly onto bone scaffolds [46]. While this strategy has shown positive outcomes in randomized clinical trials, the complexity of such procedures limits its current use as a viable treatment option for everyday dental practice. The more utilized scenario has therefore been the combination of bone grafting materials with the use of biological agents/growth factors capable of speeding new bone formation including BMPs, enamel matrix derivative, or platelet-derived growth factor [22,47,48]. Of this group, it has been especially demonstrated that BMP2 has the most potent ability to induce new bone formation, which has been commercially available with FDA approval [44,49–53]. Interestingly, PRP and PRF have also been investigated as bioactive modifiers as potential sources of growth factors for bone regeneration. The rest of this chapter focuses specifically on the use of PRF during GBR procedures.

11.11 Recent surgical approaches using PRF in combination with GBR

To date, there exist two methods to combine PRF with GBR procedures. The first acts as a barrier membrane, whereby the PRF scaffolds can be flattened into natural autologous barrier membranes with a resorption time of between 10 to 14 days and serves to provide additional wound healing properties to the overlaying soft tissues (Figure 11.3). The second aim is to supply bone-grafting particles with PRF by cutting PRF membranes into small "fragments" and thereafter mixing them with bone-grafting materials. This has been shown to improve the handling properties of bone grafts by making them "stickier" but also additionally provides the proteins and growth factors responsible for facilitating angiogenesis of bone biomaterials. Below we highlight these two separate techniques in case reports.

11.12 PRF as a barrier membrane in GBR procedures

As expressed in previous sections of this chapter, the main principles of GBR are to protect the slower growing bone tissues from fast-growing soft tissues. To accomplish this task, a variety of barrier membranes have been brought to market especially in recent years. While initially PRF was utilized for a variety of biological procedures in dentistry, it became clear that its main effects on soft tissues led to the hypothesis that PRF could potentially serve as a barrier membrane in GBR procedures. It is now well understood that PRF is able to accomplish both soft-tissue regeneration of overlaying tissue, protect the underlying bone tissues from incoming pathogens (due to its accumulation of host-defense immune cells such as leukocytes), and facilitate angiogenesis to the underlying bone structure.

A first case presents a typical PRF membrane following centrifugation (Figure 11.7). It may easily be compressed in a PRF box to produce flattened PRF membranes that may thereafter be used as a replacement to commonly utilized collagen barrier membranes. This may therefore serve as a barrier in simple or complex cases of GBR either utilized around bone grafts but also in combination with advanced implant placement (Figure 11.8). One of the common questions that frequently arises is whether PRF should be utilized alone, or concurrently combined with a collagen barrier membrane. Furthermore, if combined with a collagen membrane, should PRF be placed overtop or underneath this collagen membrane? Following years of research and in agreement with a recent consensus report, PRF membranes may be utilized alone for GBR procedures when re-entry is not expected. The advantages are that the periosteum, which additionally contains a number of progenitor cells, is in contact with living cells from the PRF matrix as opposed to being entirely blocked by a non-living collagen membrane. Interestingly, however, if re-entry is expected and due to the expected attachment occurring between the periosteum and PRF, raising a subsequent periosteal flap following use of PRF is more easily accomplished when PRF is utilized in combination with a collagen barrier membrane. Therefore, if a two-stage surgery is expected, PRF should be utilized in combination with a collagen barrier membrane whereby the collagen barrier membrane is placed directly adjacent to the bone-grafting material to facilitate re-entry,

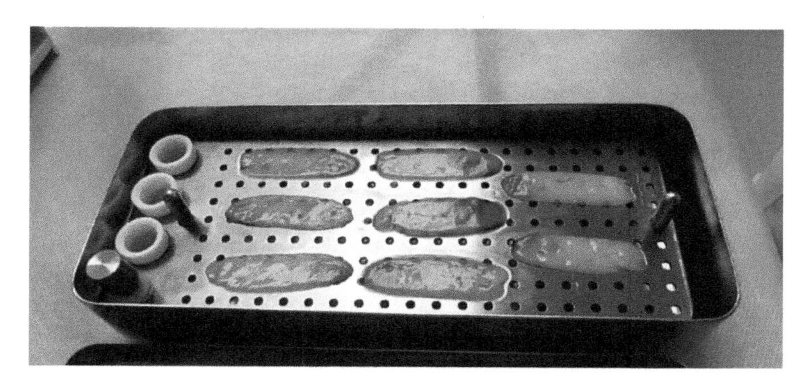

Figure 11.7 Platelet rich fibrin (PRF) scaffolds that have been flattened to be later utilized as barrier membranes during GBR procedures.

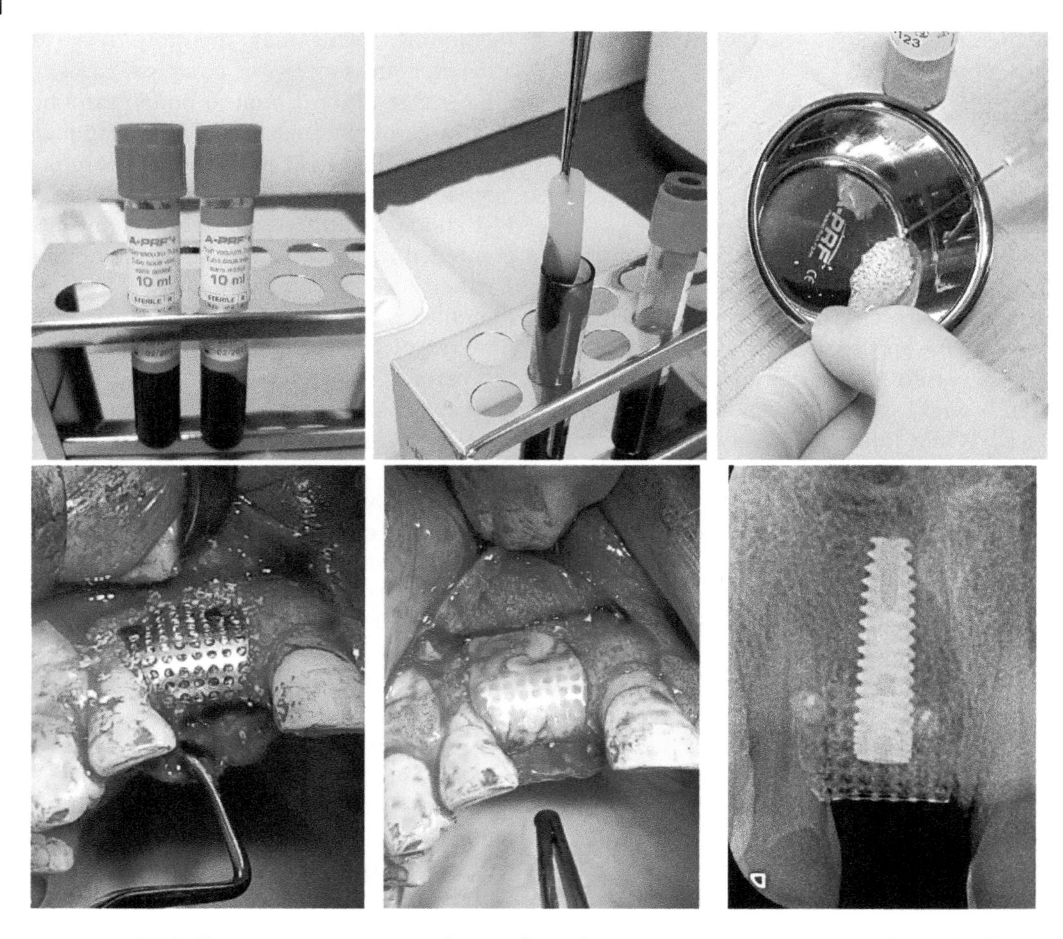

Figure 11.8 Guided bone regenerative procedure performed on a missing upper incisors performed with a bone-grafting material in combination with liquid PRF. Thereafter, a GBR procedure was performed with a titanium mesh to protect the graft from pressure (Case performed by Dr. Adina Manuela Hahaianu).

and the PRF membrane placed overtop and in contact with the soft tissues where it has a more pronounced effect [4]. In this way collagen barrier membranes are additionally protected from membrane exposure leading to a potential risk of infection.

11.13 PRF in combination with bone-grafting materials

More recently, PRF has been cut into small fragments and mixed with bone-grafting materials. While the effects of platelet concentrates on bone-forming osteoblast behavior have been long debated, it is now generally accepted that PRF acts mainly by facilitating angiogenesis of bone tissues, a highly relevant and critical factor during bone regeneration. For these reasons, two PRF membranes are seen in Figure 11.9 cut into small fragments and thereafter mixed with an equal volume of bone-grafting materials. Similarly, the additional use of an injectable liquid PRF can thereafter be combined with bone grafts to improve the stability of the bone graft by acting as a "sticky" matrix. One issue that has been reported in the literature has been whether the combination of PRF into bone grafts has

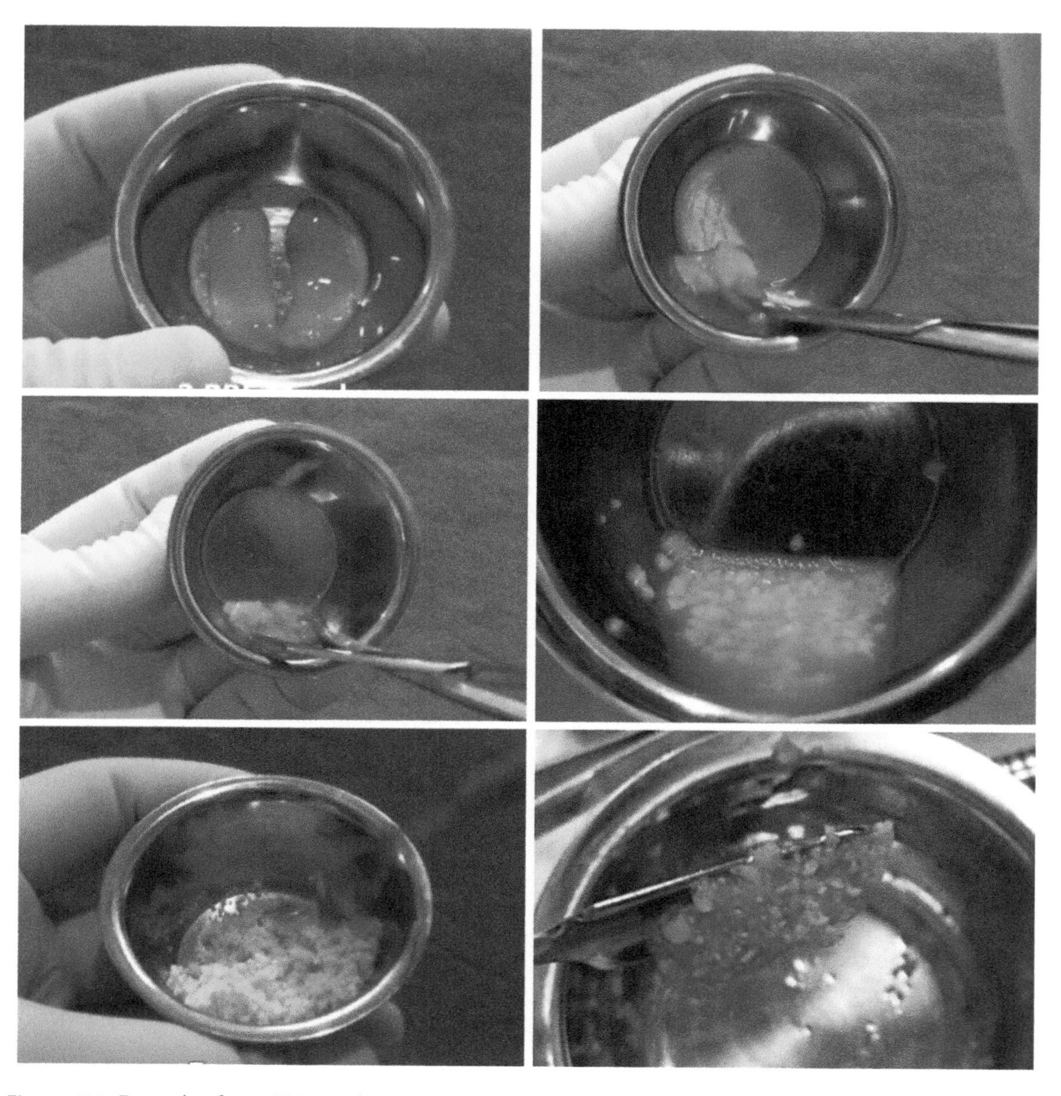

Figure 11.9 Example of two PRF membranes that are cut with surgical scissors and thereafter mixed with particulate bone grafts. Notice the sticky consistency and the better handling properties of bone grafts following this combination approach.

the potential to act as a bone-inducing agent. While PRF alone is not considered osteoinductive by its ability to form ectopic bone formation, its combination with progenitor cells improves the osteoinductive potential of stem cells [54]. Therefore, given the right milieu for bone regeneration, its combination may improve bone regeneration. Below we summarize studies on this topic accordingly.

11.14 Studies investigating PRF for GBR

While PRF has been utilized often in various studies investigating dimensional changes post extraction [3,55–59], much less research has investigated the influence of PRF on pure bone regeneration during GBR procedures. In fact, all studies investigating histologically or radiographically the effect of PRF on GBR have been performed in animal studies with one clinical study investigating implant stability following regeneration with PRF (Table 11.3). In a first study by Liao *et al.* (2011), PRF was examined when combined with MSCs and a GBR membrane to verify the osteogenic potential of bone substitutes. It was found that PRF + MSCs have good potential for bone regeneration, although no valuable controls were investigated supporting the use of PRF [60]. Thereafter, Ozdemir *et al.* (2013) investigated in 24 adult male New Zealand rabbit's calvarium 1) empty, 2) PRF, 3) anorganic bovine bone (ABB, BioOss), and 4) biphasic calcium phosphate (BCP) at 1 and 3 months of healing. It was found that significantly more new bone area was noted in the PRF alone group than in the control group, however, no statistically significant differences were found among PRF, BCP, and ABB groups after 1 month. PRF and ABB had superior new bone formation when compared to the control and the BCP group after 3 months [61]. Yoon *et al.* (2014) investigated the influence of PRF on angiogenesis and osteogenesis in GBR procedures using a xenogenic bone graft in rabbit cranial defects at 1, 2, and 4 months. Each of the experimental sites received bovine bone with PRF, and each of the control sites received bovine bone alone; therefore, a direct comparison was possible. At all experimental time points, immunostaining intensity for VEGF was consistently higher when PRF was utilized when compared to the control group. However, the differences between the control group and the experimental group were not statistically significant in the histomorphometrical and immunohistochemical examinations for new bone formation [62]. Therefore, PRF did not additionally improve new bone formation in this study.

Angelo *et al.* (2014) reported in the only clinical study the biomechanical stability of augmented sites in maxillary bone when bone grafts were used with or without the addition of PRF [63]. Eighty-two patients with horizontal atrophy of the anterior maxillary crest were treated with biphasic (60% HA/40% bTCP) or monophasic (100% bTCP) bone grafts with or without addition of PRF [63]. In total, 109 implants were inserted into the augmented sites with an 8.3 month follow-up and the insertion-torque-value (ITV) was measured as a clinical indication of the (bio)mechanical stability of the augmented bone. The results from this study concluded that the use of PRF did not influence late stability of implants in sites augmented with a bone-grafting material with/without PRF [63].

Knapen *et al.* (2015) investigated the effect of PRF in a total of 72 hemispheres created in the calvaria of 18 rabbits and filled with three different bone fillers: PRF, bovine hydroxyapatite (BHA), BHA + PRF. Empty hemisphere were used as controls (Figure 11.10) [64]. Six rabbits were sacrificed at three distinct time points including at 1 week, 5 weeks, and 12 weeks, and thereafter, histological and histomorphometrical analyses were carried out. It was found that although at the early phase of bone regeneration (1 week), a higher proportion of connective tissue colonized the regeneration chamber in the two groups containing BHA particles, no statistical differences were found within the four groups in terms of bone quantity and quality at each timepoint ($p = .3623$) (Figure 11.11) [64]. According to the present study, PRF did not seem to provide any additional effect on the kinetics or quantity of bone in the present model for GBR [64].

Ezirganli *et al.* (2015) assessed the effects of PRF, BioOss, and BCP bone grafts on total volume resorption levels following bone augmentation in nine New Zealand rabbits [65]. Computed tomography was performed at 90, 120, 150, and 180 days. Statistically significant differences between groups DBBG and BCP were not found; however, statistically significantly lower values were found between bone BioOss/BCP and PRF ($P < 0.001$). While this study did not investigate if bone regeneration could be improved when combined with PRF, it demonstrated that GBR alone with PRF is not sufficient [65].

Table 11.3 Use of Platelet Rich Fibrin (PRF) during various procedures of guided bone regeneration (GBR) in animals and human studies. (GTR = guided tissue regeneration; MSC = mesenchymal stem cells; BCP = bicalcium phosphate bone graft).

Author	Defect	Healing Period	Groups	Main Outcomes
Liao *et al.* (2011)	Guided Osteogenesis in dogs	2 and 4 months	1) GTR + PRF, 2) PRF MSC, 3) GTR alone, 4) empty	Autologous PRF plus osteoinductive MSCs have good potential for bone regeneration.
Ozdemir *et al.* (2013)	rabbits, GBR calvaria	1, 3 months	1) control, 2) PRF, 3) BioOss, 4) BCP	Significantly more new bone area was noted in the PRF alone group than in the control group, no statistically significant differences were found among PRF, BCP, and ABB groups after 1 month. PRF and ABB also had superior effects in new bone formation area control to the BCP group after 3 months.
Yoon *et al.* (2014)	rabbit, calvarial circular defects	1, 2, 4 weeks	1) BioOss, 2) BioOss + PRF	At all experimental time points, immunostaining intensity for VEGF was consistently higher in the experimental group than in the control group. However, PRF along with xenogenic bone substitutes does not show a significant effect on bony regeneration.
Angelo *et al.* (2015)	Biomechanic stability after augmented maxillary	8 months	1) bone graft, 2) bone graft + PRF	The use of PRF did not influence late stability of implants in sites augmented with a bone grafting material with/without PRF.
Knapen *et al.* (2015)	72 hemispheres in rabbits	1, 5 and 12 weeks	1) empty, 2) PRF, 3) BIoOss, 4) BioOss + PRF	According to the present study, L-PRF does not seem to provide any additional effect on the kinetics, quality, and quantity of bone in the present model of guided bone regeneration.
Ezirganly *et al.* (2015)	18 bone defects in rabbits	90, 120, 150, 180 days	1) PRF, BioOss, 3) BCP	According to the total volume on the 90th and 180th days, statistically significant differences between groups BioOss and BCP were not found; however, statistically significant differences were found between group PRF and the others groups ($P < 0.001$).
Kawase *et al.* (2015)	mice, subcutaneous defects	10-21 days	1) PRF, 2) iron-heated PRF	The heat-compression technique doubled the resorption rates (21 days) when compared to standard PRF (10 day resorption in mice)

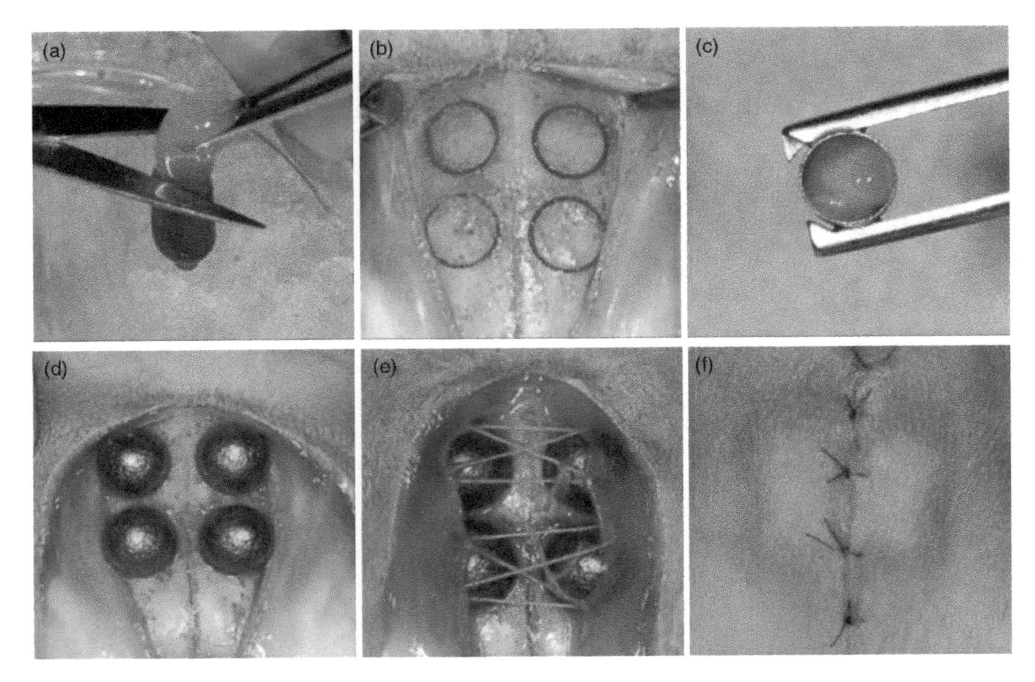

Figure 11.10 Animal experiment investigating new bone formation utilizing PRF with a bone-grafting material. (A) PRF preparation, the red cell clot is removed; (B) the partial osteotomies; (C) PRF placed in the hemisphere; (D) the hemispheres inserted in the partial osteotomies; (E) periosteal closure; (F) wound closure. Source: Knapen *et al.* 2015 [64]. Reproduced with permission of John Wiley & Sons.

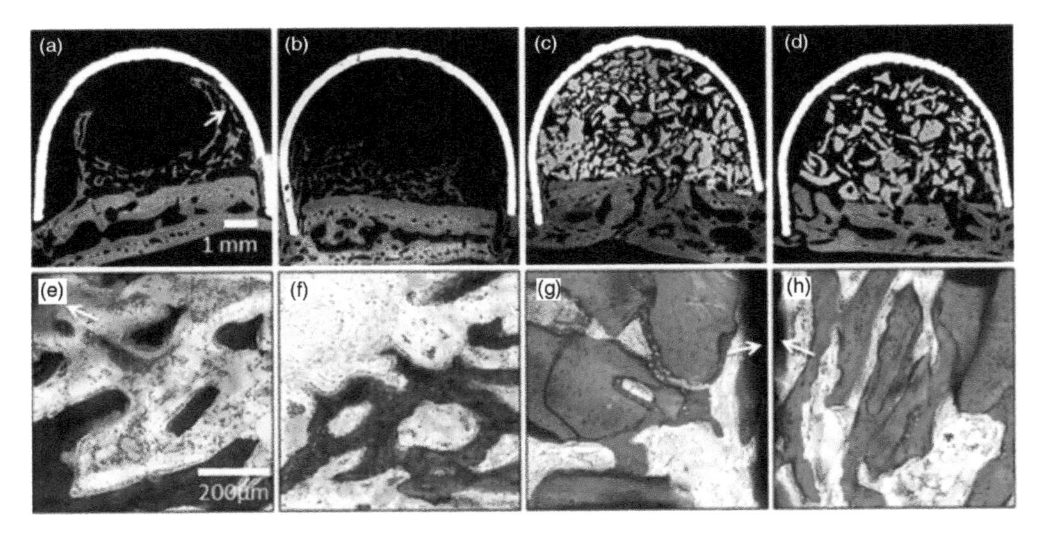

Figure 11.11 Study published demonstrating that PRF did not facilitate new bone formation when combined with a bone grafting material. The same scale was used for A, B, C, D, and E, F, G, H, respectively. SEM pictures at the 5-week time point: (A) empty hemisphere, the white arrow shows the bone growing against the wall; (B) L-PRF hemisphere; (C) BHA hemisphere; (D) BHA + L-PRF hemisphere. Methylene blue/basic fusine pictures: (E) empty hemisphere, the white arrow indicates a massive blood clot; (F) L-PRF hemisphere; (G) BHA hemisphere, the white arrow indicates the titan wall; (H) BHA + L-PRF hemisphere, the white arrow indicates the titan wall. BHA = bovine hydroxyapatite; L-PRF = leukocyte- and platelet rich fibrin; SEM = scanning electron microscopy. Source: Knapen *et al.* 2015 [64]. Reproduced with permission of John Wiley & Sons.

In a final study by Kawase *et al.* (2015), it was observed that the resorption properties of PRF membranes could be altered by heating, although the use of such a technique has not been brought to clinical practice [66].

In conclusion, it may be reported that 1) PRF alone cannot be used to increase horizontal or vertical bone and must be combined with bone grafting materials. 2) PRF has mild potential to enhance new bone formation for GBR procedures as a result of 3) enhancement on early vascularization of bone tissues, important for new bone formation in complex regenerative cases. Therefore, and based on the presented literature, there is limited data with much further research needed to further characterize the use of PRF in GBR in humans.

11.15 Discussion and future research

Despite the increasing popularity of PRF and its use in regenerative dentistry, it remains interesting to point out that there is limited availability of studies (especially clinical) that support its effectiveness during GBR. Data from soft tissues regenerated with PRF strongly support its use [4]. Therefore, the use of PRF as a barrier membrane is hypothesized to strongly contribute to tissue regeneration in GBR procedures yet no study to date has characterized its regenerative potential. This missing study is therefore greatly needed. As potential for future research, it becomes imminent to further characterize the soft-tissue wound healing parameters in well-controlled studies when PRF is utilized as a barrier membrane for GBR procedures.

Interestingly, research has now shown that PRF acts to promote new bone formation post-extraction. Therefore, more research determining why under one clinical scenario, PRF leads to enhanced new bone formation in extraction sockets, whereas during GBR procedures, the data is limited. PRF for extraction socket management has ultimately been shown to preserve the quality and density of the residual ridge, reduce infection rates and operation time. These benefits are increasingly associated with a low cost of operation and a minimal or no risk of infection. In a recent systematic review article, it was concluded by a group of 20 leading experts that there remains a great necessity to further study the effects of PRF during new bone formation. While collagen barrier membranes are standard during such procedures, additional use or replacement altogether with PRF may provide further regenerative advantages when compared to collagen barrier membranes alone. Future studies are thus necessary to validate these potential advantages.

Another area of research where PRF could potentially show some benefit is following GBR procedures with either autologous/allogeneic bone blocks or in combination with titanium meshes. For instance, one reported problem in the literature while using autogenous and more specifically allogenic bone blocks has been the risk of exposure (Figure 11.12). For these reasons, it may be worthwhile to completely cover autogenous bone blocks with PRF membranes to favor revascularization of these tissues and reduce risk of block exposure/infection. A similar risk of exposure has also been observed while utilizing titanium meshes during GBR procedures [67]. Therefore, attempts have been made to cover titanium meshes with PRF membranes either with/without additional collagen membranes (Figure 11.13). While this strategy has been adapted more frequently by many clinicians, few studies have published the long-term results to determine if the rate of exposure is in fact reduced.

It must also be mentioned that since PRF stimulates tissues mainly due to its angiogenic properties, it has the potential to increase the regeneration of many tissues simultaneously as opposed to one specific tissue. PRF has therefore been shown to affect many cell types by stimulating the recruitment and proliferation of endothelial

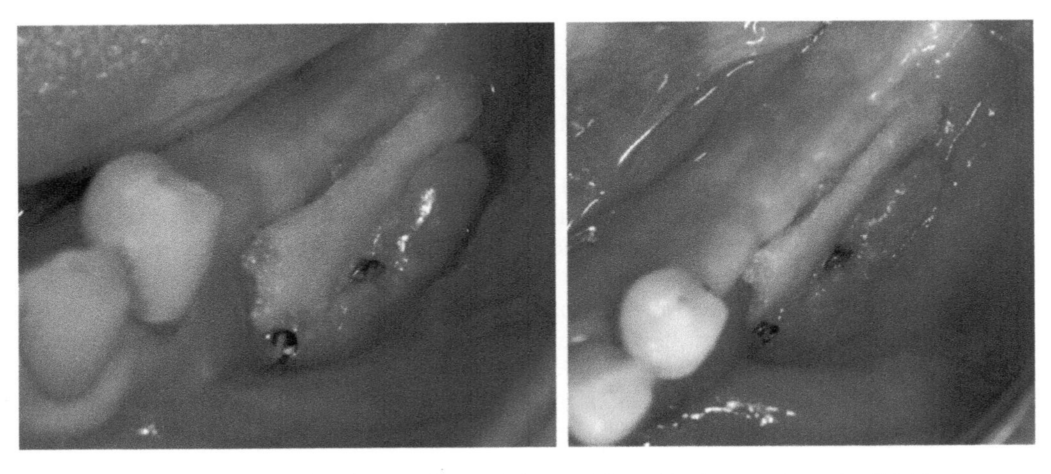

Figure 11.12 GBR procedures with either autologous/allogeneic bone blocks pose the potential risk of exposure following surgery (Case corrected by Dr. Michael A. Pikos).

cells, gingival fibroblast, chondrocytes, and osteoblasts thereby heavily promoting tissue repair and angiogenesis at the site of injury [68,69]. It remains to be investigated what effect the use of local autologous growth factors found in PRF compared to the growing use of recombinant growth factors such as PDGF or BMP may play in regeneration of various tissues in the oral cavity [42,70–72]. Since the main blood protein found in PRF is also PDGF, it remains of interest to compare the wound healing properties of both rhPDGF to PRF in standardized defects in well-controlled studies. Although recombinant proteins have a well-documented regenerative potential [73–75], many biological limitations to their use, including low stability, fast degradation rates, coupled with extremely high costs, might favor the use of PRF. Future research should therefore compare the half-life and bioactivity of the growth factors found in PRF in comparison to recombinant growth factors.

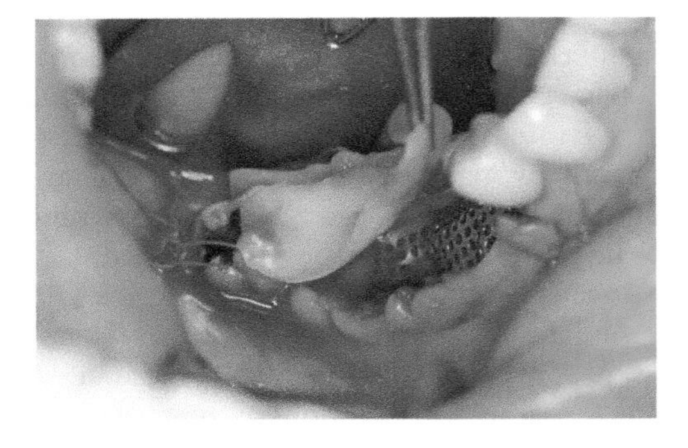

Figure 11.13 GBR procedures demonstrating the use of a PRF membrane to cover a titanium mesh to reduce the risk of exposure (Case performed by Dr. Michael A. Pikos).

One additional area of research highly relevant to the PRF field that has gained much attention in recent years has been that of personalized medicine. It remains interesting to point out that based on the authors personal experience, it is well understood that not all centrifugation protocols are equivalent and lead to the same amount of growth factor concentrations. This is mainly due to the patient's individual variability with respect to their hematocrit values as well as other factors such as patient age, patient sex, patient medical history, and patient medication. It remains virtually unknown how any of these parameters may affect PRF clot formation/stability and growth factor release over time. Therefore, future research investigating patient differences/variability, most notably hematocrit values may further play a role in the centrifugation protocols utilizing PRF.

In conclusion, the literature seems to point to the fact that the use of PRF for regenerative procedures seems to favor soft-tissue regeneration when compared to hard tissues. To date, only a limited supply of available study support the ability for PRF to improve new bone formation and therefore future study is eminently needed. Overall, studies do demonstrate that use of PRF favors rapid angiogenesis of tissues, an area highly relevant to bone regeneration. Additionally, the handling properties of bone grafts may be further improved when combining PRF to bone particles, particularly favoring graft stability. Future research investigating PRF as a barrier membrane and as a replacement to standard collagen membranes seem to be a potential future use of PRF during GBR procedures.

References

1 Gottlow J, Nyman S, Karring T, Lindhe J. New attachment formation as the result of controlled tissue regeneration. J Clin Periodontol. 1984;11(8):494–503.
2 Choukroun J, Adda F, Schoeffler C, Vervelle A. Une opportunité en paro-implantologie: le PRF. Implantodontie. 2001;42(55):e62.
3 Hoaglin DR, Lines GK. Prevention of localized osteitis in mandibular third-molar sites using platelet-rich fibrin. International journal of dentistry. 2013; 2013:875380.
4 Miron RJ, Fujioka-Kobayashi M, Bishara M, Zhang Y, Hernandez M, Choukroun J. Platelet-Rich Fibrin and Soft Tissue Wound Healing: A Systematic Review. Tissue engineering Part B, Reviews. 2016.
5 Jung RE, Fenner N, Hammerle CH, Zitzmann NU. Long-term outcome of implants placed with guided bone regeneration (GBR) using resorbable and non-resorbable membranes after 12-14 years. Clinical oral implants research. 2013; 24(10):1065–73.
6 Dahlin C, Linde A, Gottlow J, Nyman S. Healing of bone defects by guided tissue regeneration. Plast Reconstr Surg. 1988; 81(5):672–6.
7 Buser D, Dula K, Belser U, Hirt HP, Berthold H. Localized ridge augmentation using guided bone regeneration. 1. Surgical procedure in the maxilla. The International journal of periodontics & restorative dentistry. 1993;13(1):29–45.
8 Buser D, Dahlin C, Schenk R. Guided bone regeneration. Chicago: Quintessence. 1994.
9 Hardwick R, Dahlin C. Healing pattern of bone regeneration in membrane-protected defects: a histologic study in the canine mandible. The International journal of oral & maxillofacial implants. 1994;9(1):13–29.
10 Fujihara K, Kotaki M, Ramakrishna S. Guided bone regeneration membrane made of polycaprolactone/calcium carbonate composite nano-fibers. Biomaterials. 2005;26(19):4139–47.
11 Toffler M. Guided bone regeneration (GBR) using cortical bone pins in combination with leukocyte-and platelet-rich fibrin (L-PRF). Compend Contin Educ Dent. 2014;35(3):192–8.
12 Salata LA, Hatton PV, Devlin AJ, Craig GT, Brook IM. In vitro and in vivo evaluation of e-PTFE and alkali-cellulose membranes for guided bone regeneration. Clinical oral implants research. 2001;12(1):62–8.
13 Carbonell J, Martín IS, Santos A, Pujol A, Sanz-Moliner J, Nart J. High-density polytetrafluoroethylene membranes in guided bone and tissue regeneration procedures: a literature review. International journal of oral and maxillofacial surgery. 2014;43(1):75–84.
14 Sigurdsson TJ, Hardwick R, Bogle GC, Wikesjö UM. Periodontal repair in dogs: space provision by reinforced ePTFE membranes enhances bone and cementum regeneration in large supraalveolar defects.

Journal of periodontology. 1994;65(4): 350–6.

15 Sculean A, Donos N, Brecx M, Reich E, Karring T. Treatment of intrabony defects with guided tissue regeneration and enamel-matrix-proteins. Journal of clinical periodontology. 2000;27(7):466–72.

16 Chiapasco M, Zaniboni M. Clinical outcomes of GBR procedures to correct peri-implant dehiscences and fenestrations: a systematic review. Clinical oral implants research. 2009;20(s4): 113–23.

17 Kuchler U, Chappuis V, Gruber R, Lang NP, Salvi GE. Immediate implant placement with simultaneous guided bone regeneration in the esthetic zone: 10-year clinical and radiographic outcomes. Clinical oral implants research. 2016;27(2): 253–7.

18 Zitzmann NU, Naef R, Schärer P. Resorbable versus nonresorbable membranes in combination with Bio-Oss for guided bone regeneration. International Journal of Oral & Maxillofacial Implants. 1997;12(6).

19 Zhang Y, Zhang X, Shi B, Miron R. Membranes for guided tissue and bone regeneration. Annals of Oral & Maxillofacial Surgery. 2013;1(1):10.

20 Gentile P, Chiono V, Tonda-Turo C, Ferreira AM, Ciardelli G. Polymeric membranes for guided bone regeneration. Biotechnology Journal. 2011;6(10): 1187–97.

21 Rakhmatia YD, Ayukawa Y, Furuhashi A, Koyano K. Current barrier membranes: titanium mesh and other membranes for guided bone regeneration in dental applications. Journal of prosthodontic research. 2013;57(1):3–14.

22 Nguyen TT, Mui B, Mehrabzadeh M, Chea Y, Chaudhry Z, Chaudhry K, et al. Regeneration of Tissues of the Oral Complex: Current. J Can Dent Assoc. 2013; 79:d1.

23 AlGhamdi AS, Ciancio SG. Guided tissue regeneration membranes for periodontal regeneration–a literature review. Journal of the International Academy of Periodontology. 2009;11(3):226–31.

24 Rakhmatia YD, Ayukawa Y, Furuhashi A, Koyano K. Current barrier membranes: Titanium mesh and other membranes for guided bone regeneration in dental applications. J Prosthodont Res. 2013;57(1): 3–14.

25 Thoma DS, Halg GA, Dard MM, Seibl R, Hammerle CH, Jung RE. Evaluation of a new biodegradable membrane to prevent gingival ingrowth into mandibular bone defects in minipigs. Clin Oral Implants Res. 2009;20(1):7–16.

26 Sculean A, Nikolidakis D, Schwarz F. Regeneration of periodontal tissues: combinations of barrier membranes and grafting materials - biological foundation and preclinical evidence: a systematic review. J Clin Periodontol. 2008; 35(8 Suppl):106–16.

27 Del Corso M, Vervelle A, Simonpieri A, Jimbo R, Inchingolo F, Sammartino G, et al. Current knowledge and perspectives for the use of platelet-rich plasma (PRP) and platelet-rich fibrin (PRF) in oral and maxillofacial surgery part 1: Periodontal and dentoalveolar surgery. Current pharmaceutical biotechnology. 2012;13(7): 1207–30.

28 Simonpieri A, Del Corso M, Vervelle A, Jimbo R, Inchingolo F, Sammartino G, et al. Current knowledge and perspectives for the use of platelet-rich plasma (PRP) and platelet-rich fibrin (PRF) in oral and maxillofacial surgery part 2: Bone graft, implant and reconstructive surgery. Current pharmaceutical biotechnology. 2012;13(7):1231–56.

29 Marx RE. Platelet-rich plasma: evidence to support its use. Journal of oral and maxillofacial surgery. 2004;62(4):489–96.

30 Marx RE, Carlson ER, Eichstaedt RM, Schimmele SR, Strauss JE, Georgeff KR. Platelet-rich plasma: growth factor enhancement for bone grafts. Oral Surgery, Oral Medicine, Oral Pathology, Oral Radiology, and Endodontology. 1998;85(6): 638–46.

31 Choukroun J, Diss A, Simonpieri A, Girard MO, Schoeffler C, Dohan SL, et al. Platelet-rich fibrin (PRF): a second-generation platelet concentrate. Part IV: clinical effects on tissue healing. Oral surgery, oral medicine, oral pathology, oral radiology, and endodontics. 2006; 101(3):e56–60.
32 Dohan DM, Choukroun J, Diss A, Dohan SL, Dohan AJ, Mouhyi J, et al. Platelet-rich fibrin (PRF): a second-generation platelet concentrate. Part I: technological concepts and evolution. Oral surgery, oral medicine, oral pathology, oral radiology, and endodontics. 2006;101(3):e37–44.
33 Dohan DM, Choukroun J, Diss A, Dohan SL, Dohan AJ, Mouhyi J, et al. Platelet-rich fibrin (PRF): a second-generation platelet concentrate. Part II: platelet-related biologic features. Oral surgery, oral medicine, oral pathology, oral radiology, and endodontics. 2006;101(3):e45–50.
34 Dohan DM, Choukroun J, Diss A, Dohan SL, Dohan AJ, Mouhyi J, et al. Platelet-rich fibrin (PRF): a second-generation platelet concentrate. Part III: leucocyte activation: a new feature for platelet concentrates? Oral surgery, oral medicine, oral pathology, oral radiology, and endodontics. 2006;101(3): e51–5.
35 Choukroun J, Diss A, Simonpieri A, Girard MO, Schoeffler C, Dohan SL, et al. Platelet-rich fibrin (PRF): a second-generation platelet concentrate. Part V: histologic evaluations of PRF effects on bone allograft maturation in sinus lift. Oral surgery, oral medicine, oral pathology, oral radiology, and endodontics. 2006; 101(3):299–303.
36 Miron RJ, Saulacic N, Buser D, Iizuka T, Sculean A. Osteoblast proliferation and differentiation on a barrier membrane in combination with BMP2 and TGFbeta1. Clinical oral investigations. 2013;17(3): 981–8.
37 Miron RJ, Sculean A, Shuang Y, Bosshardt DD, Gruber R, Buser D, et al. Osteoinductive potential of a novel biphasic calcium phosphate bone graft in comparison with autographs, xenografts, and DFDBA. Clinical oral implants research. 2016;27(6):668–75.
38 Giannoudis PV, Dinopoulos H, Tsiridis E. Bone substitutes: an update. Injury. 2005; 36(3):S20–S7.
39 Fretwurst T, Gad LM, Nelson K, Schmelzeisen R. Dentoalveolar reconstruction: modern approaches. Current opinion in otolaryngology & head and neck surgery. 2015;23(4): 316–22.
40 Sanz M, Vignoletti F. Key aspects on the use of bone substitutes for bone regeneration of edentulous ridges. Dental Materials. 2015;31(6):640–7.
41 Donos N, Kostopoulos L, Tonetti M, Karring T, Lang NP. The effect of enamel matrix proteins and deproteinized bovine bone mineral on heterotopic bone formation. Clinical oral implants research. 2006;17(4):434–8.
42 Miron RJ, Zhang YF. Osteoinduction: a review of old concepts with new standards. Journal of dental research. 2012;91(8): 736–44.
43 Lioubavina-Hack N, Carmagnola D, Lynch SE, Karring T. Effect of Bio-Oss® with or without platelet-derived growth factor on bone formation by "guided tissue regeneration": a pilot study in rats. Journal of clinical periodontology. 2005;32(12): 1254–60.
44 Zhang Y, Yang S, Zhou W, Fu H, Qian L, Miron RJ. Addition of a Synthetically Fabricated Osteoinductive Biphasic Calcium Phosphate Bone Graft to BMP2 Improves New Bone Formation. Clinical implant dentistry and related research. 2015.
45 Hämmerle CH, Giannobile WV. Biology of soft tissue wound healing and regeneration–Consensus Report of Group 1 of the 10th European Workshop on Periodontology. Journal of clinical periodontology. 2014;41(s15).
46 Kaigler D, Pagni G, Park CH, Braun TM, Holman LA, Yi E, et al. Stem cell therapy for craniofacial bone regeneration: a

randomized, controlled feasibility trial. Cell transplantation. 2013;22(5):767–77.

47 Turri A, Elgali I, Vazirisani F, Johansson A, Emanuelsson L, Dahlin C, et al. Guided bone regeneration is promoted by the molecular events in the membrane compartment. Biomaterials. 2016;84: 167–83.

48 Shuang Y, Yizhen L, Zhang Y, Fujioka-Kobayashi M, Sculean A, Miron RJ. In vitro characterization of an osteoinductive biphasic calcium phosphate in combination with recombinant BMP2. BMC Oral Health. 2016;17(1):35.

49 Ryoo H-M, Lee M-H, Kim Y-J. Critical molecular switches involved in BMP-2-induced osteogenic differentiation of mesenchymal cells. Gene. 2006;366(1): 51–7.

50 Wang D, Tabassum A, Wu G, Deng L, Wismeijer D, Liu Y. Bone regeneration in critical-sized bone defect enhanced by introducing osteoinductivity to biphasic calcium phosphate granules. Clinical oral implants research. 2016.

51 Torrecillas-Martinez L, Monje A, Pikos MA, Ortega-Oller I, Suarez F, Galindo-Moreno P, et al. Effect of rhBMP-2 upon maxillary sinus augmentation: a comprehensive review. Implant dentistry. 2013;22(3):232–7.

52 Misch CM, Jensen OT, Pikos MA, Malmquist JP. Vertical bone augmentation using recombinant bone morphogenetic protein, mineralized bone allograft, and titanium mesh: a retrospective cone beam computed tomography study. International Journal of Oral & Maxillofacial Implants. 2015;30(1).

53 Misch C, Wang H-L. Clinical applications of recombinant human bone morphogenetic Protein-2 for bone augmentation before dental implant placement. Clinical Advances in Periodontics. 2011;1(2):118–31.

54 Wang Z, Weng Y, Lu S, Zong C, Qiu J, Liu Y, et al. Osteoblastic mesenchymal stem cell sheet combined with Choukroun platelet-rich fibrin induces bone formation at an ectopic site. Journal of biomedical materials research Part B, Applied biomaterials. 2015;103(6):1204–16.

55 Girish Rao S, Bhat P, Nagesh KS, Rao GH, Mirle B, Kharbhari L, et al. Bone regeneration in extraction sockets with autologous platelet rich fibrin gel. Journal of maxillofacial and oral surgery. 2013; 12(1):11–6.

56 Suttapreyasri S, Leepong N. Influence of platelet-rich fibrin on alveolar ridge preservation. The Journal of craniofacial surgery. 2013;24(4):1088–94.

57 Hauser F, Gaydarov N, Badoud I, Vazquez L, Bernard JP, Ammann P. Clinical and histological evaluation of postextraction platelet-rich fibrin socket filling: a prospective randomized controlled study. Implant dentistry. 2013;22(3):295–303.

58 Anwandter A, Bohmann S, Nally M, Castro AB, Quirynen M, Pinto N. Dimensional changes of the post extraction alveolar ridge, preserved with Leukocyte- and Platelet Rich Fibrin: A clinical pilot study. Journal of dentistry. 2016;52:23–9.

59 Temmerman A, Vandessel J, Castro A, Jacobs R, Teughels W, Pinto N, et al. The use of leucocyte and platelet-rich fibrin in socket management and ridge preservation: a split-mouth, randomized, controlled clinical trial. Journal of clinical periodontology. 2016;43(11):990–9.

60 Liao HT, Chen CT, Chen CH, Chen JP, Tsai JC. Combination of guided osteogenesis with autologous platelet-rich fibrin glue and mesenchymal stem cell for mandibular reconstruction. The Journal of trauma. 2011;70(1):228–37.

61 Ozdemir H, Ezirganli S, Isa Kara M, Mihmanli A, Baris E. Effects of platelet rich fibrin alone used with rigid titanium barrier. Archives of oral biology. 2013; 58(5):537–44.

62 Yoon JS, Lee SH, Yoon HJ. The influence of platelet-rich fibrin on angiogenesis in guided bone regeneration using xenogenic bone substitutes: a study of rabbit cranial defects. Journal of cranio-maxillo-facial surgery : official publication of the

European Association for Cranio-Maxillo-Facial Surgery. 2014;42(7):1071–7.

63 Angelo T, Marcel W, Andreas K, Izabela S. Biomechanical Stability of Dental Implants in Augmented Maxillary Sites: Results of a Randomized Clinical Study with Four Different Biomaterials and PRF and a Biological View on Guided Bone Regeneration. BioMed research international. 2015;2015:850340.

64 Knapen M, Gheldof D, Drion P, Layrolle P, Rompen E, Lambert F. Effect of leukocyte- and platelet-rich fibrin (L-PRF) on bone regeneration: a study in rabbits. Clinical implant dentistry and related research. 2015;17 Suppl 1:e143–52.

65 Ezirganli S, Kazancioglu HO, Mihmanli A, Sharifov R, Aydin MS. Effects of different biomaterials on augmented bone volume resorptions. Clinical oral implants research. 2015;26(12):1482–8.

66 Kawase T, Kamiya M, Kobayashi M, Tanaka T, Okuda K, Wolff LF, et al. The heat-compression technique for the conversion of platelet-rich fibrin preparation to a barrier membrane with a reduced rate of biodegradation. Journal of biomedical materials research Part B, Applied biomaterials. 2015;103(4):825–31.

67 Louis PJ, Gutta R, Said-Al-Naief N, Bartolucci AA. Reconstruction of the maxilla and mandible with particulate bone graft and titanium mesh for implant placement. Journal of Oral and Maxillofacial Surgery. 2008;66(2):235–45.

68 Roy S, Driggs J, Elgharably H, Biswas S, Findley M, Khanna S, et al. Platelet-rich fibrin matrix improves wound angiogenesis via inducing endothelial cell proliferation. Wound repair and regeneration : official publication of the Wound Healing Society [and] the European Tissue Repair Society. 2011;19(6):753–66.

69 Chen FM, Wu LA, Zhang M, Zhang R, Sun HH. Homing of endogenous stem/progenitor cells for in situ tissue regeneration: Promises, strategies, and translational perspectives. Biomaterials. 2011;32(12):3189–209.

70 Steed DL, Donohoe D, Webster MW, Lindsley L. Effect of extensive debridement and treatment on the healing of diabetic foot ulcers. Diabetic Ulcer Study Group. J Am Coll Surg. 1996;183(1):61–4.

71 Wieman TJ, Smiell JM, Su Y. Efficacy and safety of a topical gel formulation of recombinant human platelet-derived growth factor-BB (becaplermin) in patients with chronic neuropathic diabetic ulcers. A phase III randomized placebo-controlled double-blind study. Diabetes care. 1998; 21(5):822–7.

72 White AP, Vaccaro AR, Hall JA, Whang PG, Friel BC, McKee MD. Clinical applications of BMP-7/OP-1 in fractures, nonunions and spinal fusion. International orthopaedics. 2007;31(6):735–41.

73 Young CS, Ladd PA, Browning CF, Thompson A, Bonomo J, Shockley K, et al. Release, biological potency, and biochemical integrity of recombinant human platelet-derived growth factor-BB (rhPDGF-BB) combined with Augment(TM) Bone Graft or GEM 21S beta-tricalcium phosphate (beta-TCP). Journal of controlled release : official journal of the Controlled Release Society. 2009;140(3):250–5.

74 Park YJ, Lee YM, Lee JY, Seol YJ, Chung CP, Lee SJ. Controlled release of platelet-derived growth factor-BB from chondroitin sulfate-chitosan sponge for guided bone regeneration. J Control Release. 2000;67(2-3):385–94.

75 Wissink MJ, Beernink R, Poot AA, Engbers GH, Beugeling T, van Aken WG, et al. Improved endothelialization of vascular grafts by local release of growth factor from heparinized collagen matrices. J Control Release. 2000;64(1-3):103–14.

12

Modern Approach to Full Arch Immediate Loading: The Simonpieri Technique with PRF and i-PRF

Alain Simonpieri

Abstract

The dental rehabilitation of patients with complete edentulism remains a prominent challenge for the daily practitioner. It is now estimated that over 20% of the population aged 65 and older has complete tooth loss and it is further estimated that with an increasingly aging population, this number will only continue to rise. While conventional dentures have been utilized over decades as a means to restore function in edentulous patients, dental implants have played a significant role in both patient quality of life and patient satisfaction by providing stable and fixed anchorage of dentures. For these reasons, a number of full arch dental restorative techniques with implants have more frequently been utilized in modern dentistry with various advantages/disadvantages based on patient anatomy, financial means, and criteria for inclusion. During immediate loading, the survival rate is often based on the outcomes of osseointegration with little regard for final aesthetic outcomes. While the main goal is to achieve osseointegration and aesthetics in order to maintain long-term stability, very few have focused on the stability of bone around implants over long-healing periods or focused on soft-tissue thickness, whereby failure in either of these two factors will induce the loss of the second factor.

This chapter focuses on the requirements needed to achieve and maintain long-term stability by utilizing autologous platelet rich fibrin (PRF) as a biological agent capable of inducing early vascularization of tissues. Furthermore, anatomical and surgical considerations are discussed to optimize implant placement and positioning (Fast Guide, sub-crestal insertion, platform switching). Lastly, the prosthetic requirements are discussed as essential criteria for long-term aesthetics as a guidance for soft-tissue design (rigid and screwed provisional prosthesis). This chapter reports on over 14 years of clinical experiments utilizing PRF for more than 1100 full arch immediate implant cases with over 7500 documented implants.

Highlights

- Full arch immediate implant placement and loading
- Introduction to the Fast Guide system with parallel and symmetrical implant placement
- The use of PRF and an injectable PRF to improve graft stability in large bone augmentation procedures
- Discussion over the biological, anatomical, surgical, and prosthetic requirements for long-term success of full arch immediate loading

Platelet Rich Fibrin in Regenerative Dentistry: Biological Background and Clinical Indications, First Edition.
Edited by Richard J. Miron and Joseph Choukroun.

12.1 Introduction

Full edentulism remains a prominent challenge in dentistry [1]. While national epidemiological surveys conducted throughout the world have suggested that the percentage of fully edentulous patients has gradually decreased over time [1], the drastic rise in the aging population predicts more fully edentulous patients by 2020 than ever before encountered [1,2]. Other national surveys in third-world countries now estimate over 30% of the population aged 65 and over are fully edentulous [3]. In 2012, Eke *et al.* estimated the prevalence, severity, and extent of periodontitis in the adult U.S. population [4]. It was found that over 47% of the population (representing over 60 million adults in the U.S. alone) had periodontitis, distributed as 8.7%, 30.0%, and 8.5% with mild, moderate, and severe cases, respectively. Adults aged 65 years and older had even poorer results with 64% having either moderate or severe periodontitis [4]. Unfortunately, tooth loss is a prominent endpoint for such patients.

Interestingly, it has now been shown that due in large part to the aging "baby boomers," over 14% of the world's total population is 65+ years of age with an edentulous rate ranging from 20% to 30% in this population. It is estimated that between 200 and 300 million people worldwide will require full dentures. While the classical full arch denture is most frequently utilized, it has numerous reported drawbacks documented over the years including poor denture stability, difficulty eating, and pain associated with areas of discomfort [5]. Furthermore, lack of salivary flow, decreased muscle motor control, and reduced bite forces have also been commonly reported problems [6–10]. Masticatory forces for patients wearing complete dentures report less than 20% of original bite forces registered when compared to the natural dentition [11,12].

For these reasons a number of rehabilitation procedures have been introduced over the past three decades making use of dental implants as anchorage devices in order to improve the stability and support of full arch dentures [1]. While original studies focused on the long-term survival of implants loaded following delayed periods, more recent research has aimed at complete rehabilitation of the edentulous patient utilizing immediate-functional loading of fixed prostheses supported by implants [13–19]. These reports are highlighted by high long-term survival rates after complete rehabilitation [13–19].

Noteworthy, however, are the few investigators who have more recently attempted to successfully load full arch immediate implants into fresh extraction sites, drastically reducing the total surgical time needed to fully restore patient oral function [20–26]. While various protocols have been enhanced by modifying implant design, implant length, implant size, and/or angulation of implants, very little study has focused on long-term aesthetic outcomes or long-term soft- and hard-tissue stability over time, an equally important parameter for the longevity of implant success and prevention of future peri-implant tissue disease [27]. While the majority of research in implant dentistry has focused on hard-tissue osseointegration, it is well known that for long-term survival of dental implants, regeneration of soft tissues also carries vast importance [28].

This chapter focuses on results from over 7500 implants placed immediately into fresh extraction sockets loaded immediately in over 1100 full arch cases. A 98% success rate has been achieved in these cases with important surgical concepts being key parameters later discussed throughout this chapter. Discussion over the use of platelet rich fibrin (PRF), either as an injectable-PRF or as a PRF fibrin matrix have been the driving force propelling soft-tissue wound healing and angiogenesis at earlier time points. Below, I summarize my experiences with PRF during full arch immediate implant placement and loading.

12.2 Immediate loading in implant dentistry—what is success?

It has been well-documented in the literature that immediate loading has short- and long-term survival rates of greater than 95% [29–33]. In full arch restorations, however, this does not necessary correspond to success especially as it relates to aesthetics. Figure 12.1 demonstrates numerous examples of full arch immediate implants that maintain their osseointegration, however, the facial aesthetic outcomes in each of these cases may easily be characterized as extremely poor. Therefore, true success in such cases should be defined by not only the osseointegration of dental implants but also the final aesthetic outcomes (Figure 12.2). It has been reported by the International Team for Implantology at the ITI Consensus Conference that soft-tissue stability is an essential criterion for long-term stability of implants and essential for bone volume [34]. Nevertheless, it is also known that soft-tissue stability depends on bone volume.

They are, therefore, both requirements for one another [35–37]. Simply stated: "If you lose bone, you will lose soft tissue. If you lose soft tissue, you will lose bone" (Figure 12.2).

The field of immediate implant dentistry has gradually evolved over time and we now

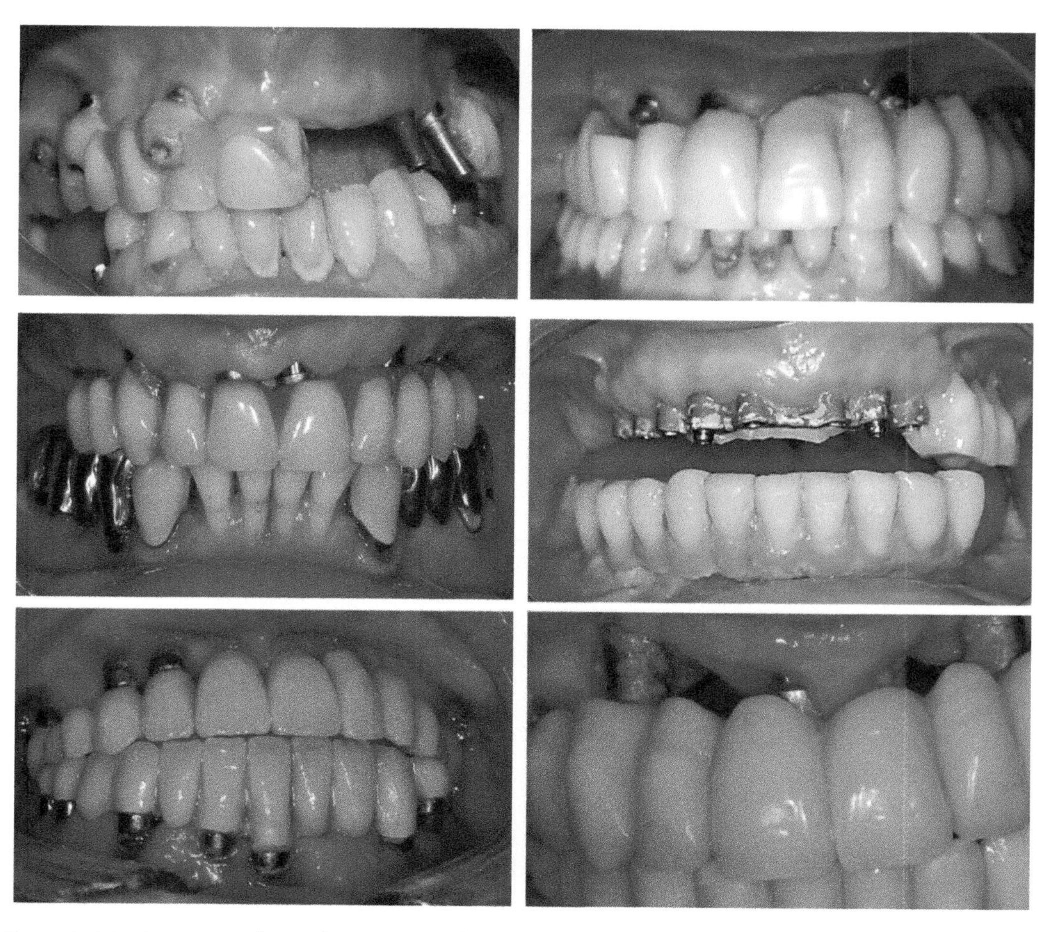

Figure 12.1 Various cases of osseointegrated implants with insufficient aesthetic outcomes.

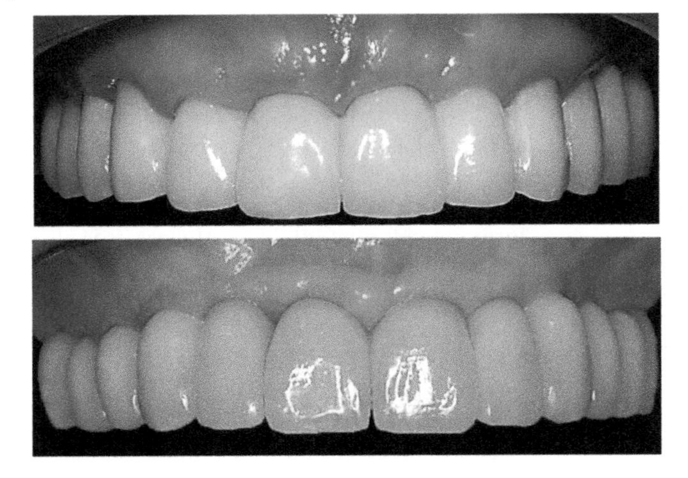

Figure 12.2 Definition of true aesthetic outcomes with both soft-tissue contours and thickness with underlying bone.

know that a triad of requirements must be fulfilled in order to improve the success of these complex protocols (Figure 12.3). These include a) biological requirements, b) anatomical and surgical requirements, and c) prosthetic requirements. This triad of requirements is absolutely essential and provides the guidelines and framework for long-term stability as discussed below.

12.3 Biological requirements

In many senses, of primordial importance for any tissue to grow is an adequate blood supply [38]. It has been shown that by simply adding blood to bone biomaterials, a drastic and marked increase in new vessel ingrowth is observed [39]. Two key concepts important for all surgery is that a) bone density is directly related to blood vessel density [40], and b) tissue tension negatively impacts tissue angiogenesis [41]. For these reasons, tension-free flap closure has been a reported concept in many surgical disciplines in dentistry [42]. Other important factors include patient systemic conditions, including the negative influence of diabetes, cholesterol levels, and vitamin D deficiencies on wound healing [43–50]. Other biological factors that may potentially speed tissue regeneration include the use of growth factors and bone grafting materials with collagen-incorporation being a key

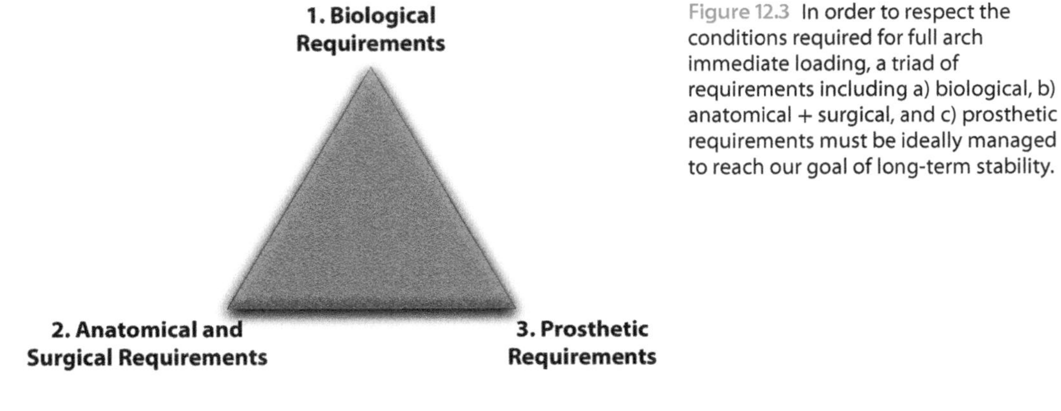

Figure 12.3 In order to respect the conditions required for full arch immediate loading, a triad of requirements including a) biological, b) anatomical + surgical, and c) prosthetic requirements must be ideally managed to reach our goal of long-term stability.

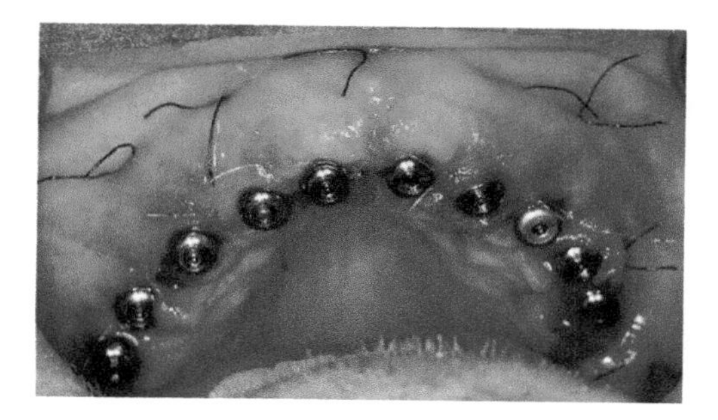

Figure 12.4 Keys to improve revascularization of tissues is by reducing pressure by utilizing tension-free flap closure, specific flap management, and the use of an apical mattress suturing technique.

factor [51–56]. A last avenue that has tremendously helped in the biological realm of regeneration is the ability to naturally derive growth factors from blood via platelet concentrates [57–60]. Platelet rich fibrin contains an array of growth factors along with a naturally derived three-dimensional fibrin matrix. This combination has drastically improved the ability for oral tissues to be revascularized favoring future tissue regeneration. Nevertheless, tension-free flap closure, specific flap management, and apical mattress sutures are all requirements and help by reducing pressure on these revascularized tissues (Figure 12.4).

12.4 Anatomical and surgical requirements

12.4.1 Implant placement

One advancing area of research where a great deal has been learned over the past decade has been the effect of implant placement on aesthetic outcomes [61]. When single teeth are replaced by immediate implant placement in their natural position, it was found that buccal mucosal recession was often encountered with implants threads being often left exposed [62,63]. This is further complicated in the aesthetic zone where the remaining facial bone is less than 1 mm in the majority of cases [64]. For these reasons,

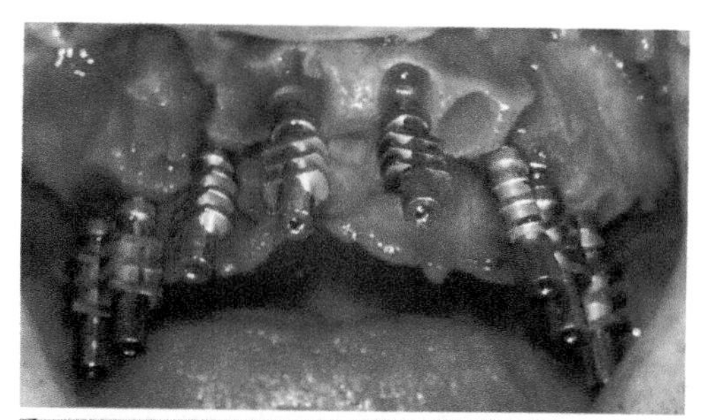

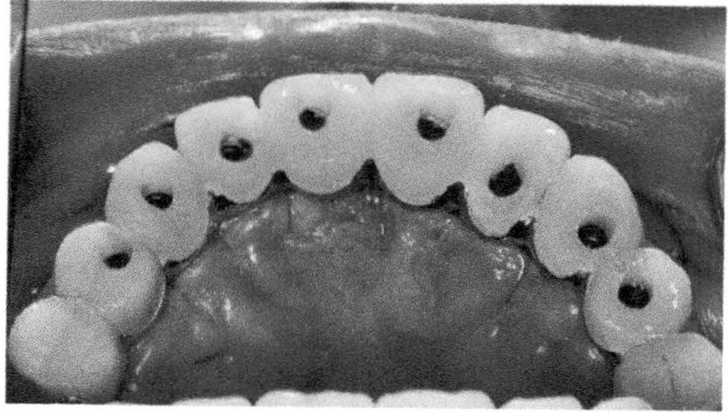

Figure 12.5 During immediate implant placement and for implants placed in general, a palatal placement of implants is generally advised in order to maintain/reconstruct the thin facial wall as well as to allow for screw retained fixed prosthetics.

the International Team for Implantology and others adapted a more palatal approach to implant placement being a crucial key factor for long-term stability. This is equally and potentially more important in immediate implant full arch restorations. As depicted in Figure 12.5, implants are always placed palatally in the prosthetic corridor favoring screw-retained prosthetics. More recently and with additional surgical experience, it has further been shown that the axis of implant preparation and placement is a key component to the long-term aesthetic success. For these reasons, a variety of surgical procedures including digital planning, and surgical guides have been developed to facilitate this task. Interestingly, one of the most natural ways to plan ideal axis of implant placement is to follow the naso-palatal foramen (Figure 12.6). It therefore remains possible to simply place a nasopalatal pin into the foramen as part of a fast guide surgical kit to better guide axial inclinations during implant placement (Figures 12.7 and 12.8). The pin may

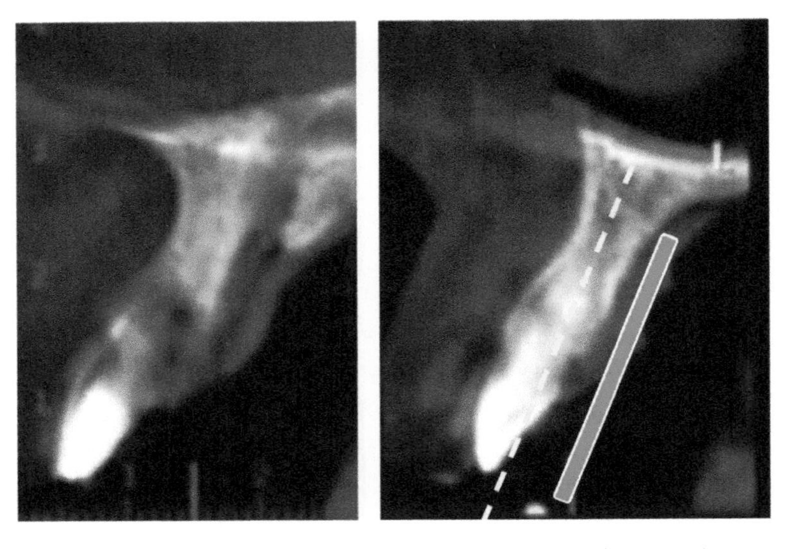

Figure 12.6 Logically, one of the most natural ways to plan for the ideal axis of implant placement is by following the naso-palatal foramen, which follows the natural axis of the central incisors.

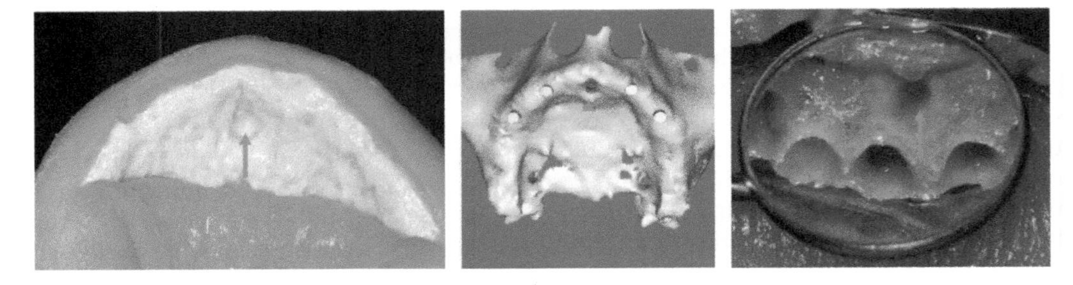

Figure 12.7 Several methods now exist to choose the ideal implant axis including digital planning systems as well as surgical guides. However, the most ideal way is to follow the natural anatomy by utilizing the axis of the nasopalatal foramen.

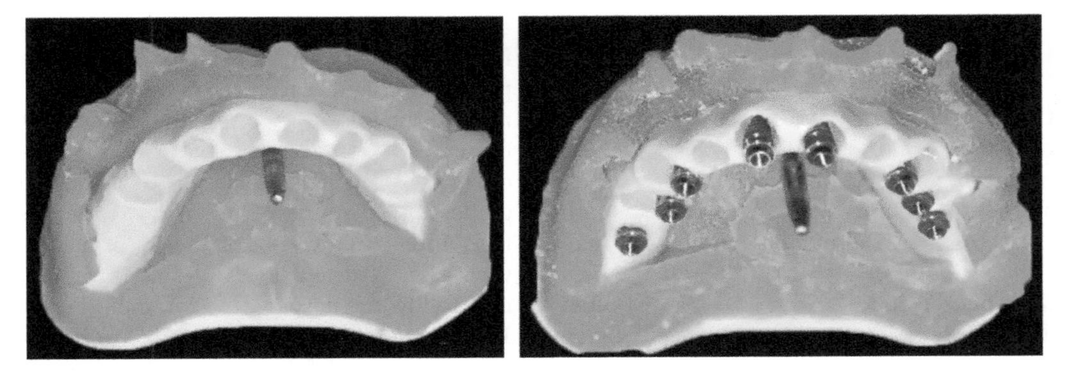

Figure 12.8 Model demonstration of the nasopalatal pin being placed in the naso-palatal foramen. Notice the ease of placement and the axis of insertion ideal for subsequent implant placement.

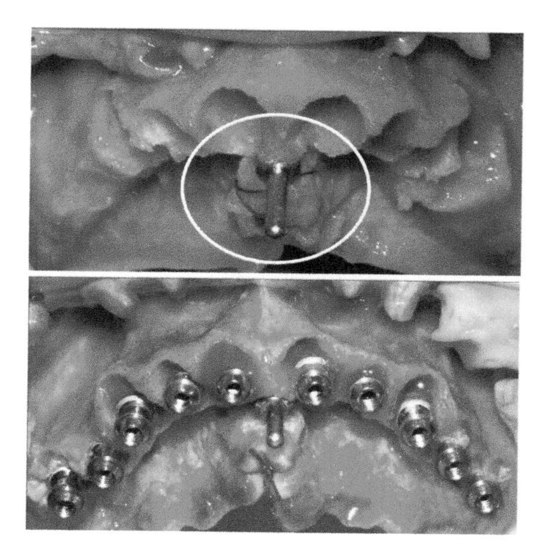

Figure 12.9 Clear demonstration of the nasopalatal pin being placed in the naso-palatal foramen. Notice the ease of placement and the axis of insertion ideal for subsequent implant placement.

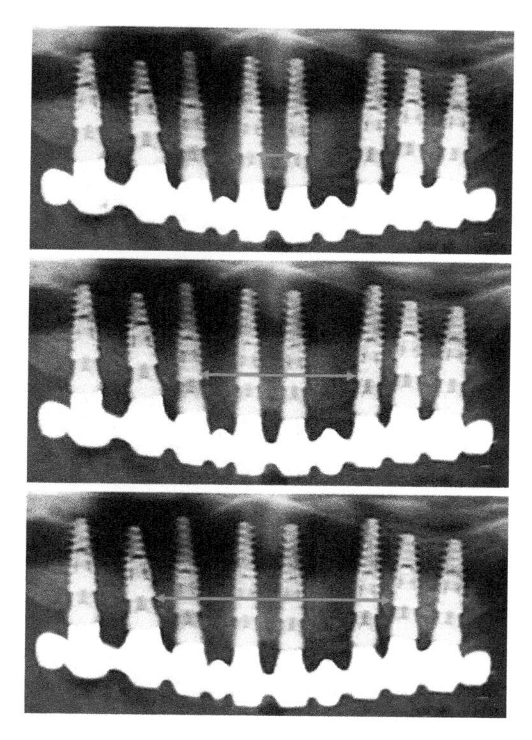

Figure 12.10 Implant placement utilizing this technique must place implants with a symmetry of the incisors, canines, premolars, and so on.

thereafter be followed surgically during implant placement in a linear axis with the pin (Figure 12.9). All implants can therefore be placed with the same axis and with the same result.

It is equally as important for ideal aesthetics to obtain symmetry (Figure 12.10). This concept has long been forgotten especially in full arch implant dentistry where implants are commonly placed at different heights and distances. As part of my full arch technique utilizing the Fast Guide System, it remains essential that all implants be

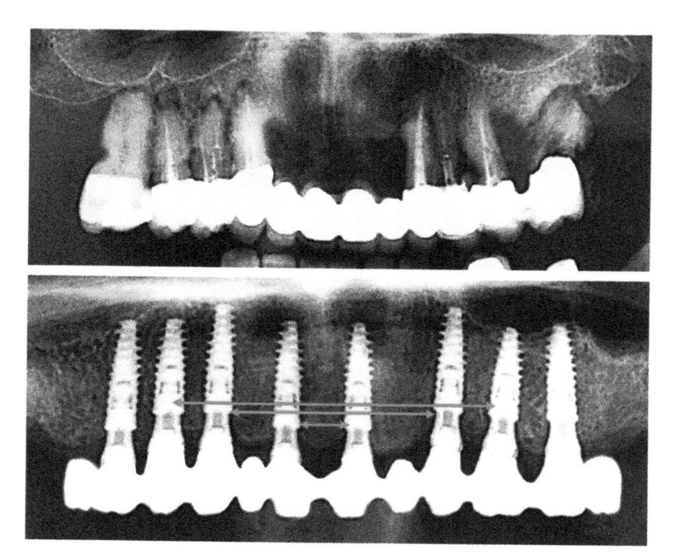

Figure 12.11 Implant placement utilizing this technique was first achieved during conventional implant therapy, but has since been most frequently utilized during immediate implant placement.

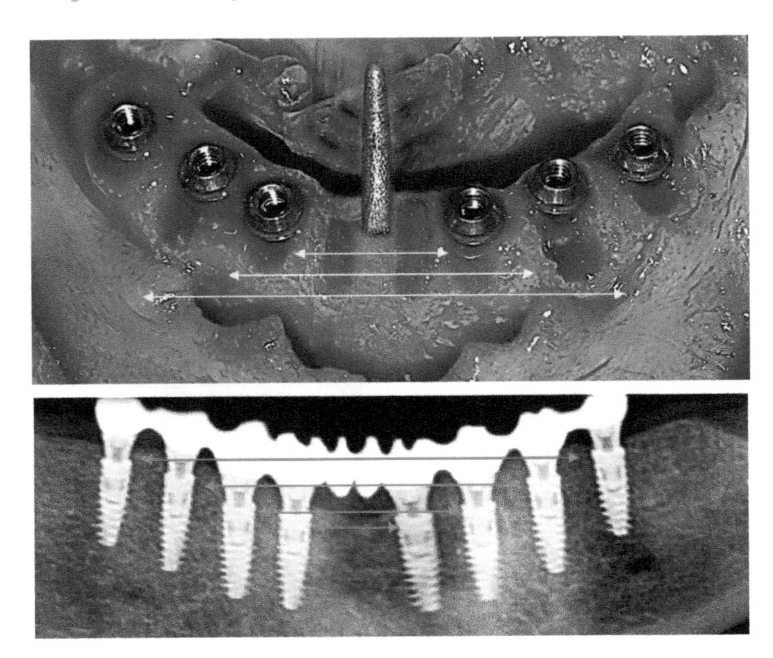

Figure 12.12 This technique can be achieved in both the maxilla but also the mandible. Once again, symmetry of implant placement, distance and depth is a critical factor for the long-term aesthetic outcome of such cases.

placed at the same depth, with symmetry of the collars at an ideal distance of 7 mm between implants (Figure 12.11). This technique can be achieved either in the maxilla or the mandible (Figure 12.12). All implants are placed 2 mm sub-crestally to avoid pressure on the cortical bone. Therefore, empty spaces around the abutments are noted with the use of platform switching being utilized to further minimize crestal bone loss. By utilizing these principles, it is easy to obtain adequate height of interproximal bone papilla with a 2 mm sub-crestal approach avoiding engagement of the cortical bone (thereby avoiding possible resorption) (Figure 12.13).

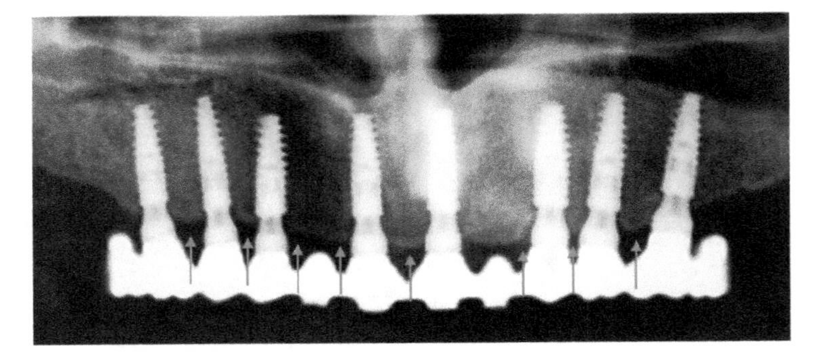

Figure 12.13 Implants are placed in a sub-crestal position at 2 mm. Platform connections are utilized in order to maintain the bone above the implants as depicted in this figure. Furthermore, no pressure is placed directly on the cortical bone. By utilizing this method, it is much more possible to obtain easy formation of the interproximal bone and respective papilla.

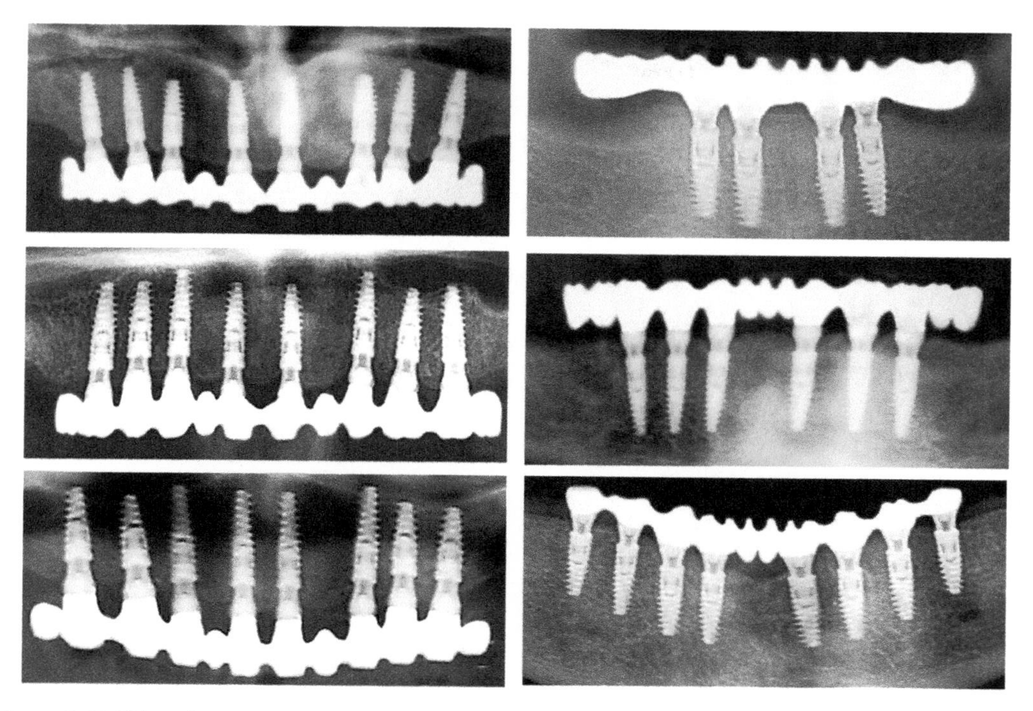

Figure 12.14 This technique requires placing between 8 to 10 implants in the maxilla and 4 to 8 in the mandible depending on the patient morpho-type and occlusal function.

Another interesting feature that has been modified over time especially with the development of newer implants, is the concept of utilizing implants with a narrow diameter. Recent research has shown how titanium alloys and/or incorporation of various metals such as zirconia have allowed more strength in implants facilitating the use of smaller diameter implants [65,66]. Narrower implants are able to generate less bone trauma and less vessel damage/loss, and therefore, more bone is achieved and maintained around smaller implants. Furthermore, narrow implants allow less marginal bone loss around the implants as a 3 mm recommended distance can be maintained [67]. Typically, this procedure is performed by placing 8 to 10 implants in the maxilla and 4 to 8 in the mandible depending on the patient morpho-type and occlusal function (Figure 12.14).

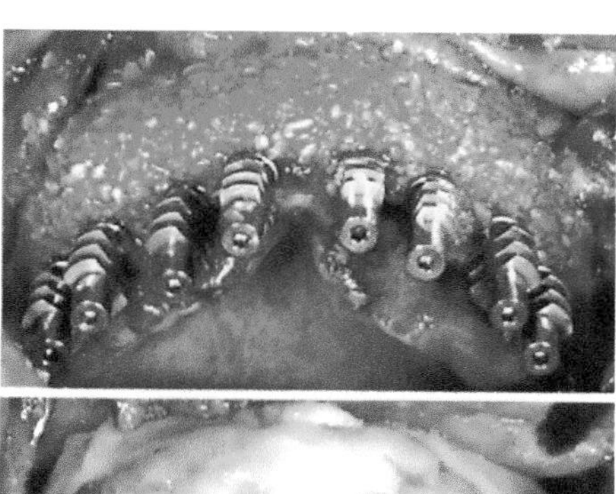

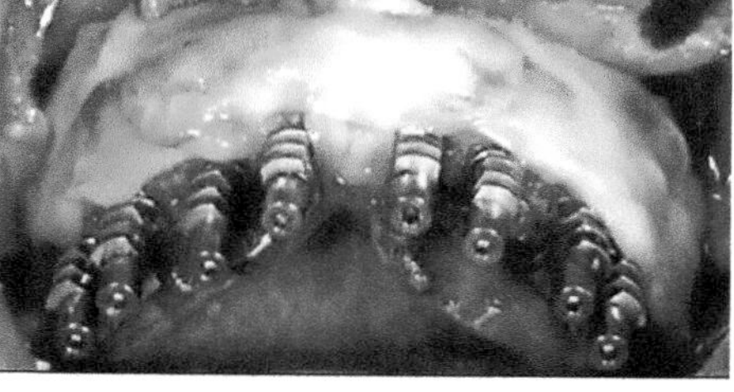

Figure 12.15 Following bone augmentation of the buccal wall with FDBA in combination with an injectable-PRF, an overlaying advanced matrix of PRF (A-PRF) is applied to provide additional wound healing to the soft tissues and to increase overall vascularization.

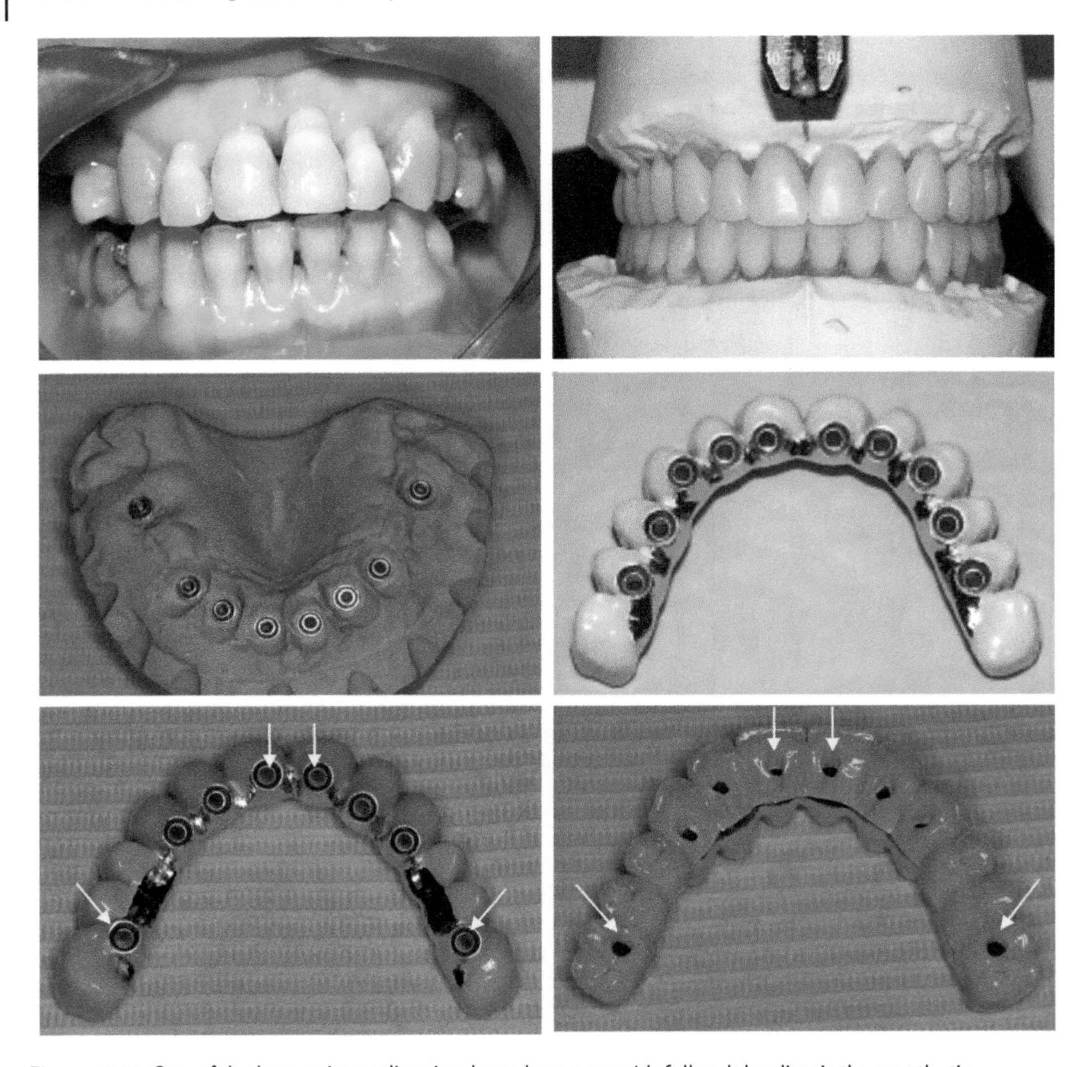

Figure 12.16 One of the keys to immediate implant placement with full arch loading is the prosthetic requirements. A provisional is designed purely from metals for strength. In this way, a reduction in mechanical stress exerted on each implant can be minimized with prevention of micro-movements. Furthermore, and very important for the provisional restoration, the design is made to guide the future gum profile.

12.4.2 Systematic apposition graft

One of the key requirements of full arch immediate implant placement and loading is the necessity of utilizing bone-grafting materials during surgery. Due to the complexity of such cases, it is well known that many patients present themselves with severe bone loss and complex diseased periodontal tissues throughout the maxilla and mandible. Furthermore, and additionally complicating the regenerative surgeries, many present themselves to our dental clinics in France and Italy where smoking is of higher prevalence [68,69]. It has therefore been recommended that in order to augment missing bone, and prevent further bone resorption following tooth loss, a 2 to 4 mm buccal thickness

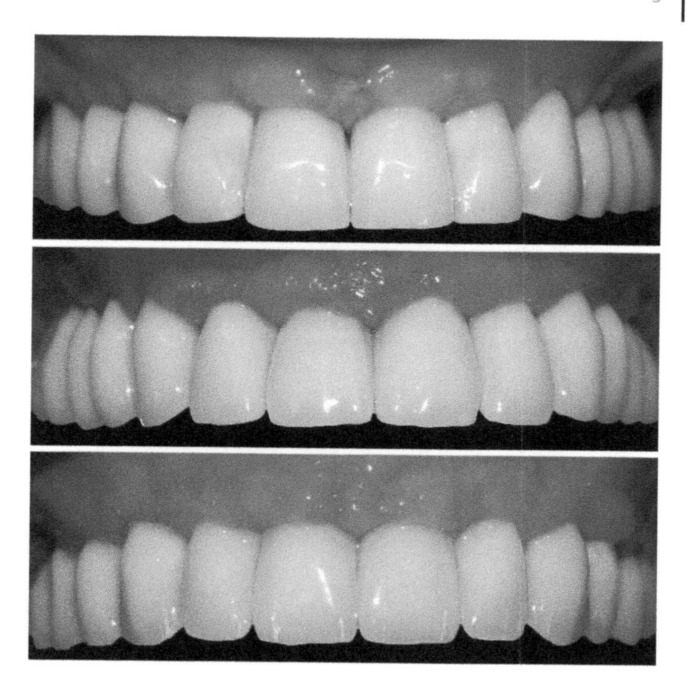

Figure 12.17 Profile of soft tissues after only 6 or 7 days of healing. Notice the excellent adaptation of tissues to the fixed provisional prosthesis with excellent contouring at very early time points. Notice the excellent vascularization of tissues with little evidence of surgical intervention.

is recommended for aesthetic reasons. In these cases and due to poor vascularization, two critical components are required. First, bone grafts containing accessible collagen such as freeze-dried bone allograft (FDBA) are always utilized. Second, the use of an injectable-PRF with an overlaying matrix of PRF is combined with surgery to improve vascularization (Figure 12.15). Therefore, this concept may be explained with two key concepts including the "Generous Bone Graft" concept and with additional use of PRF to re-introduce blood flow immediately into these complicated defects.

12.4.3 Flap management and suture technique

Another key component for not only this technique but all surgical approaches is to utilize tension-free flap closure. This is achieved by two methods, by flap preparation (incision in the periosteum, low tension, flap mobility) and also by utilizing the apical mattress suture technique. The advantages of utilizing the apical mattress suture technique are that it provides a tension-free closure of the flap with full immobilization. For this technique to be successful, the penetration of the needle must occur at least 1 cm from the margin to allow adequate tension-free closure (Figure 12.14). Sutures are routinely performed with monofilament glycolon with an expected resorption time of 3 to 4 weeks.

12.5 Prosthetic requirements

Equally as important for the long-term success of immediate implant placement and loading of full arches is prosthetic planning. Excellent collaboration with equally skilled team members is key to predictable success. Surgery should never begin without ideal planning. In all our cases, provisional restorations are placed at 4 to 8 days following surgery and must be rigid and screw retained [70]. Interestingly, Hruska *et al.* placed 1300 immediate implants and found that the success rates achieved over 21 years was 99.3%

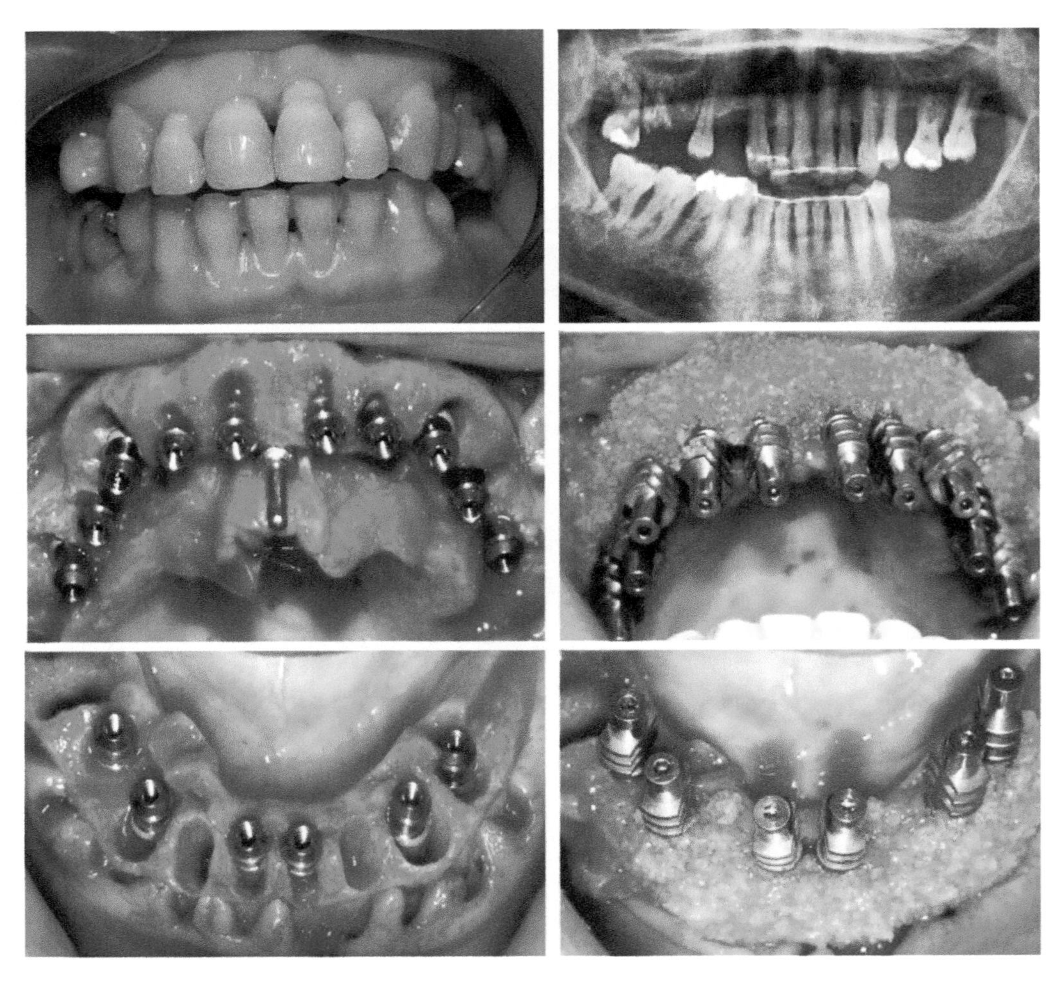

Figure 12.18 Demonstration of another example of a bi-maxillary case treated utilizing this protocol. Once again a 2 to 4 mm buccal bone graft is created using i-PRF followed by a provisional restorations respecting the same principles presented in the previous sections.

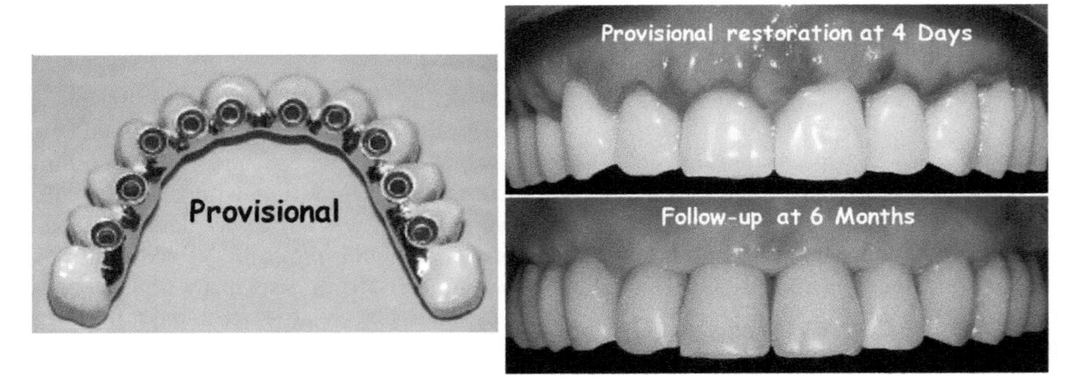

Figure 12.19 Provisional prosthetic component fabricated with rigid metals with a 4-day and 6-month follow-up. Notice the soft tissue adaptation around the provisional at 6 months.

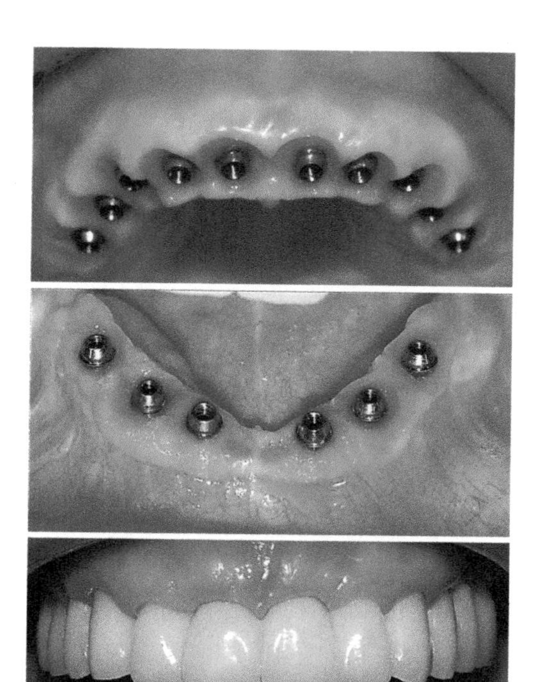

Figure 12.20 Final ceramic restoration in the bi-maxillary case presented in Figures 12.18 and 12.19.

with the intraoral welding machine, 98.3% with the provisional plastic prosthesis with metal frame, 97.9% with metal wings, and 88.02% with provisional plastic prosthesis. Therefore, the use of plastic provisional prosthesis has been discontinued due to these significantly lower results [70]. In this way, a reduction in mechanical stress exerted on each implant can be minimized with prevention of micro-movements [71,72]. Furthermore, and very important for the provisional restoration, the design should guide the future gum profile (Figure 12.16).

Thereafter, post-operatory visits are recommended at 1 week. In Figure 12.17, observe the wound healing after 6 days of post-operation following application with PRF. The additional use of PRF in this technique greatly enhances soft-tissue healing via vascularization of these tissues. Furthermore, the absence of having to use a collagen barrier membrane allows for the periosteum to interact within 10 to 14 days with the underlying bone tissue since the PRF membranes are fully replaced by host tissues within this time frame. Notice the soft-tissue healing in all cases, the symmetry of the tissues, and also the ability for the papilla to gradually creep coronally and fill the voids creating a naturally looking final restoration.

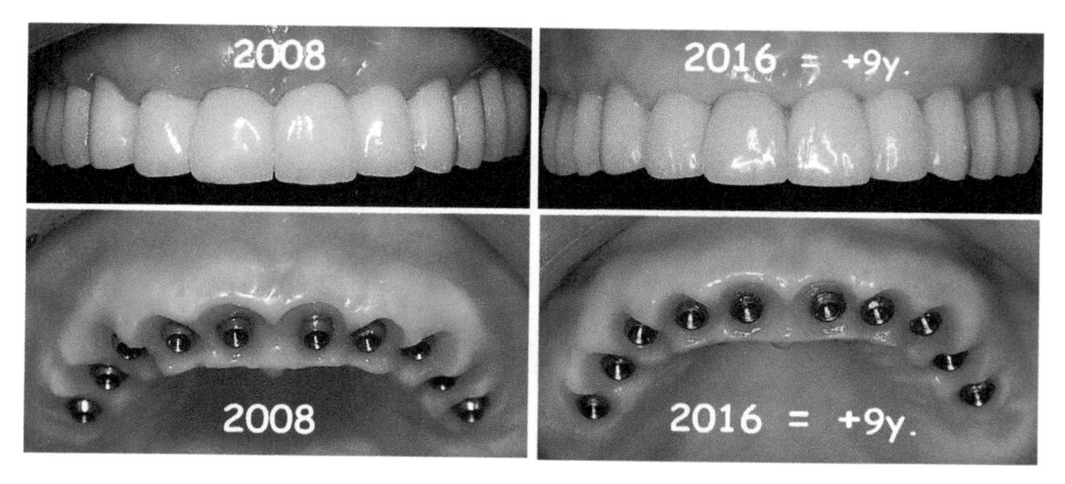

Figure 12.21 One of the long-term concerns with immediate implant placement is the long-term aesthetic results. Notice the improvements in soft tissues over time utilizing this technique with platelet concentrates being added to speed soft-tissue wound healing.

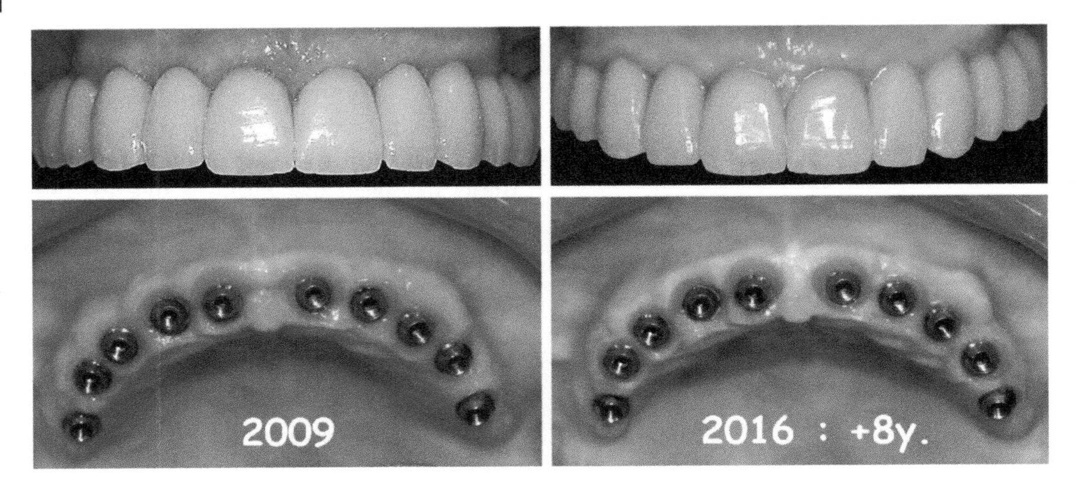

Figure 12.22 Another case demonstrating long-term improvements utilizing full arch immediate implant placement with immediate loading over an 8-year period with gains in soft-tissue thickness.

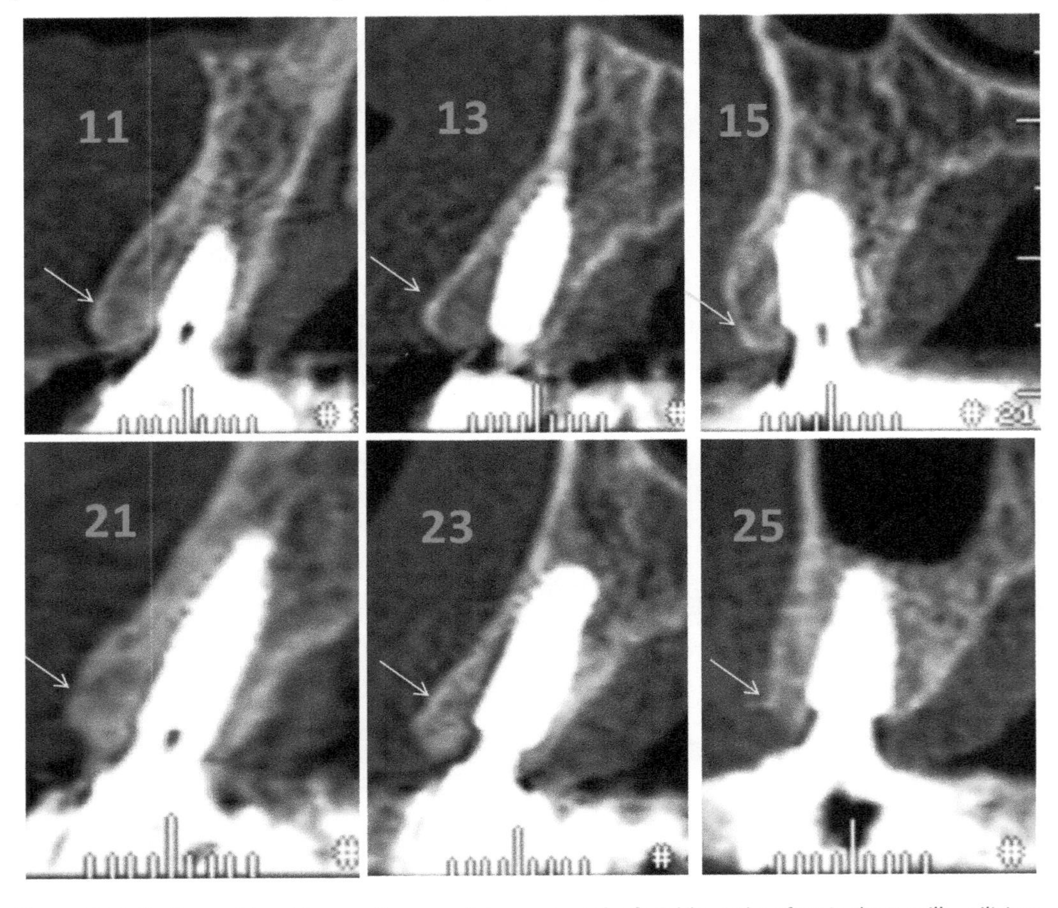

Figure 12.23 Radiographic evidence of bone maintenance on the facial/buccal surface in the maxilla utilizing immediate implant placement with FDBA. Implants were placed the day of surgery with a 2 to 4 mm buccal bone thickness created using FDBA. Results depict the radiographic evidence following 7 years.

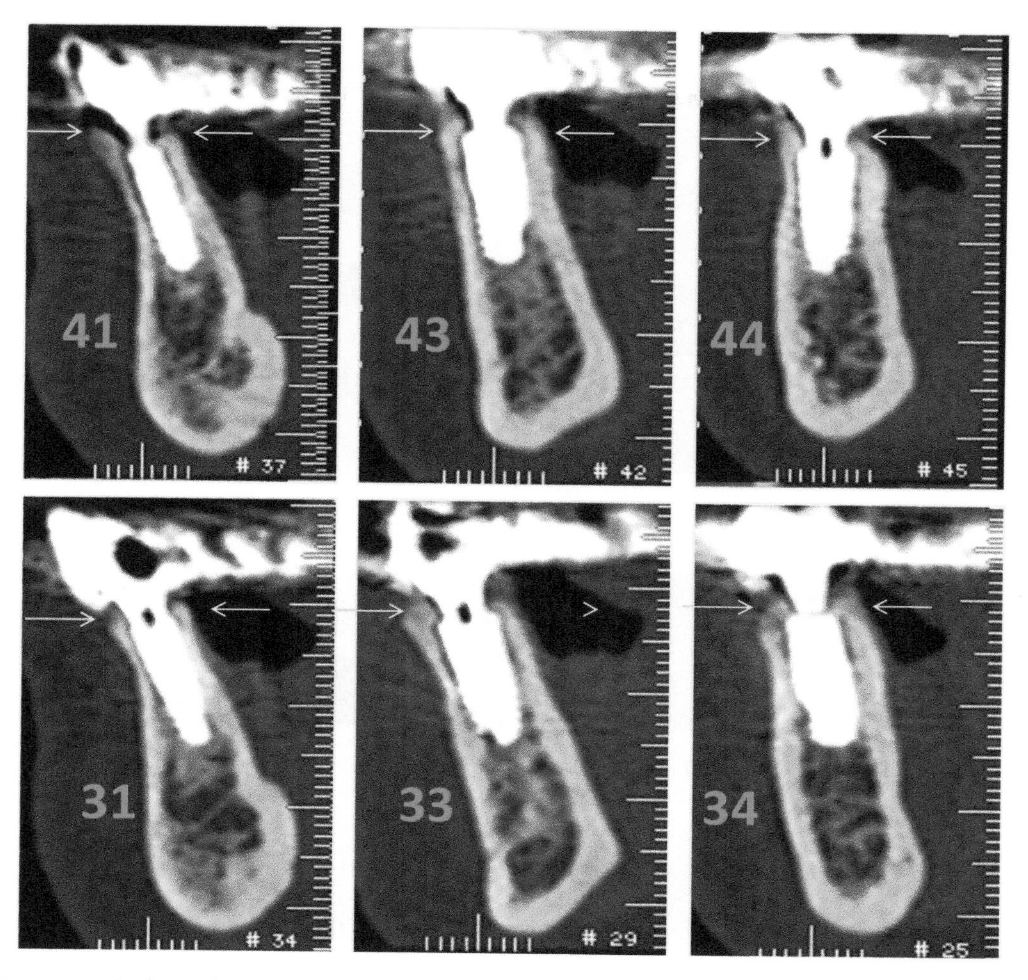

Figure 12.24 Radiographic evidence of bone maintenance on the facial/buccal surface in the mandible utilizing immediate implant placement with FDBA. Implants were placed the day of surgery with a 2 to 4 mm buccal bone thickness. Results depict the radiographic evidence following 7 years.

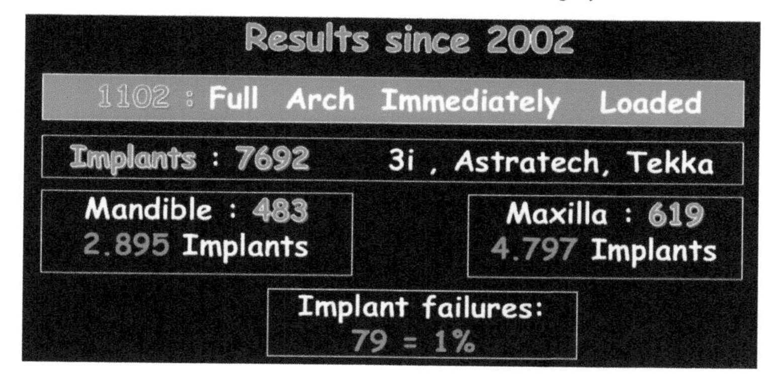

Figure 12.25 My long-term results utilizing immediate implant placement with immediate loading of full arches. Over 1100 documented cases have been performed with approximately 7700 implants. Only 79 implants were lost throughout this entire period.

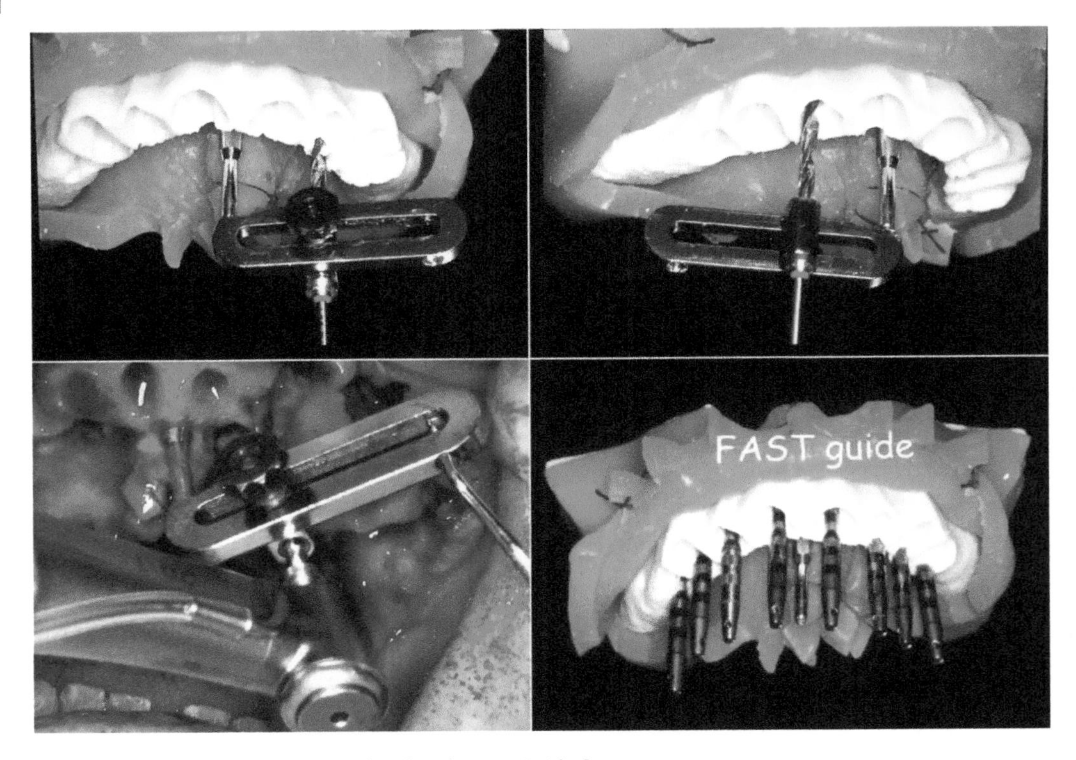

Figure 12.26 Components contained within the Fast Guide System.

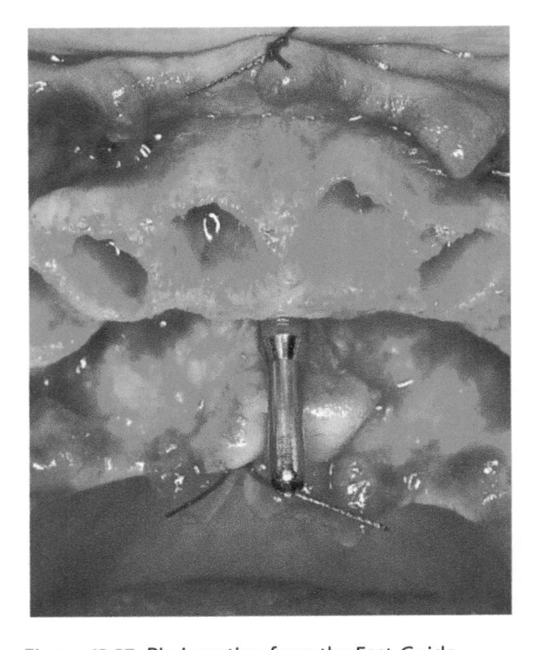

Figure 12.27 Pin insertion from the Fast-Guide System into the naso-palatal foramen.

12.6 Final results

By utilizing this set of principles, it brings great pleasure to report the long-term outcomes of these cases that have been documented over the past 15 years. Figure 12.18 demonstrates another example of a bimaxillary case treated using the same protocol. Once again a 2 to 4 mm buccal bone graft is created using i-PRF followed by a provisional restoration respecting the same principles presented in the previous sections. Figure 12.19 demonstrates the provisional restorations at 6 days and 6 months. Notice the ability for soft tissues to heal and also the bone papilla to create adequate soft-tissue design with indexed papillae for the final restoration (Figure 12.20). When this is achieved, the final ceramics can easily be inserted and maintained over a long period.

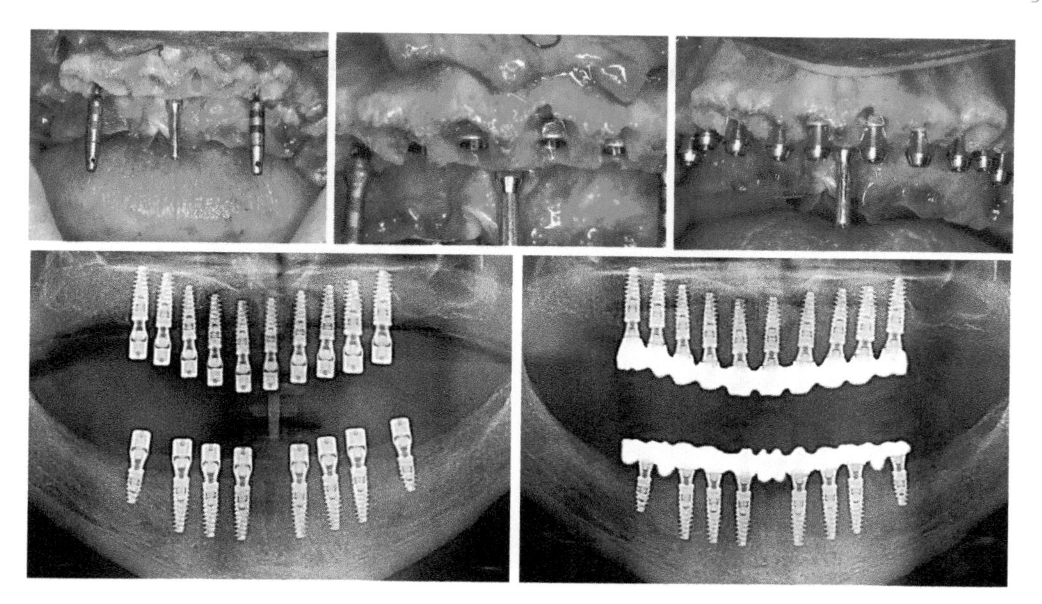

Figure 12.28 The main advantage of using the Fast Guide System is that implants are placed with a parallel axis with symmetry between quadrants 1 and II or III and IV.

12.7 Documented long-term stability

Most important during immediate implant placement is the long-term stability. Many reports have now documented how immediate implant placement leads to soft-tissue mucosal recession, lower keratinized tissues followed by peri-implant infection and possible loss of implants. Figure 12.21 demonstrates a case performed in 2008. Interestingly, observe this same case 9 years later in 2016. Notice the long-term increase in soft-tissue keratinization with excellent stability. One might even consider this long-term improvement over time. Figure 12.22 demonstrates another such case with excellent stability over time. One of the reasons for these successful outcomes is the ability to easily maintain these tissues with adequate cleaning. After performing over 1000 full arch cases, it becomes evident that both soft tissue is necessary for bone maintenance and bone tissue is necessary for soft-tissue maintenance. Furthermore and interestingly, notice that despite the fact that FDBA grafts were

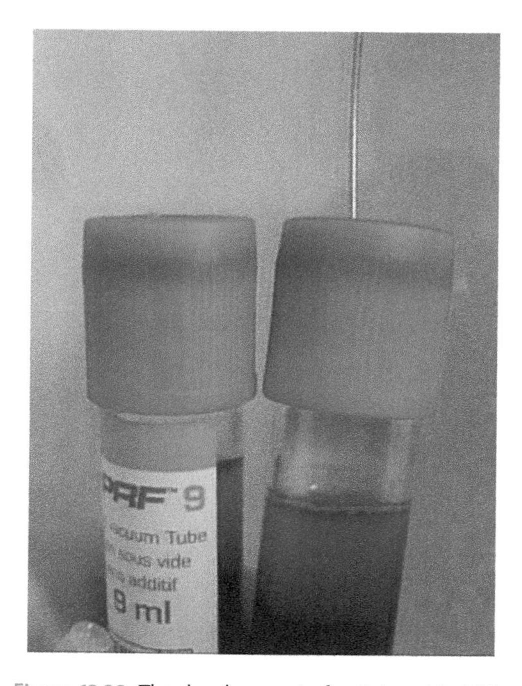

Figure 12.29 The development of an injectable-PRF allows for the top 1mL of a 10mL blood collection to be utilized following a 3-minute centrifuge at 700 rpm (60G). This formulation of i-PRF contains proportionally a higher number of leukocytes and growth factors.

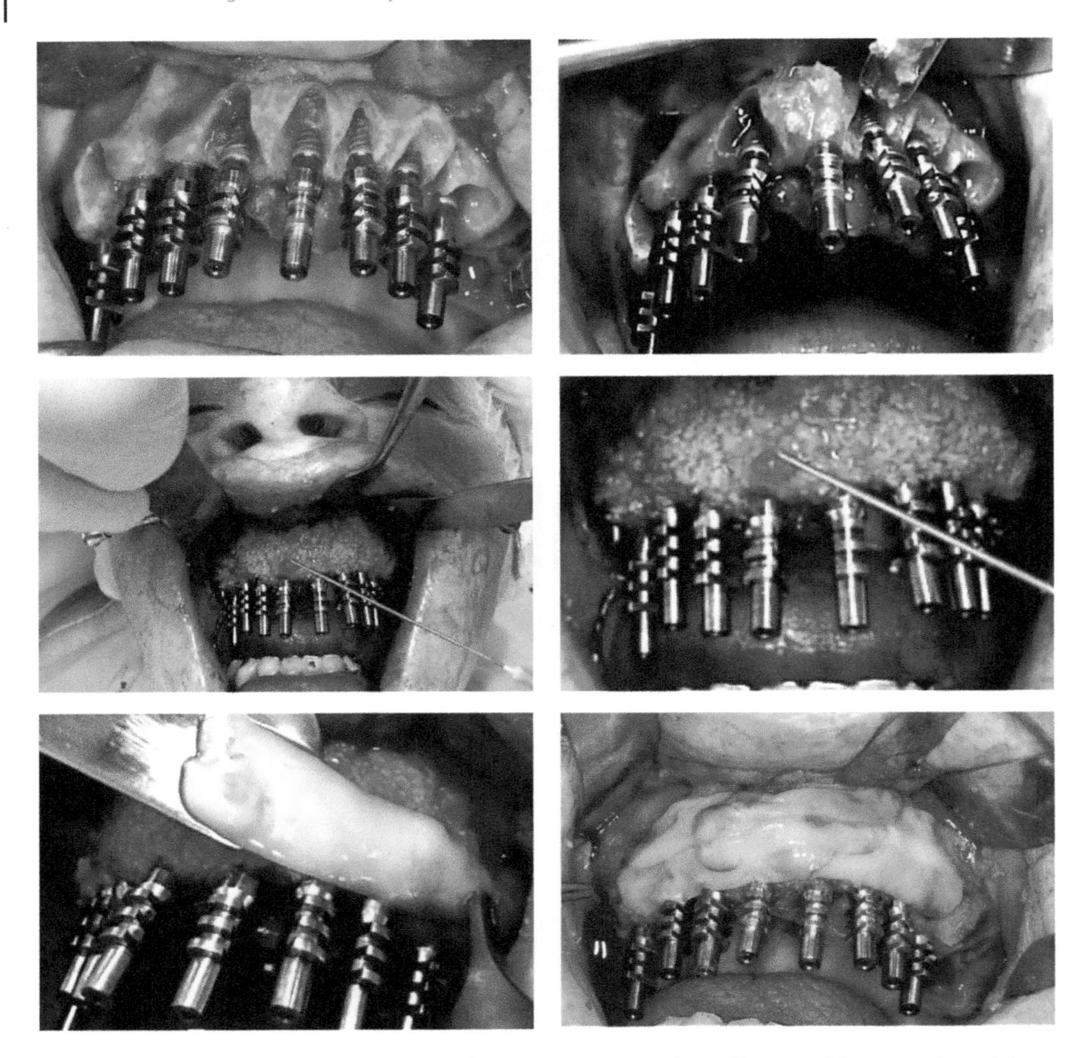

Figure 12.30 Immediate implant placement followed by a 2 to 4 mm buccal bone grafting procedure with FDBA. Afterward, an injectable-PRF is utilized to adsorb fibrin i-PRF onto the graft to provide stability following a 1- to 2-minute clotting period. Thereafter, advanced-PRF membranes are utilized over the bone grafting material and implants.

utilized in all cases, bone stability is maintained even years after surgery due to the fact a 2 to 4 mm buccal bone augmentation was utilized without risk of resorption (Figure 12.23). This protocol is used in the mandible with similar long-term success (Figure 12.24).

12.8 Long-term statistical results: full arch immediate implant placement and loading

Since 2002, over 1100 cases have been performed utilizing this technique with over

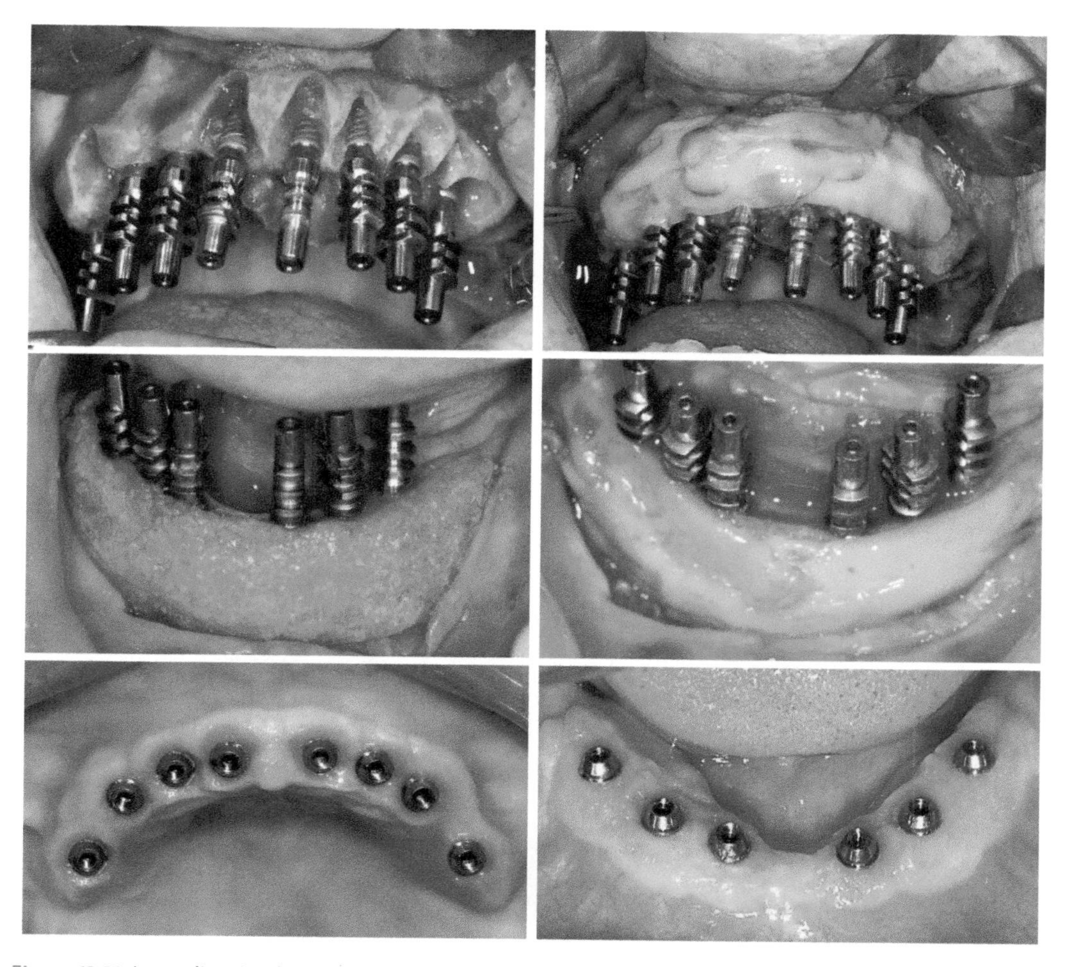

Figure 12.31 Immediate implant placement in a compromised case utilizing both i-PRF and PRF in both the maxilla and mandible. Notice the excellent healing at 6 months (bottom row) in these initial severely compromised cases utilizing this technique with immediate implant placement.

7700 implants placed (Figure 12.25). Of the 7700 implants, only a 1% failure rate has been reported. Almost all implants were lost in the posterior maxillary region. Interestingly, almost all failures occurred before the year 2009 (between 2002 and 2008) where the failure rate was roughly 2%. Based on my personal experiences, the following protocols were adapted:

1. Stopped immediately loading implants placed in the sinus when less then 4 mm of crestal bone was remaining.
2. Conscience effort to evaluate biological factors such as vitamin D and cholesterol prior to implant placement.
3. Introduction of the apical matrix suturing technique has improved re-vascularization of tissues by reducing tension on bone and soft tissues.
4. Improved experience with immediate implant placement and loading since 2002.

Furthermore, around the year 2014, three additional improvements have been made

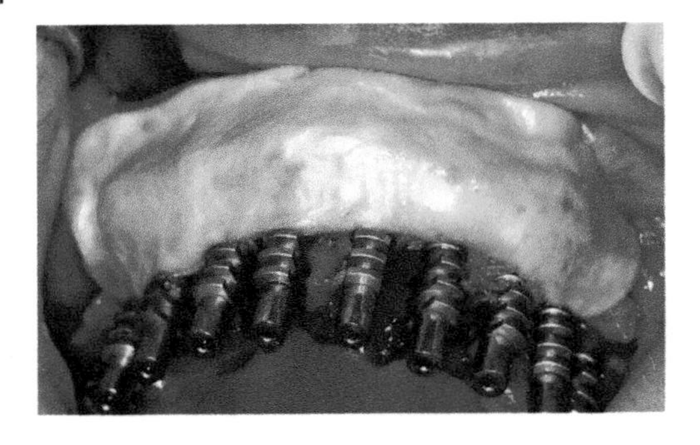

Figure 12.32 Development of a Twin Matrix has allowed for more keratinized tissue formation in compromised cases. This matrix acts as both a barrier membrane for soft tissues as well as a matrix for soft-tissue regeneration, thereby increasing keratinized tissues.

that have all contributed to the regenerative outcomes utilizing this approach:

1. The Fast Guide has been introduced that allowed for better parallel implant placement.
2. An injectable PRF (i-PRF) was developed that helped stabilize bone grafts and induce vascularization of these tissues.
3. A collagen Twin Matrix has been developed to further help complex cases by facilitating keratinized tissues over time.

12.8.1 The "Fast Guide" System for immediate implant placement

One of the pioneering abilities to improve surgical full arch immediate implant placement has been the development of a "Fast Guide" system that I helped co-develop. Figure 12.26 illustrates the components that revolve around inserting a pin into the naso-palatal canal to provide an axis of future implant placement. This atraumatic instrument may be utilized to improve parallel implant placement with optimal implant symmetry. Figure 12.27 demonstrates the Fast Guide System, which is placed in the naso-palatal foramen to guide implant axis in

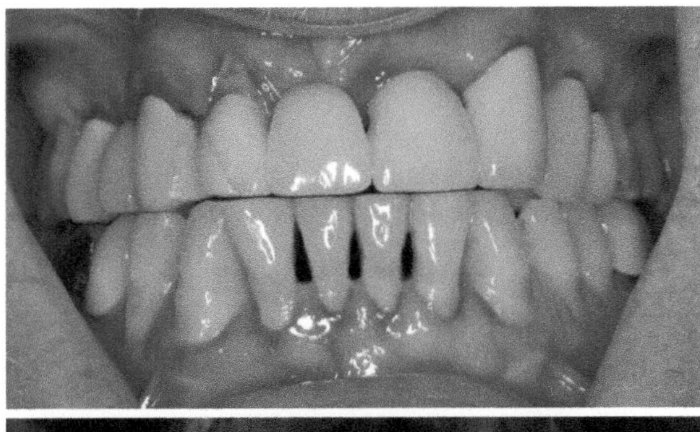

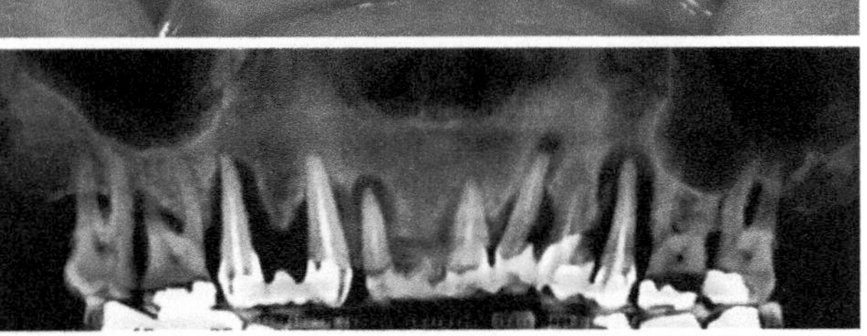

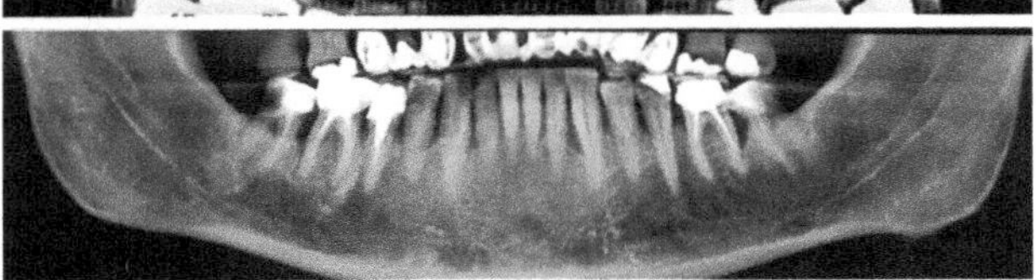

Figure 12.33 Clinical and radiographic images of a case of chronic periodontitis. Figures 12.34 through 12.36 illustrate how immediate implant placement and loading can be achieved in such compromised cases with excellent aesthetic results following healing.

the maxilla. The main advantage of using this system is that implants are placed with a parallel axis with symmetry between quadrants I and II or III and IV (Figure 12.28).

12.8.2 An injectable-PRF (i-PRF) for adequate graft stability and compaction

One often-neglected factor is the impact of graft stability on graft consolidation. The literature has routinely shown that for block grafts, an adequate primary stability of bone blocks via the use of screws is necessary for the successful integration of autogenous bone grafts into host tissues [73–75]. Therefore, despite using autologous bone tissues, it remains interesting to point out the necessity to stabilize these grafts adequately to prevent micro-motion. Since the development of an injectable PRF (i-PRF) in 2014, many possibilities now exist since i-PRF is harvested in liquid formulation that quickly coagulates following contact with bone-grafting materials (Figure 12.29). Therefore, its use has vastly improved the potential of these surgeries with no unnatural additives being utilized. Figure 12.30 demonstrates how i-PRF and PRF are used in combination for regenerative procedures. Figure 12.31 confirms the use of both techniques even in severely compromised cases.

12.8.3 The collagen Twin Matrix

The last regenerative biomaterial that has greatly facilitate immediate implant placement in full arches has been the development of a thick collagen Twin Matrix utilized for soft-tissue regeneration to increase keratinized tissues (Figure 12.32). This matrix acts as both a barrier membrane for soft tissues as well as simultaneously acts as a matrix for soft-tissue regeneration and increasing keratinized tissues.

12.8.4 Can we get more soft tissue?

In Figure 12.33, observe how a loss of bone due to periodontitis has resulted in loss of soft tissue with a resulting disastrous case. In this scenario, very limited regenerative options are available. Figure 12.34 demonstrates the use of PRF and Twin Matrix simultaneously to improve the regenerative outcomes. Figure 12.35 demonstrates the final provisional full arch immediate restoration following implant placement. Notice the 6-month restorative outcomes utilizing this strategy (Figure 12.36).

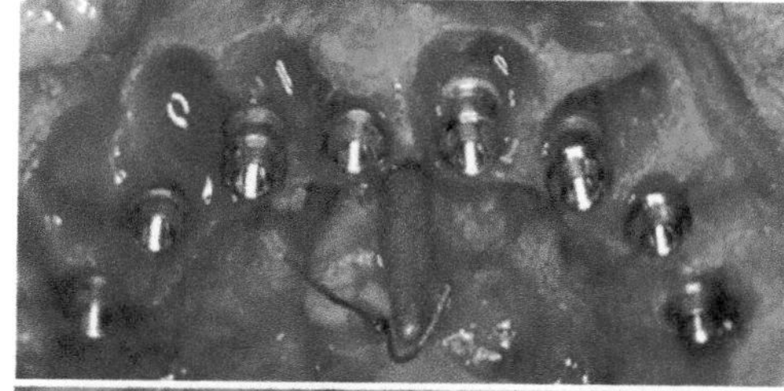

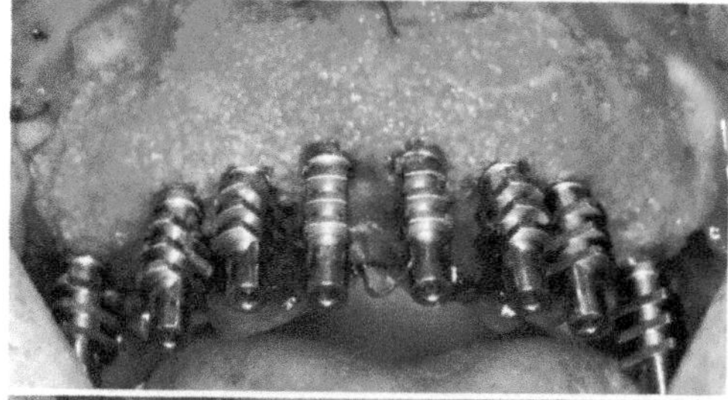

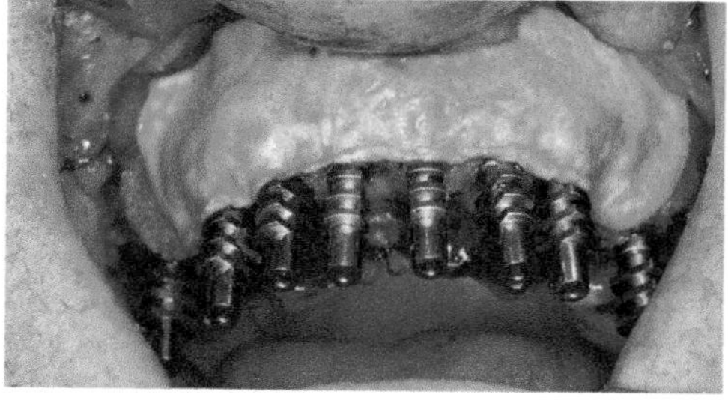

Figure 12.34 Immediate implant placement in the case presented in Figure 12.33 utilizing i-PRF and a Twin Matrix.

12.8.5 Potential wound healing: example of aesthetic failure without management of tension and regeneration with a Twin Matrix and PRF

This section is to further supplement the concept of biological healing using platelet

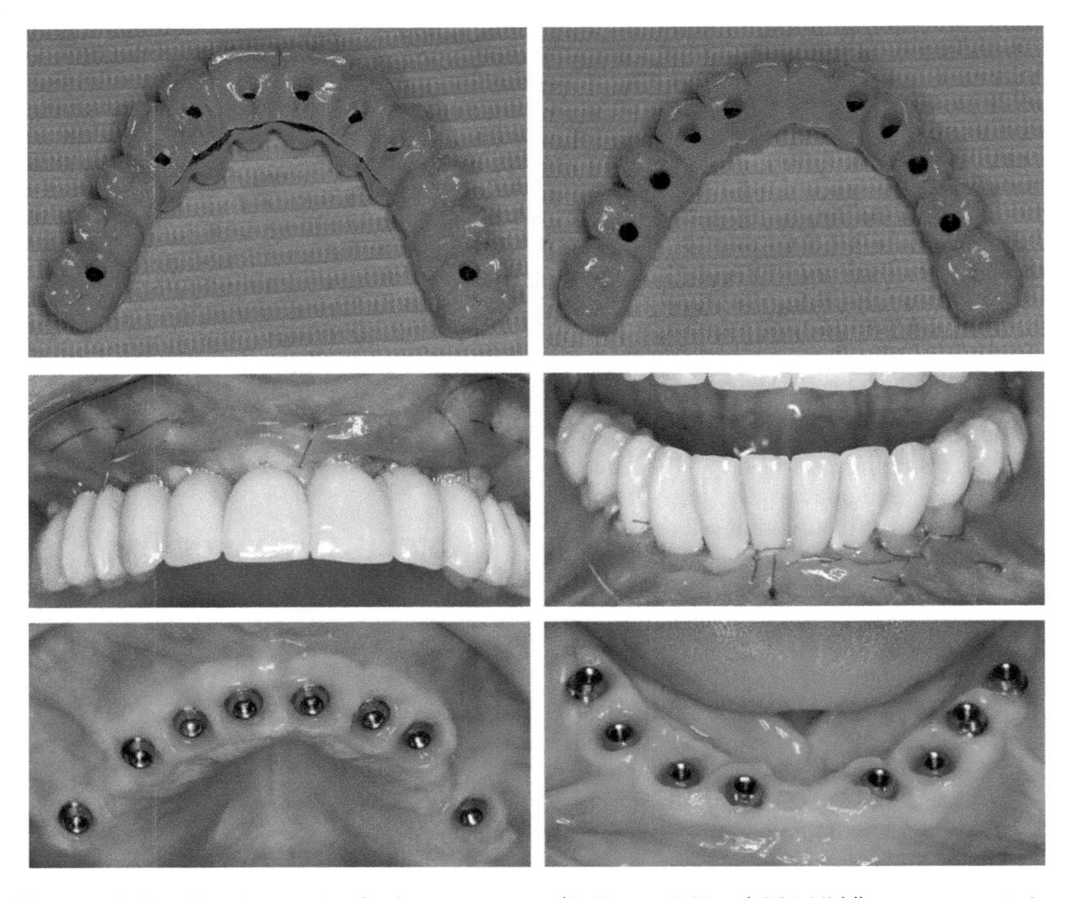

Figure 12.35 Provisional restoration for the case presented in Figures 12.33 and 12.34. Middle row represents 4 days post-surgery. Bottom row represents 6 months post-surgery.

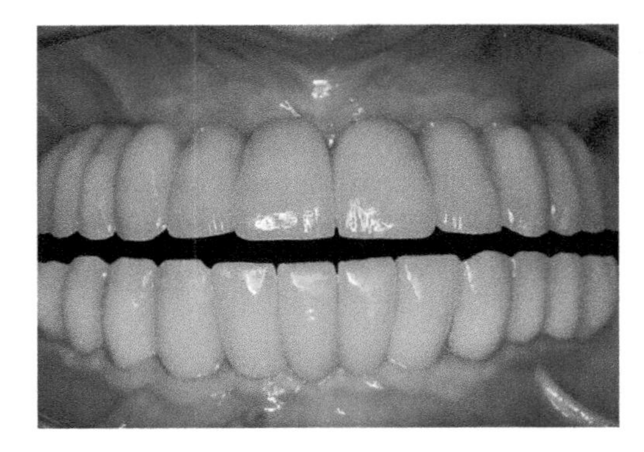

Figure 12.36 Final restoration of the severe periodontitis case presented in Figure 12.33. Notice the soft-tissue healing as well as the ability for keratinized tissue to form with papilla after 6 months.

concentrates. Figure 12.37 demonstrates a case with high tension resulting in aesthetic failure. Such a case requires a retreatment to reach sufficient aesthetic outcome but remains extremely complex to regenerate due to the shallow vestibule.

In a first step of the surgery, the tension was removed by creating a split incision into the vestibule below the keratinized tissue (Figure 12.38). Ideally the goal was to create more keratinized tissue, however, such cases are not routinely performed and thus long-term outcomes have not been documented. In this case, an equine collagen matrix was placed (Figure 12.38) with eight PRF membranes to cover this matrix followed by suturing

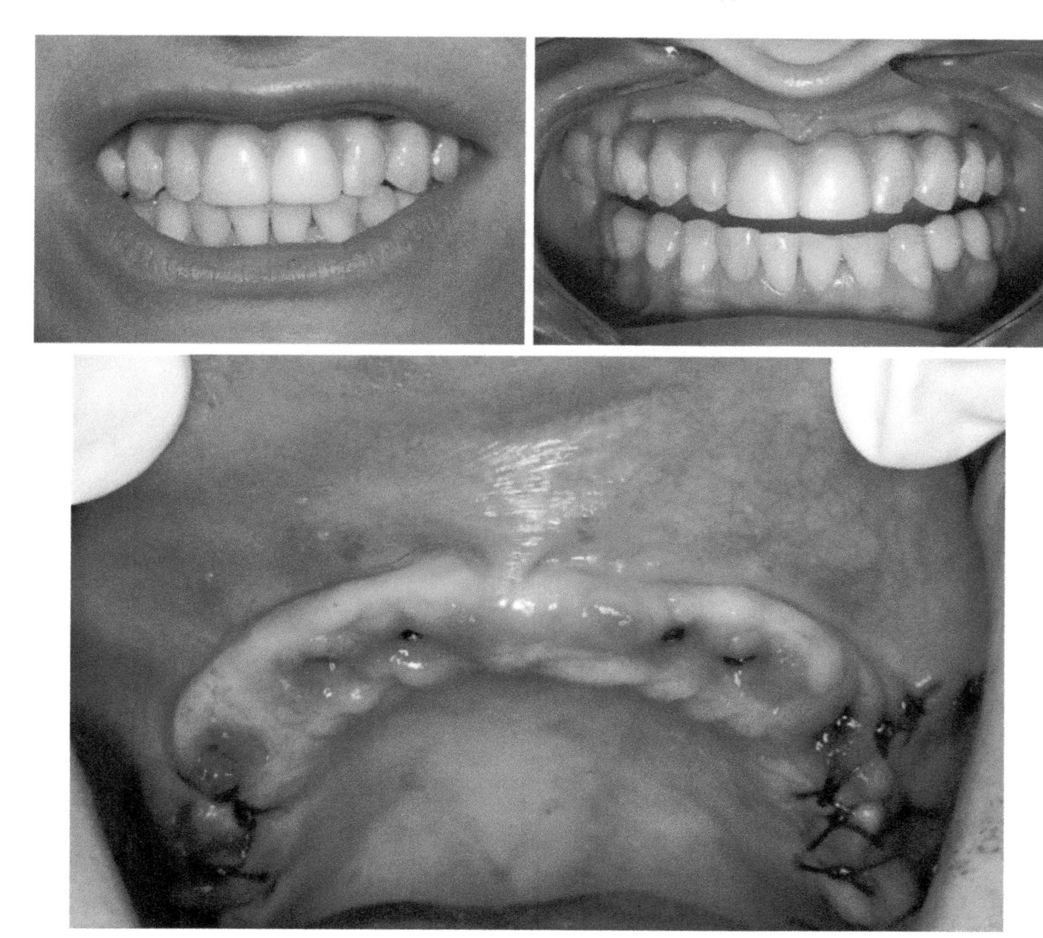

Figure 12.37 This case presents with high tension resulting in aesthetic failure. Such a case requires a retreatment to reach sufficient aesthetic outcome but remains extremely complex to regenerate due to the shallow vestibule.

to maintain stability of the PRF membranes (Figure 12.38). Since PRF contains an abundance of immune defense cells (leukocytes), it may therefore be left exposed in the oral cavity. Such a case could not be performed with an acellular collagen matrix due to risk of exposure and risk of infection. What's interesting about this case is the remarkable tissue healing that occurred after only 15 days (Figure 12.39). The keratinized tissue was once again further increased by 6 months. Figure 12.40 shows the before and after case of the final restoration. Most noticeably, observe the soft- tissue healing. We, therefore, can conclude the potent regenerative potential of PRF and i-PRF and most notably the ideal wound healing properties facilitating the aesthetic outcomes in this case.

12.9 Conclusion

Fourteen years of full arch immediate implant placement and immediate loading have allowed an established protocol with success rates over 98%. The long-term

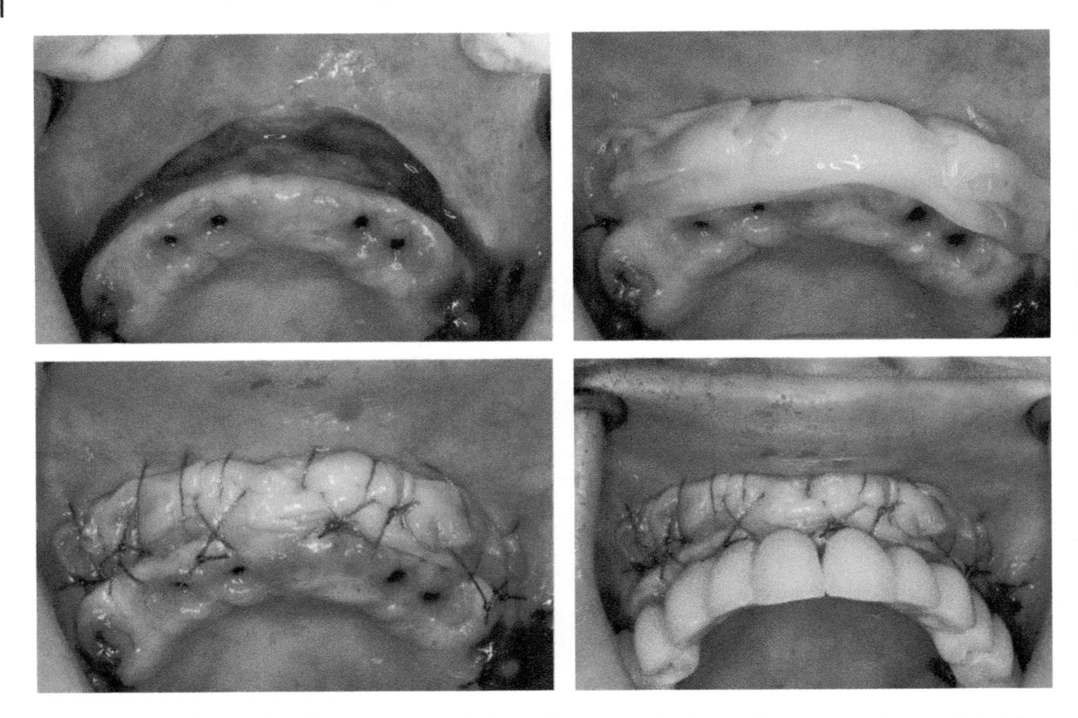

Figure 12.38 The first goal of this case was to eliminate the tension in the vestibule by creating a split incision below the keratinized tissue. Thereafter, an equine collagen matrix was placed followed by 8 PRF membranes. Thereafter, immediate loading of the full arch restoration was placed.

aesthetic outcomes in over 7700 placed implants and 1100 full arches testifies to soft- and hard-tissue healing properties of this technique. Many technical aspects have been optimized and studied including the necessity for optimal 1) biological requirements, 2) anatomical and surgical requirements, and 3) prosthetic requirements. We have also introduced surgical guides and biomaterials such as the "Fast Guide System" that facilitate implant placement. We've introduced i-PRF and a collagen matrix as biomaterials that further support vascularization and keratinized soft tissues, respectively. In conclusion, the use of PRF has made such a technique possible by further promoting wound healing and graft stability with excellent long-term follow-up.

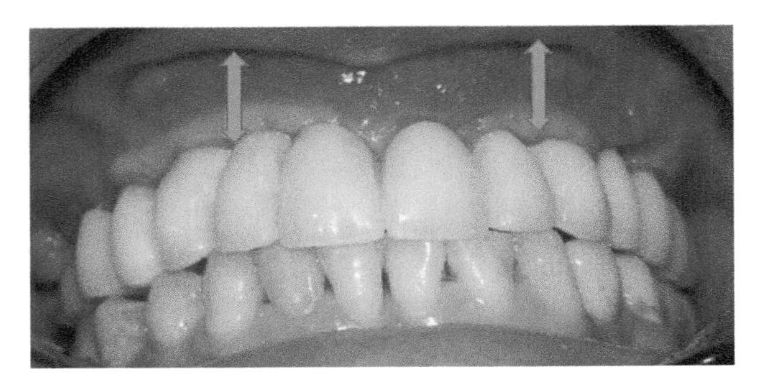

Figure 12.39 Healing of the widened vestibule after only 15 days. Notice the gain in soft tissue by utilizing this technique for expanding the vestibule.

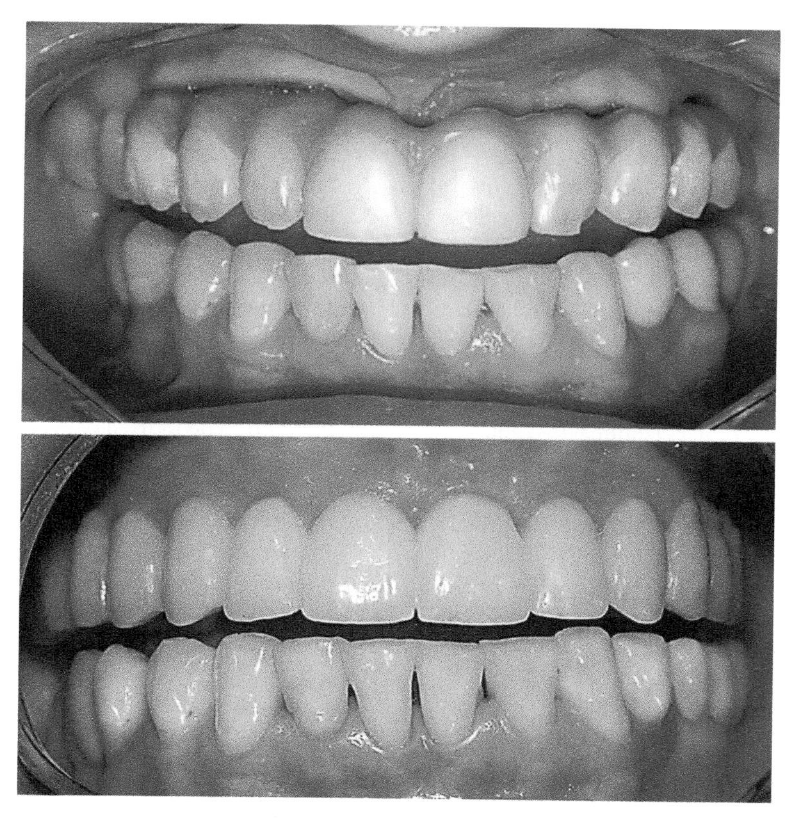

Figure 12.40 Before and after case of this aesthetic failure with a low vestibule. After 6 months of healing, notice the new formation of keratinized tissue utilizing PRF.

References

1 Turkyilmaz I, Company AM, McGlumphy EA. Should edentulous patients be constrained to removable complete dentures? The use of dental implants to improve the quality of life for edentulous patients. Gerodontology. 2010;27(1):3–10.
2 Douglass CW, Shih A, Ostry L. Will there be a need for complete dentures in the United States in 2020? J Prosthet Dent. 2002;87(1):5–8.
3 Medina-Solis CE, Perez-Nunez R, Maupome G, Avila-Burgos L, Pontigo-Loyola AP, Patino-Marin N, et al. National survey on edentulism and its geographic distribution, among Mexicans 18 years of age and older (with emphasis in WHO age groups). Journal of oral rehabilitation. 2008;35(4):237–44.
4 Eke PI, Dye BA, Wei L, Thornton-Evans GO, Genco RJ. Prevalence of periodontitis in adults in the United States: 2009 and 2010. Journal of dental research. 2012; 91(10):914–20.
5 Allen PF, McMillan AS. A longitudinal study of quality of life outcomes in older adults requesting implant prostheses and complete removable dentures. Clinical oral implants research. 2003;14(2):173–9.
6 Wolff A, Gadre A, Begleiter A, Moskona D, Cardash H. Correlation between patient satisfaction with complete dentures and denture quality, oral condition, and flow

rate of submandibular/sublingual salivary glands. Int J Prosthodont. 2003;16(1):45–8.

7 Ikebe K, Matsuda K, Morii K, Furuya-Yoshinaka M, Nokubi T, Renner RP. Association of masticatory performance with age, posterior occlusal contacts, occlusal force, and salivary flow in older adults. Int J Prosthodont. 2006; 19(5):475–81.

8 Ishijima T, Koshino H, Hirai T, Takasaki H. The relationship between salivary secretion rate and masticatory efficiency. Journal of oral rehabilitation. 2004;31(1):3–6.

9 Koshino H, Hirai T, Ishijima T, Ikeda Y. Tongue motor skills and masticatory performance in adult dentates, elderly dentates, and complete denture wearers. J Prosthet Dent. 1997;77(2):147–52.

10 Koshino H, Hirai T, Ishijima T, Tsukagoshi H, Ishigami T, Tanaka Y. Quality of life and masticatory function in denture wearers. Journal of oral rehabilitation. 2006;33(5): 323–9.

11 Kapur KK, Soman SD. Masticatory performance and efficiency in denture wearers. 1964. J Prosthet Dent. 2006;95(6): 407–11.

12 Heath MR. The effect of maximum biting force and bone loss upon masticatory function and dietary selection of the elderly. International dental journal. 1982; 32(4):345–56.

13 Esposito M, Grusovin MG, Maghaireh H, Worthington HV. Interventions for replacing missing teeth: different times for loading dental implants. The Cochrane database of systematic reviews. 2013;3: Cd003878.

14 Schnitman PA, Wohrle PS, Rubenstein JE, DaSilva JD, Wang NH. Ten-year results for Branemark implants immediately loaded with fixed prostheses at implant placement. The International journal of oral & maxillofacial implants. 1997;12(4): 495–503.

15 Balshi TJ, Wolfinger GJ. Immediate loading of Branemark implants in edentulous mandibles: a preliminary report. Implant dentistry. 1997;6(2):83–8.

16 Froberg KK, Lindh C, Ericsson I. Immediate loading of Branemark System Implants: a comparison between TiUnite and turned implants placed in the anterior mandible. Clinical implant dentistry and related research. 2006;8(4):187–97.

17 Randow K, Ericsson I, Nilner K, Petersson A, Glantz PO. Immediate functional loading of Branemark dental implants. An 18-month clinical follow-up study. Clinical oral implants research. 1999;10(1):8–15.

18 Degidi M, Piattelli A. 7-year follow-up of 93 immediately loaded titanium dental implants. The Journal of oral implantology. 2005;31(1):25–31.

19 Malo P, Rangert B, Nobre M. All-on-4 immediate-function concept with Branemark System implants for completely edentulous maxillae: a 1-year retrospective clinical study. Clinical implant dentistry and related research. 2005;7 Suppl 1:S88–94.

20 Daas M, Assaf A, Dada K, Makzoume J. Computer-Guided Implant Surgery in Fresh Extraction Sockets and Immediate Loading of a Full Arch Restoration: A 2-Year Follow-Up Study of 14 Consecutively Treated Patients. International journal of dentistry. 2015; 2015:824127.

21 Meloni SM, De Riu G, Pisano M, Dell'aversana Orabona G, Piombino P, Salzano G, et al. Computer-assisted implant surgery and immediate loading in edentulous ridges with dental fresh extraction sockets. Two years results of a prospective case series study. European review for medical and pharmacological sciences. 2013;17(21):2968–73.

22 Mozzati M, Arata V, Gallesio G, Mussano F, Carossa S. Immediate postextraction implant placement with immediate loading for maxillary full-arch rehabilitation: A two-year retrospective analysis. Journal of the American Dental Association (1939). 2012;143(2):124–33.

23 Mozzati M, Arata V, Gallesio G, Mussano F, Carossa S. Immediate postextractive dental implant placement with immediate

loading on four implants for mandibular-full-arch rehabilitation: a retrospective analysis. Clinical implant dentistry and related research. 2013;15(3): 332–40.

24 Pellicer-Chover H, Penarrocha-Oltra D, Bagan L, Fichy-Fernandez AJ, Canullo L, Penarrocha-Diago M. Single-blind randomized clinical trial to evaluate clinical and radiological outcomes after one year of immediate versus delayed implant placement supporting full-arch prostheses. Medicina oral, patologia oral y cirugia bucal. 2014;19(3):e295–301.

25 Penarrocha M, Boronat A, Garcia B. Immediate loading of immediate mandibular implants with a full-arch fixed prosthesis: a preliminary study. Journal of oral and maxillofacial surgery : official journal of the American Association of Oral and Maxillofacial Surgeons. 2009; 67(6):1286–93.

26 Romanos GE, Gupta B, Gaertner K, Nentwig GH. Distal cantilever in full-arch prostheses and immediate loading: a retrospective clinical study. The International journal of oral & maxillofacial implants. 2014;29(2):427–31.

27 Wang Y, Zhang Y, Miron RJ. Health, Maintenance, and Recovery of Soft Tissues around Implants. Clinical implant dentistry and related research. 2015.

28 Sculean A, Gruber R, Bosshardt DD. Soft tissue wound healing around teeth and dental implants. Journal of clinical periodontology. 2014;41 Suppl 15:S6–22.

29 Crespi R, Cappare P, Crespi G, Lo Giudice G, Gastaldi G, Gherlone E. Immediate Implant Placement in Sockets with Asymptomatic Apical Periodontitis. Clinical implant dentistry and related research. 2016.

30 Han CH, Mangano F, Mortellaro C, Park KB. Immediate Loading of Tapered Implants Placed in Postextraction Sockets and Healed Sites. The Journal of craniofacial surgery. 2016;27(5):1220–7.

31 Peron C, Romanos G. Immediate Placement and Occlusal Loading of Single-Tooth Restorations on Partially Threaded, Titanium-Tantalum Combined Dental Implants: 1-Year Results. The International journal of periodontics & restorative dentistry. 2016;36(3):393–9.

32 Ketabi M, Deporter D, Atenafu EG. A Systematic Review of Outcomes Following Immediate Molar Implant Placement Based on Recently Published Studies. Clinical implant dentistry and related research. 2016.

33 Xu L, Wang X, Zhang Q, Yang W, Zhu W, Zhao K. Immediate versus early loading of flapless placed dental implants: a systematic review. The Journal of prosthetic dentistry. 2014;112(4):760–9.

34 Proceedings of the Third ITI (International Team for Implantology) Consensus Conference. Gstaad, Switzerland, August 2003. The International journal of oral & maxillofacial implants. 2004;19 Suppl: 7–154.

35 Puisys A, Linkevicius T. The influence of mucosal tissue thickening on crestal bone stability around bone-level implants. A prospective controlled clinical trial. Clinical oral implants research. 2015;26(2): 123–9.

36 Fu JH, Lee A, Wang HL. Influence of tissue biotype on implant esthetics. The International journal of oral & maxillofacial implants. 2011;26(3):499–508.

37 Lee A, Fu JH, Wang HL. Soft tissue biotype affects implant success. Implant dentistry. 2011;20(3):e38–47.

38 Ghanaati S, Unger RE, Webber MJ, Barbeck M, Orth C, Kirkpatrick JA, et al. Scaffold vascularization in vivo driven by primary human osteoblasts in concert with host inflammatory cells. Biomaterials. 2011;32(32):8150–60.

39 Barbeck M, Najman S, Stojanovic S, Mitic Z, Zivkovic JM, Choukroun J, et al. Addition of blood to a phycogenic bone substitute leads to increased in vivo vascularization. Biomedical materials (Bristol, England). 2015;10(5):055007.

40 Udagawa A, Sato S, Hasuike A, Kishida M, Arai Y, Ito K. Micro-CT observation of

angiogenesis in bone regeneration. Clinical oral implants research. 2013;24(7):787–92.
41 Mammoto A, Connor KM, Mammoto T, Yung CW, Huh D, Aderman CM, et al. A mechanosensitive transcriptional mechanism that controls angiogenesis. Nature. 2009;457(7233):1103–8.
42 Park JC, Kim CS, Choi SH, Cho KS, Chai JK, Jung UW. Flap extension attained by vertical and periosteal-releasing incisions: a prospective cohort study. Clinical oral implants research. 2012;23(8):993–8.
43 Annibali S, Pranno N, Cristalli MP, La Monaca G, Polimeni A. Survival Analysis of Implant in Patients With Diabetes Mellitus: A Systematic Review. Implant dentistry. 2016;25(5):663–74.
44 King S, Klineberg I, Levinger I, Brennan-Speranza TC. The effect of hyperglycaemia on osseointegration: a review of animal models of diabetes mellitus and titanium implant placement. Archives of osteoporosis. 2016;11(1):29.
45 Zhang J, Shirai M, Yamamoto R, Yamakoshi Y, Oida S, Ohkubo C, et al. Effect of Nerve Growth Factor on Osseointegration of Titanium Implants in Type 2 Diabetic Rats. The International journal of oral & maxillofacial implants. 2016;31(5):1189–94.
46 Du Z, Xiao Y, Hashimi S, Hamlet SM, Ivanovski S. The effects of implant topography on osseointegration under estrogen deficiency induced osteoporotic conditions: Histomorphometric, transcriptional and ultrastructural analysis. Acta Biomater. 2016;42:351–63.
47 Giro G, Chambrone L, Goldstein A, Rodrigues JA, Zenobio E, Feres M, et al. Impact of osteoporosis in dental implants: A systematic review. World journal of orthopedics. 2015;6(2):311–5.
48 Siebert T, Jurkovic R, Statelova D, Strecha J. Immediate Implant Placement in a Patient With Osteoporosis Undergoing Bisphosphonate Therapy: 1-Year Preliminary Prospective Study. The Journal of oral implantology. 2015;41 Spec No: 360–5.
49 Choukroun J, Khoury G, Khoury F, Russe P, Testori T, Komiyama Y, et al. Two neglected biologic risk factors in bone grafting and implantology: high low-density lipoprotein cholesterol and low serum vitamin D. The Journal of oral implantology. 2014;40(1):110–4.
50 Javed F, Malmstrom H, Kellesarian SV, Al-Kheraif AA, Vohra F, Romanos GE. Efficacy of Vitamin D3 Supplementation on Osseointegration of Implants. Implant dentistry. 2016;25(2):281–7.
51 Salata LA, Franke-Stenport V, Rasmusson L. Recent outcomes and perspectives of the application of bone morphogenetic proteins in implant dentistry. Clinical implant dentistry and related research. 2002;4(1):27–32.
52 Kim NH, Lee SH, Ryu JJ, Choi KH, Huh JB. Effects of rhBMP-2 on Sandblasted and Acid Etched Titanium Implant Surfaces on Bone Regeneration and Osseointegration: Spilt-Mouth Designed Pilot Study. BioMed research international. 2015;2015: 459393.
53 Lee SW, Hahn BD, Kang TY, Lee MJ, Choi JY, Kim MK, et al. Hydroxyapatite and collagen combination-coated dental implants display better bone formation in the peri-implant area than the same combination plus bone morphogenetic protein-2-coated implants, hydroxyapatite only coated implants, and uncoated implants. Journal of oral and maxillofacial surgery : official journal of the American Association of Oral and Maxillofacial Surgeons. 2014;72(1):53–60.
54 Wang J, Zheng Y, Zhao J, Liu T, Gao L, Gu Z, et al. Low-dose rhBMP2/7 heterodimer to reconstruct peri-implant bone defects: a micro-CT evaluation. Journal of clinical periodontology. 2012;39(1):98–105.
55 Zhang Y, Yang S, Zhou W, Fu H, Qian L, Miron RJ. Addition of a Synthetically Fabricated Osteoinductive Biphasic Calcium Phosphate Bone Graft to BMP2 Improves New Bone Formation. Clinical implant dentistry and related research. 2015.

56 Fujioka-Kobayashi M, Schaller B, Saulacic N, Zhang Y, Miron RJ. Growth Factor Delivery of BMP9 Utilizing a Novel Natural Bovine Bone Graft with Integrated Atelo-Collagen Type I: Biosynthesis, Characterization and Cell Behavior. Journal of biomedical materials research Part A. 2016.

57 Dohan DM, Choukroun J, Diss A, Dohan SL, Dohan AJ, Mouhyi J, et al. Platelet-rich fibrin (PRF): a second-generation platelet concentrate. Part II: platelet-related biologic features. Oral surgery, oral medicine, oral pathology, oral radiology, and endodontics. 2006;101(3):e45–50.

58 Fujioka-Kobayashi M, Miron RJ, Hernandez M, Kandalam U, Zhang Y, Choukroun J. Optimized Platelet Rich Fibrin With the Low Speed Concept: Growth Factor Release, Biocompatibility and Cellular Response. Journal of periodontology. 2016:1–17.

59 Ghanaati S, Booms P, Orlowska A, Kubesch A, Lorenz J, Rutkowski J, et al. Advanced platelet-rich fibrin: a new concept for cell-based tissue engineering by means of inflammatory cells. The Journal of oral implantology. 2014;40(6): 679–89.

60 Miron R, Fujioka-Kobayashi M, Bishara M, Zhang Y, Hernandez M, Choukroun J. Platelet Rich Fibrin and Soft Tissue Wound Healing: A Systematic Review. Tissue engineering Part B, Reviews. 2016.

61 Chappuis V, Engel O, Shahim K, Reyes M, Katsaros C, Buser D. Soft Tissue Alterations in Esthetic Postextraction Sites: A 3-Dimensional Analysis. Journal of dental research. 2015;94(9 Suppl): 187s–93s.

62 Chen ST, Buser D. Esthetic outcomes following immediate and early implant placement in the anterior maxilla–a systematic review. The International journal of oral & maxillofacial implants. 2014;29 Suppl:186–215.

63 Morton D, Chen ST, Martin WC, Levine RA, Buser D. Consensus statements and recommended clinical procedures regarding optimizing esthetic outcomes in implant dentistry. The International journal of oral & maxillofacial implants. 2014;29 Suppl:216–20.

64 Chappuis V, Buser R, Bragger U, Bornstein MM, Salvi GE, Buser D. Long-term outcomes of dental implants with a titanium plasma-sprayed surface: a 20-year prospective case series study in partially edentulous patients. Clinical implant dentistry and related research. 2013;15(6): 780–90.

65 Nelson K, Schmelzeisen R, Taylor TD, Zabler S, Wiest W, Fretwurst T. The Impact of Force Transmission on Narrow-Body Dental Implants Made of Commercially Pure Titanium and Titanium Zirconia Alloy with a Conical Implant-Abutment Connection: An Experimental Pilot Study. The International journal of oral & maxillofacial implants. 2016;31(5): 1066–71.

66 Shabanpour R, Mousavi N, Ghodsi S, Alikhasi M. Comparative Evaluation of Fracture Resistance and Mode of Failure of Zirconia and Titanium Abutments with Different Diameters. The journal of contemporary dental practice. 2015;16(8): 613–8.

67 Tarnow D, Cho S, Wallace S. The effect of inter-implant distance on the height of inter-implant bone crest. Journal of periodontology. 2000;71(4):546–9.

68 Khlat M, Sermet C, Le Pape A. Increased prevalence of depression, smoking, heavy drinking and use of psycho-active drugs among unemployed men in France. European journal of epidemiology. 2004; 19(5):445–51.

69 Ng M, Freeman MK, Fleming TD, Robinson M, Dwyer-Lindgren L, Thomson B, et al. Smoking prevalence and cigarette consumption in 187 countries, 1980-2012. Jama. 2014;311(2):183–92.

70 Hruska A, Borelli P, Bordanaro AC, Marzaduri E, Hruska KL. Immediate loading implants: a clinical report of 1301

implants. The Journal of oral implantology. 2002;28(4):200–9.

71 Degidi M, Piattelli A. Immediate functional and non-functional loading of dental implants: a 2- to 60-month follow-up study of 646 titanium implants. Journal of periodontology. 2003;74(2):225–41.

72 Degidi M, Piattelli A. Comparative analysis study of 702 dental implants subjected to immediate functional loading and immediate nonfunctional loading to traditional healing periods with a follow-up of up to 24 months. The International journal of oral & maxillofacial implants. 2005;20(1):99–107.

73 Regev E, Smith RA, Perrott DH, Pogrel MA. Maxillary sinus complications related to endosseous implants. International Journal of Oral & Maxillofacial Implants. 1995;10(4).

74 Schwartz-Arad D, Levin L, Sigal L. Surgical success of intraoral autogenous block onlay bone grafting for alveolar ridge augmentation. Implant dentistry. 2005; 14(2):131–8.

75 Barone A, Covani U. Maxillary alveolar ridge reconstruction with nonvascularized autogenous block bone: clinical results. Journal of Oral and Maxillofacial Surgery. 2007;65(10):2039–46.

13

Use of Platelet Rich Fibrin in Facial Aesthetics and Rejuvenation

Cleopatra Nacopoulos

Abstract

While this book focuses on the use of platelet rich fibrin (PRF) in dentistry, it remains remarkable to note the growing number of dental practitioners who now adopt training in facial aesthetics. As the population continues to age and are equally more concerned with their aesthetic appearances, an increasing use of products including Botox, hyaluronic acids, PDO threads and platelet rich plasma (PRP) among other materials have been utilized for facial rejuvenation procedures. It is now estimated that over 16 million aesthetic procedures are performed annually in the United States alone and this trend is only expected to continue to rise as the population ages and procedures are deemed more convenient, cost-effective, and safe. Interestingly, the development of lower centrifugation speeds for PRF has pioneered the use of a liquid PRF that can be utilized as a replacement to conventional PRP therapies, but bears the advantage of not containing any additives including anti-coagulants—known inhibitors of tissue regeneration. This chapter highlights conventional treatments for facial aesthetics and thereafter discusses the use of a liquid injectable PRF for facial rejuvenation.

Highlights

- An introduction to the field of facial aesthetics
- The increasing demand for facial aesthetics worldwide
- The currently utilized materials on the market and their disadvantages
- The natural approach with PRF
- Surgical illustrations of PRF utilized for facial rejuvenation

13.1 Introduction

Aging skin is an inevitable process that occurs as we gradually get older (Figure 13.1) [1,2]. Several factors, both genetic and environmental, such as exposure to sun and pollution, have been shown to affect skin by causing DNA damage [3]. A cluster of different physical changes to the skin including atrophy, telangiectacia, fine and deep wrinkles, yellowing (solar elastosis), and dyspigmentation can also occur. Poor diet, lack of exercise, caffeine consumption, smoking, and drugs are also known factors that speed the aging process [4]. One key issue that favors good general health is hydration. Adequate hydration is of course necessary for health in general, but hydration of the skin is related to a healthy skin barrier preventing excessive trans-epidermal water loss. From this standpoint, dehydration of skin is a major known risk factor for aging and other severities such as dryness of skin, apoptosis of epithelial cells, and excessive

Platelet Rich Fibrin in Regenerative Dentistry: Biological Background and Clinical Indications, First Edition.
Edited by Richard J. Miron and Joseph Choukroun.

AGING : process of becoming older
Youthful appearance
Optimal volume distribution
accumulation of changes in a human being over time, encompassing physical, psychological, and social change

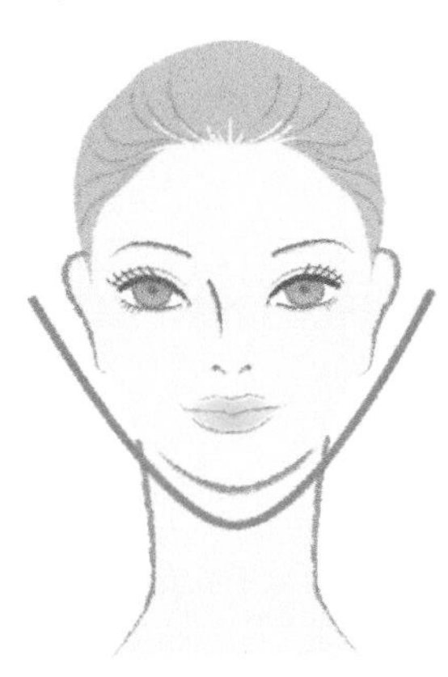

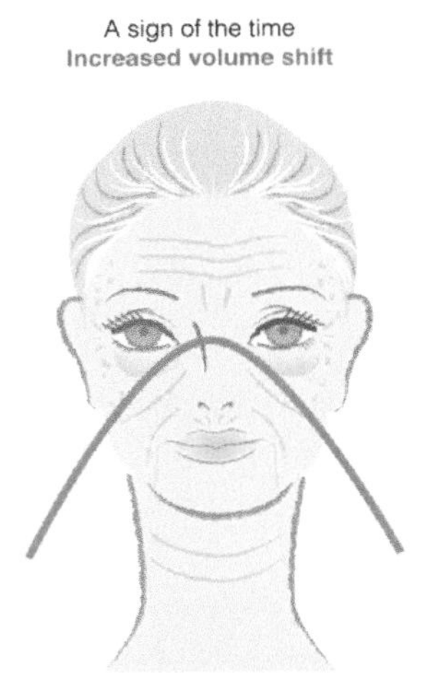

Figure 13.1 The age-related changes associated with aging skin. In young skin, volume and optimal distribution is seen through the face that begins to droop.

oil production causes a blurry and flaky skin complexion. Aging has also been associated with obvious demarcations of the face, for instance, at the corners of the mouth, cheeks, eyelids, forehead, eyebrows, and nose all affected [5]. Based on the visible differences that occur with aging, a variety of treatment procedures have therefore been proposed with the aim of favoring a youthful appearance.

One of the first known methods introduced for facial rejuvenation incorporated acupuncture into their therapies [6]. The concept was fabricated based on the fact that trauma to skin with a needle and syringe, derma pen, or derma roller could induce slight cell damage leading to new angiogenesis and growth factor release, both enhancing the healing process in the local areas. More invasive techniques were also commercialized including face lifts, aggressive laser treatments, and various forms of grafting procedures [7–9]. These were much more invasive and often left the patients in pain with longer healing periods with the added fact that many surgeries were non-reversible with possible secondary complications. Naturally, the more recent trend has been to seek alternative strategies that are more minimally-invasive and more natural by nature. Therefore, a variety of procedures were introduced including Botox, fillers (silicone, calcium hydroxyapatite, polymethylmethacrylate hyaluronic acid products, hyaluronic acid + calcium hydroxyapatite, poly-lactic acid), various laser therapies at different wavelengths/intensities, and PDO threads, among others [10–12].

These less-invasive therapies have been more commonly utilized due to the decreased risk of surgery/patient fear, as well as their associated complications. It is now estimated that roughly 16 million aesthetic procedures are performed annually in the United States alone as reported by the American Society of Plastic Surgery (Figure 13.2 and 13.3). These striking numbers describe the prominent increase in facial aesthetic procedures and the trend continues to demonstrate that less-invasive procedures are becoming the norm with biological agents that are natural. Therefore, by using natural blood, which can be centrifuged to reach supra-physiology concentrations of growth factors, one can expect a natural healing process without intentionally

Aesthetic medicine focuses on improving cosmetic appearance

- scars
- skin laxity
- wrinkles
- moles
- liver spots
- excess fat
- cellulite
- unwanted hair
- skin discoloration
- spider veins

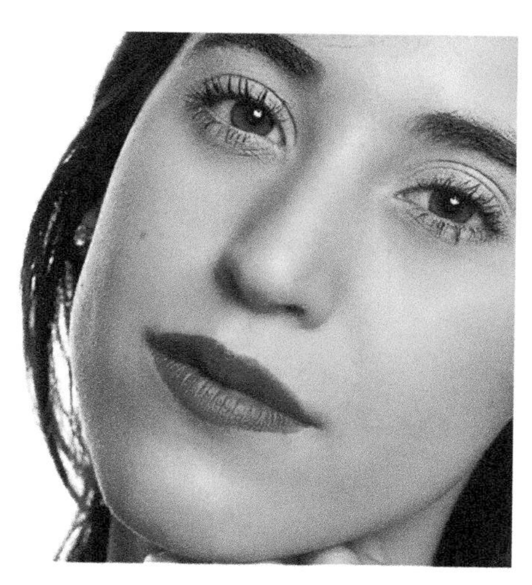

Figure 13.2 The field of aesthetic medicine focuses on improvements in physical and mental well-being by improving patient scars, skin laxity, wrinkles, moles, liver spots, excess fat, cellulite, unwanted hair, skin discoloration, and spider veins to name a few.

inducing a foreign body reaction with an unknown biomaterial such as fillers. This chapter highlights the use of PRF in aesthetic dentistry with a focus on patient selection, background and previously utilized procedures. The application of an injectable PRF is further introduced for several indications in facial aesthetics.

13.2 Features of the skin

The skin serves the main function to protect internal organs from physical biological and chemical agents as well as from ultraviolet (UV) radiation [13]. It also serves a prominent defense role in preventing dehydration by controlling the loss and gain of fluids.

Aesthetic medicine includes dermatology, reconstructive surgery and plastic surgery
Includes
Surgical:
• liposuction
• facelifts
• breast implants
• Radio frequency ablation
Non-surgical:
• mesotherapy
• radio frequency skin tightening
• non surgical liposuction
• chemical peel
• laser
Improves:
• quality of life
• psychological wellbeing
• social function

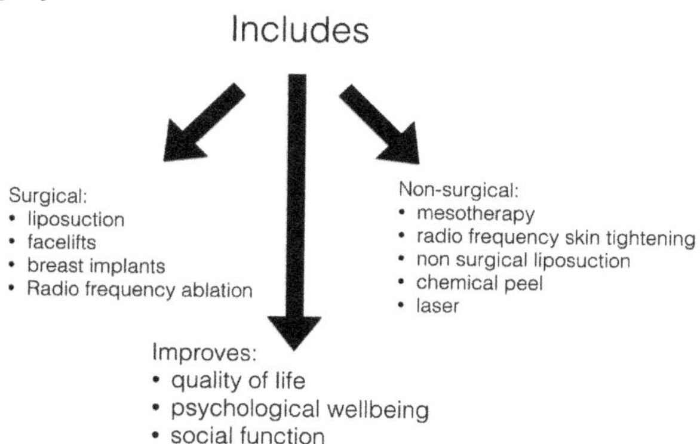

Figure 13.3 The field of aesthetic dentistry and medicine has now reached over 16 million procedures performed annually in the United States alone categorized into dermatology, reconstructive surgery, and plastic surgery.

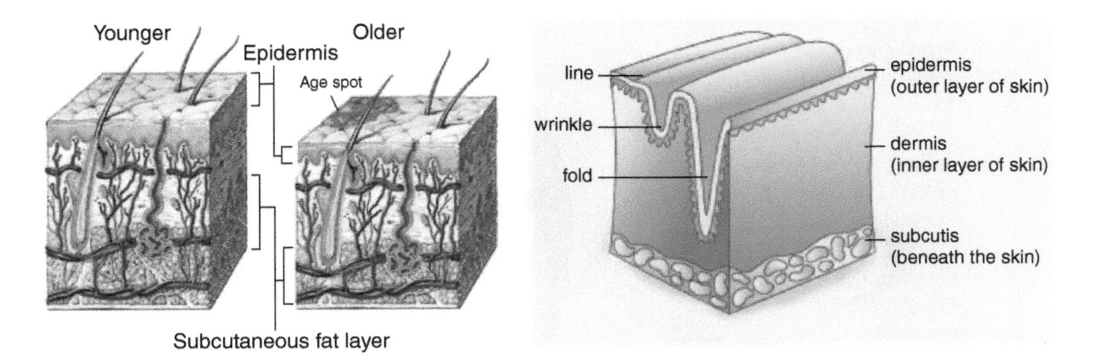

Figure 13.4 Various layers of the skin.

From a biological point of view, it comprises of two layers—an outer epidermis and an internal dermis. The function of the epidermal barrier has been described as having five primary functions including: 1) pathogen defense, 2) water-ion balance and protection against 3) mechanical, 4) chemical insults as well as 5) solar radiation. One must successfully understand the physiological functions of the epidermis to better understand the relevance of these tissues during aging and rejuvenation (Figure 13.4) [14].

The *epidermis* is made up of a stratified squamous epithelium of four to five layers of cells in thickness containing several cell types. These layers can be further classified into the strata basale (germinativum), spinosum, granulosum, lucidum (only in thick skin) and corneum, and include host cells primarily consisting of keratinocytes but also melanocytes, Langerhans cells, and Merkel cells.

The *stratum basale* is a single layer of cuboidal basal cells firmly attached to one another by cell-cell junctions called cadherins and desmosomes. When they attach to the basement membrane, cell-membrane junctions (termed hemi-desmosomes) contain integrins. One of the main functions in this layer are that keratinocytes are continuously proliferating and renewing the epidermis layer of the outermost superficial layer that are lost with epidermal turnover.

The *stratum spinosum* is the outermost layer of the stratum basale and consists of several layers of cells from the stratum basale that slowly lose contact with the basement membrane. These cells appear histologically more flattened as they move toward the outer surface and become less active over time.

The *stratum granulosum* comprises even more cells that are flattened in appearance with keratohyalin granules. These granules contain pro-filaggrin, a precursor of filaggrin that bundles the keratin filaments together.

The *stratum lucidum* is a cell layer where cells have lost their nuclei and organelles and contain a keratin-rich cytoplasm.

Lastly, the *stratus corneum* consists of dead, highly keratinized cells. Keratin filaments polymerize by forming strong disulphide bonds. Lamellar granules have been shown to discharge their lipids that fill the intercellular spaces, which contributes to the barrier properties of the epidermis.

The combination of these aforementioned layers in normal tissues provides the skin with the properties to provide host defense from incoming insults. These include desmosomes that prevent bacterial infiltration, lipid discharge from lamellar granules, and constant migration and shedding of keratinocytes.

While one might expect that the epidermal barrier serves the only function in skin, it is important to note that several other cell types are comprised within skin that have enormous aesthetic implications due to their ability to recognize foreign body materials. For example, Langerhans cells activate the adaptive immune-response by presenting antigens of T-cells [15]. Injection of foreign materials could lead to negative activation of their receptors thereby secreting an abundance of host pro-inflammatory cytokines and thereby creating an immunological barrier. Similarly, melanocytes have a role in defending the host body from incoming UV light and are expressed in different numbers in various racial populations.

13.3 Aging and the epidermal barrier function mechanisms in skin aesthetics

As the body ages, it undergoes a series of modifications that directly impacts the physiology of human tissues. This could not be more apparent in the epidermis layer, which undergoes a series of events leading to drastic modifications to the texture, hydration, and composition of the skin [16]. The pathophysiological hallmark of ageing skin is atrophy. From this sense, the dermo-epidermal junction becomes flatter. It is well known that keratinocytes lose their proliferative ability and a reduction in melanocytes and Langerhans cells is observed. Therefore, regenerative procedures have been utilized to try and reverse these changes through non-invasive techniques as well as invasive surgical procedures described later in this chapter.

Noteworthy are the clinical appearances of changes to the skin with age. These include congested skin where an increased risk of breakouts is observed due to increases in oil production to compensate for dryness. The appearance of the skin can also appear flakier as it becomes blotchier or when dehydration occurs.

In normal aging, the following changes are expected as progression occurs:

- Corners of the mouth move inferiorly resulting in a slight frown look
- Cheeks sag inferiorly resulting in the appearance of jowls
- Tissue around the eyes sag inferiorly
- Eyelids (upper and lower) sag inferiorly
- Tissue of the forehead drifts inferiorly, creating wrinkles and dropping the eyebrows downward with flatter appearances
- Nose may elongate and the tip may regress inferiorly
- Nose may develop a small to pronounced dorsal hump
- Tip of the nose may enlarge and become bulbous
- Generalized wrinkling to the face naturally occurs

Furthermore, several chronological aging disorders have been reported due to congenital syndromes such as Hutchinson-Gilford syndrome/Progeria, Werner's syndrome/Adult Progeria and Ehlers-Danlos syndrome.

As we get older, all human cells age as a result of lower cellular activity [17]. A loss of bone density, increases in fat storage, and lower production of collagen may be observed. Reduction in collagen synthesis of types I and II and its associated increases in degradation have been reported disadvantages of aging leading to a net loss of collagens contained within skin providing elasticity and health.

13.4 Pre-evaluation and patient selection

During patient selection and evaluation, all patients undergo consultation for a lengthy period of time namely to characterize exactly what patient expectations are and what they really look to accomplish (Figure 13.5). Personally, I recommend asking patients to bring photos of themselves from a time when they were more at ease with their appearance and discuss what we can achieve and expect together. It is always important to remember that the most authentic look that a patient can

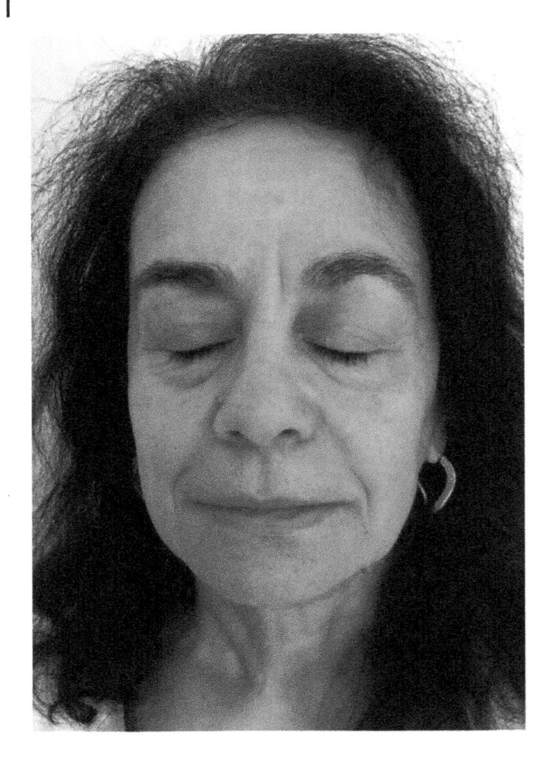

Figure 13.5 Initial patient consultation includes various aspects encompassing patient expectations, clinical photos, evaluation of the skin, and habits of the patient.

achieve is their own and that creating false-looking tissues should never be the goal of facial aesthetics.

In general, it is important to score not only the patient age, but also many other features including but not limited to general health. Skin conditions, lifestyle, smoking habits, alcohol/narcotics consumption, weight, diet, skin hydration, different skin types, sun exposure, and potential diseases or syndromes may affect the skin. From this respect, a patient whom is young (20 to 30 years of age) with less-damaged skin should expect to see improvements most noteworthy in prevention of aging. In such cases, mesotherapy is recommended, as discussed later in the chapter.

If a patient presents with medium age, [35–45] I consider seeking methods to rejuvenate deeper wrinkles, damaged skin from sun exposure, and loss of skin hydration. In such cases, the use of blood platelet derivatives is idea to penetrate the dermis of the skin in order to fill up the nasolabial folds and perform facial contouring. Additionally, mesotherapy treatment is simultaneously utilized with a liquid injectable-PRF (i-PRF) to enrich the skin with many growth factors and leukocytes in order to promote the physiological inflammatory process.

When patient age increases between 45 and 65, often the combination of therapies is required. These include platelet concentrates, potentially with lasers, fillers, PDO threads, or other materials. In such cases, it is highly recommended to combine traditional approaches of surgical therapy with less-invasive procedures utilizing PRF to augment and rejuvenate the skin.

When patients reach an age older than 65 years of age, the choice of treatment remains the combination of the above-stated treatments with more frequent visits and the use of more quantity of products. However, in such cases, it is important to understand the limitations of such procedures, especially those performed with platelet concentrates versus those performed by plastic surgeons performing face lifts. Noteworthy, in all cases, it is important at least in my practice to document all changes accordingly. In this way, doctors can maintain a track record of their work and show incoming patients their approximate expectations following therapy based on their profile and age.

13.5 Conventional therapies in facial aesthetics

Conventional therapies for facial aesthetics have a long list of currently utilized as well as failed materials that have been commercialized over the years. Perhaps those most well-known and utilized are toxins and epidermal barrier function such as botulinum toxin (Botox) [18,19]. These products have been made popular by commercialization and the

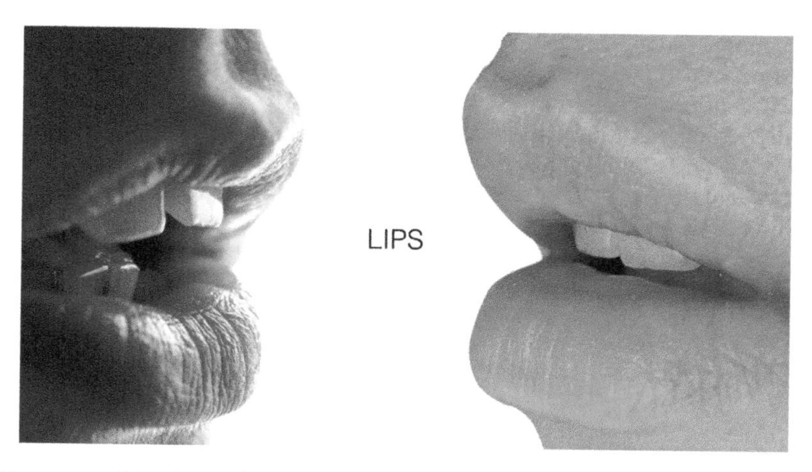

Figure 13.6 Lips are considered one of the most sought-after facial enhancement procedure.

number of celebrities routinely using these products continues to increase their popularity. There are plenty of examples that have demonstrated their successful use in various aesthetic procedures with an increase in lip volume (fillers) being one of the most aesthetic desires (Figure 13.6). It must be noted that despite some negative reported effects, medical use of Botox is generally considered safe and effective with thousands of patients having been treated with relatively few serious adverse effects.

An important point to mention, however, is that these techniques heavily rely on normal protective mechanisms of the epidermis, which can be altered or disrupted following their use. Therefore, the use of such products such as Botox have known secondary effects that may cause a cascade of reactions with (yet undetermined) consequences [20]. Furthermore, they require constant injections every 4 to 6 months or so to maintain their appearance. There has been documented evidence demonstrating that Botox may lead to the temporary denervation and relaxation of muscles for several weeks following use, by preventing the release of neurotransmitter acetylcholine at the peripheral nerve endings. While it is safe for the treatment of hyperfunctional lines and improves the general appearance of the face [21], it may cause secondary effects associated with an increased granular layer or thinning of the epidermis as a result of a foreign body reaction to this material [22,23]. Other reported secondary effects include mainly cases of muscle paresis including muscle weakness, brow ptosis, upper eye lid ptosis, lower eye lid ptosis, lateral arching of the eyebrow, double or blurred vision, loss or difficulty in voluntary closure, upper lip ptosis, uneven smile, lateral lip ptosis, lower lip flattening, orbicularis oris weakness, difficulty in chewing, dysphagia, altered voice pitch, and neck weakness. Furthermore, Botox also contains additional neurotoxin-associated proteins that may elicit intracellular responses that affect the normal physiology of the skin [24]. These have also been reported in over 40 cases of blindness caused by dermal filler injections. While it is used practically every day in the field of facial aesthetics, it is clear other materials are constantly being investigated as potential alternatives without bearing secondary side effects. The most important criteria are that the medical practitioner be well trained to reduce the number of complications. Hyaluronic acid is often a secondary choice with more biological biocompatibility with host tissues when Botox is deemed to have causes a foreign body reaction [25]. Common filler complications include but are not limited to unrealistic patient expectations, bruising/hematoma, under-correction, asymmetry, lumping, iatrogenic factors, and allergic reactions. Our intention is to replace these materials with more natural blood-derived products such as PRF for more natural healing. With fillers an immediate result may be observed but they also dissolve within a 4- to 6-month timeframe. With growth factors found in PRF, we are capable of naturally producing our own collagen and elastin in a more stable way over longer periods of time.

13.6 Lasers and epidermal barrier function

Laser therapy has also been utilized in aesthetic medicine and appears to be resurfacing as a more commonly utilized procedure to rejuvenate skin tissue with the advancements made in laser research [26,27]. This technique is certainly considered more invasive when compared to cosmeceuticals and may lead to temporary epidermal barrier function damage due to swelling and redness of skin surfaces having been over-exposed to laser therapy. Treatments including high-energy pulsed CO2 lasers and fractional CO2 laser therapies have been suggested as options for epithelium renewal by increasing the proliferation of keratinocytes [20]. Furthermore, lasers have been shown to stimulate collagen synthesis [25]. For these reasons, lasers have often been utilized alone or combined with other strategies for facial aesthetics. The treatment relies on the alteration of the function of epidermis through laser excitation. Nevertheless, secondary side effects including swelling, pigmentation, and skin irritation or infection have been reported.

13.7 Overview of utilizing platelet derivatives in facial aesthetics

Interestingly, it was proposed several years ago that platelet concentrates and most notably platelet rich plasma (PRP), could be utilized in facial aesthetics [28–30]. PRP has been shown to increase the regeneration of a variety of tissues namely by increasing blood flow to defective tissues. From this point of view, its use in facial aesthetics followed. Since then and with the advancements made with PRF, it became possible to utilize platelet concentrates without having to use anti-coagulants, known inhibitors of tissue regeneration (Figure 13.7). While acupuncture has been an ancient treatment for skin rejuvenation, the idea of utilizing other modalities such as a syringe, derma pen, and derma roller in combination with naturally derived growth factors has been more common in recent years, favoring more natural regeneration with natural products. Since PRF is totally autologous because it uses patient blood without anti-coagulants (Figure 13.8 and 13.9), it makes the procedures safer, without eliciting a foreign body reaction at low cost.

13.8 Clinical procedures utilizing PRF in facial aesthetics

The use of PRF has been utilized for a variety of aesthetic procedures in medicine that focus on improving cosmetic appearance through the treatment of conditions including scars, skin laxity, and wrinkles. Important is to understand that in the field of facial aesthetics, plastic tubes are only utilized in order to prevent coagulation into a PRF fibrin matrix. Therefore, two formulations of PRF are discussed within the present chapter: *a liquid injectable formulation of PRF centrifuged at extremely low speeds (700 RPM, 60 G for 3 minutes; i-PRF) versus PRF matrix that is utilized to enhance tissue augmentation (1300 RPM for 8 minutes; PRF matrix, A-PRF-liquid).* While various surgical procedures have been utilized, the main aim has been to improve the patient self-esteem by providing better quality of life, psychological well-being, and social function to patients and with the advancements made in PRF

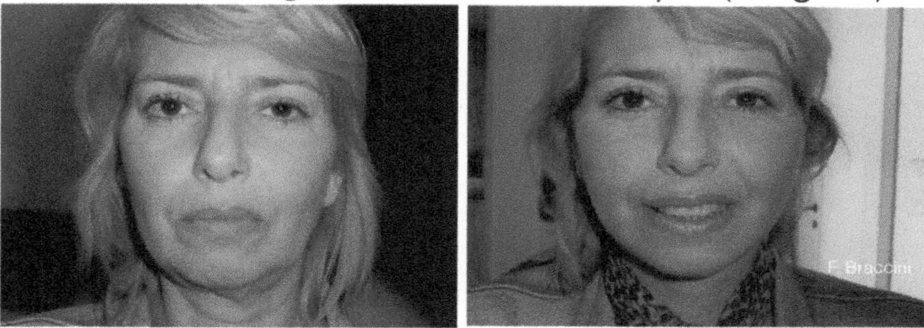

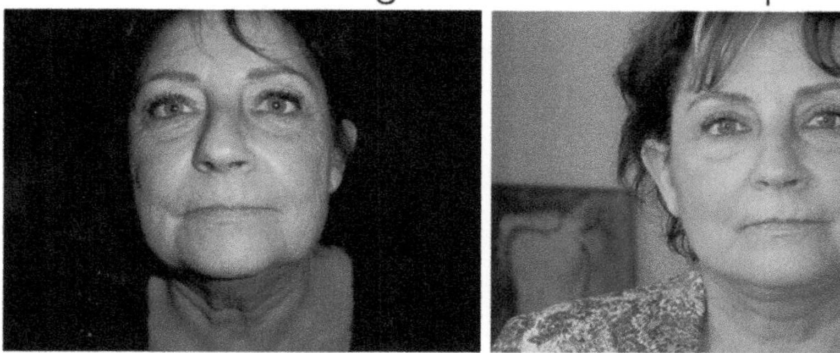

Figure 13.7 Various aesthetic procedures previously utilizing platelet rich plasma (PRP) have now been replaced with platelet rich fibrin (PRF). The major advantage is that healing may take place without anti-coagulants found in PRP.

therapy, it is now possible to do so in a natural way.

The use of PRF (1300 rpm for 8 min) or i-PRF (700 rpm for 3 min) have therefore been utilized in my practice during combination therapies to enhance aesthetic outcomes and improve patient wound healing. When preparing for regeneration with PRF,

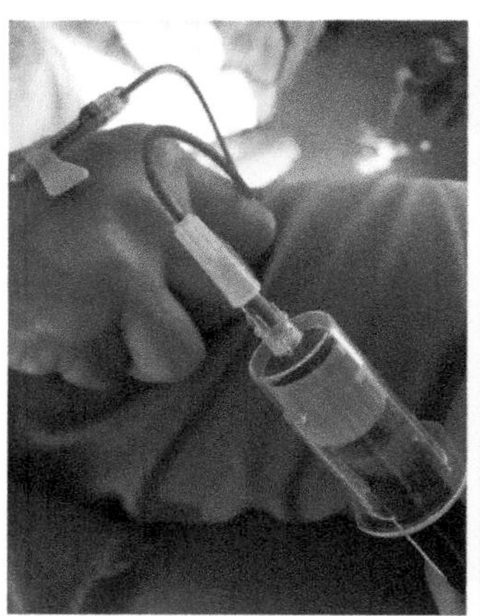

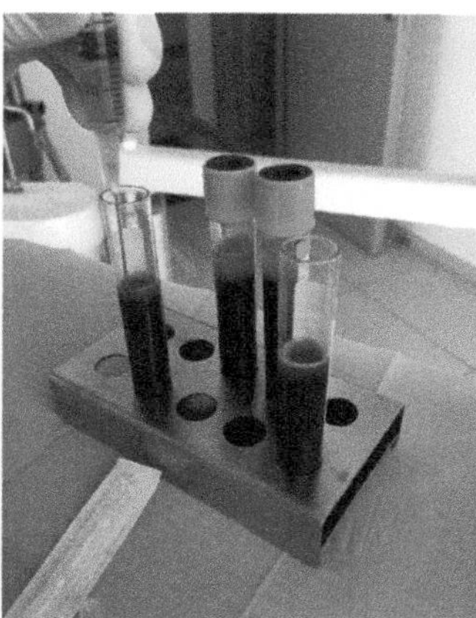

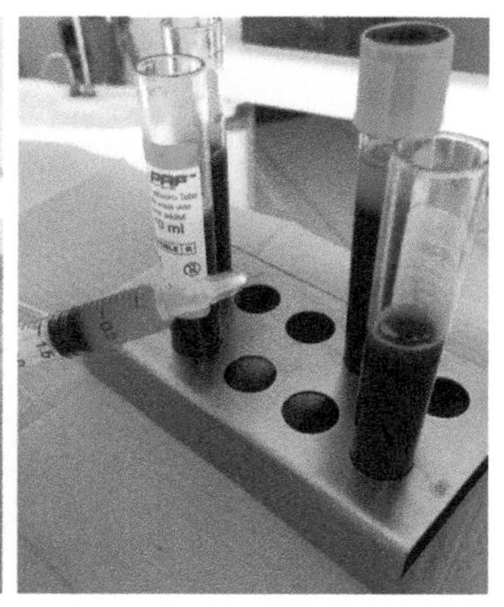

Figure 13.8 Following centrifugation at 700 rpm for 3 minutes, a layer of injectable-PRF can be observed in the upper layer of centrifugation tubes. No additives are utilized during this procedure.

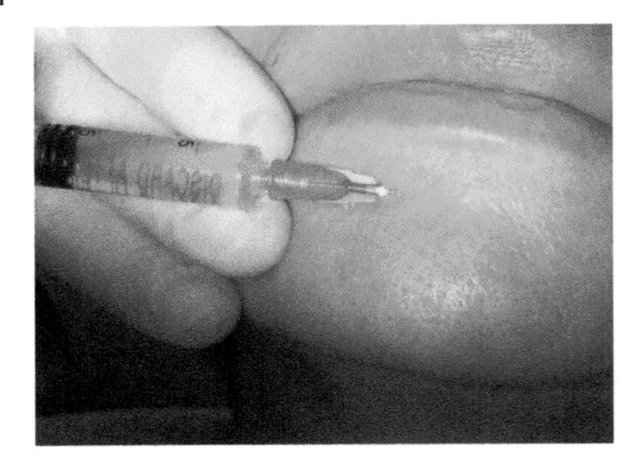

Figure 13.9 Example of a liquid injectable-PRF (i-PRF) that may be utilized to regenerate various areas of the face. i-PRF does not contain anticoagulants and therefore must be utilized within 10 minutes following blood collection.

the treating physician must first look at the skin's anatomy to evaluate the optimal choice of procedure to obtain desired end goals. Therefore, the epidermis (outer layer of skin), dermis (inner layer of skin), and subcutaneous fat layer of the skin (beneath the skin) must be fully evaluated. Furthermore, facial lines, wrinkles, and folds are also examined fully to determine the depth of damage to the skin.

When performing lip augmentation and contouring, i-PRF is utilized in combination with PRF to contour the lips. The PRF is able to provide more volume, whereas the i-PRF provides more leukocytes and a higher concentration of growth factors per volume. This procedure is typically performed once every 15 days for 60 days to ensure optimal aesthetics. In contrast, for acne scars, a derma pen (36 needles) is utilized to perform mesotherapy of damaged skin with a syringe to create multiple penetrations approximately 3 to 5 mm apart from one another to mechanically stimulate the skin during i-PRF injections. If scars are present, PRF is implanted underneath the scar in order to use the fibrin matrix to bulk the lost tissues and to create a micro-environment capable of slowly releasing growth factors over an extended period of time. Leukocytes from the i-PRF ensure and provoke the physiologic inflammation process by secreting higher leukocyte growth factors.

Many non-invasive surgical procedures have become available in which the application of filers underneath the skin during rejuvenation procedures can be achieved. When growth factors from human blood are being utilized (PRF), it is important to note that these surgical procedures are performed via the linear technique or retro-tracking technique as previously described in the literature (Figures 13.10). These

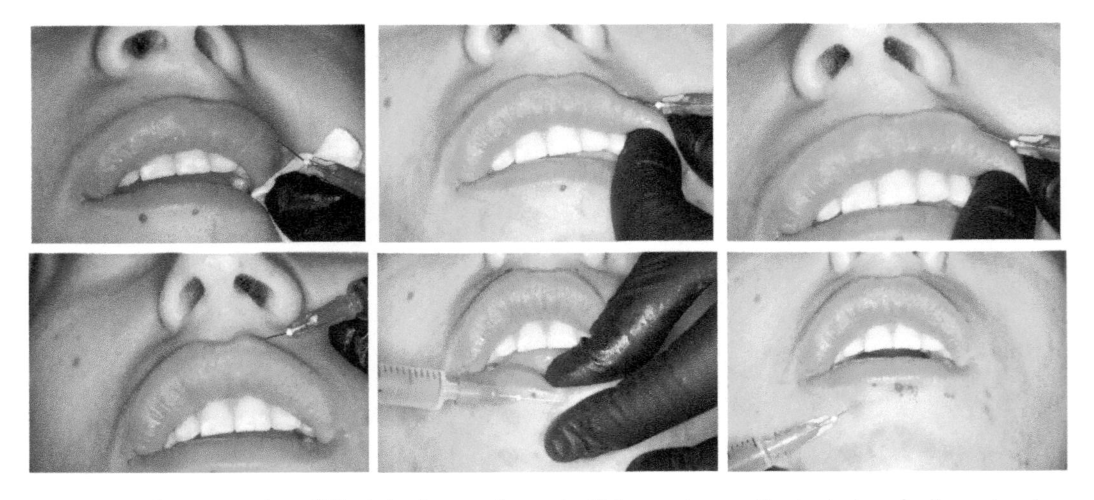

Figure 13.10 Demonstration of filler injections performed utilizing a retro-grading technique for lip contouring.

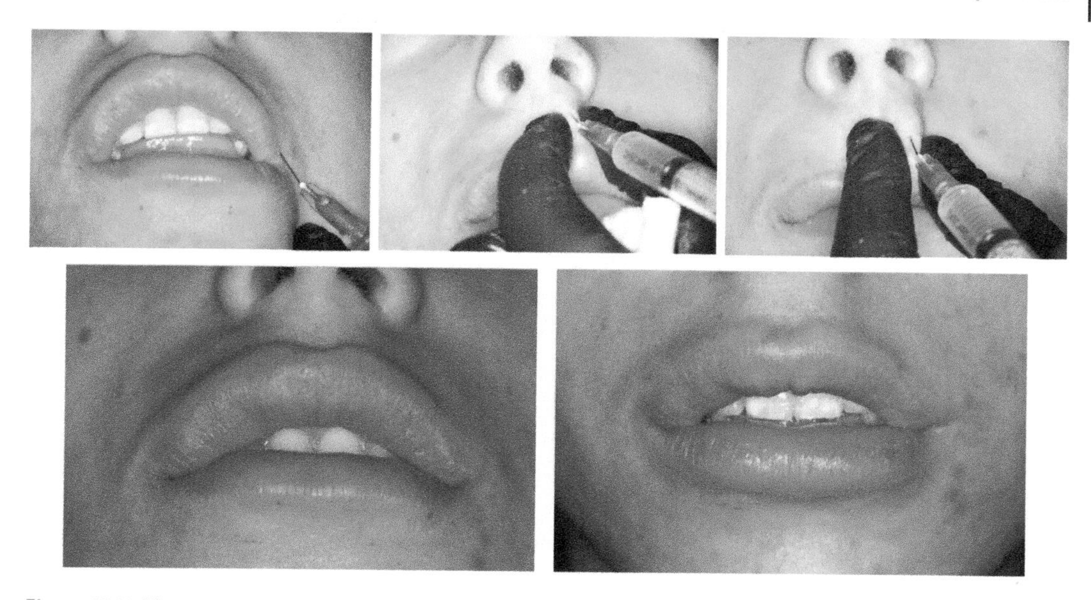

Figure 13.11 Lip augmentation procedure with outer injections performed to augment soft-tissue volume of the lip.

techniques may be applied for linear wrinkles (superficial, medium, and deep), lip and facial contouring (Figures 13.11, Figure 13.12, and Figure 13.13), forehead frowns (Figure 13.14 and Figure 13.15), glabellar, nose, tear trough, nasolabial folds, and marionette lines (Figure 13.16).

Similarly, when performing mesotherapy, two techniques are commonly utilized. The first is the micro papular technique that is

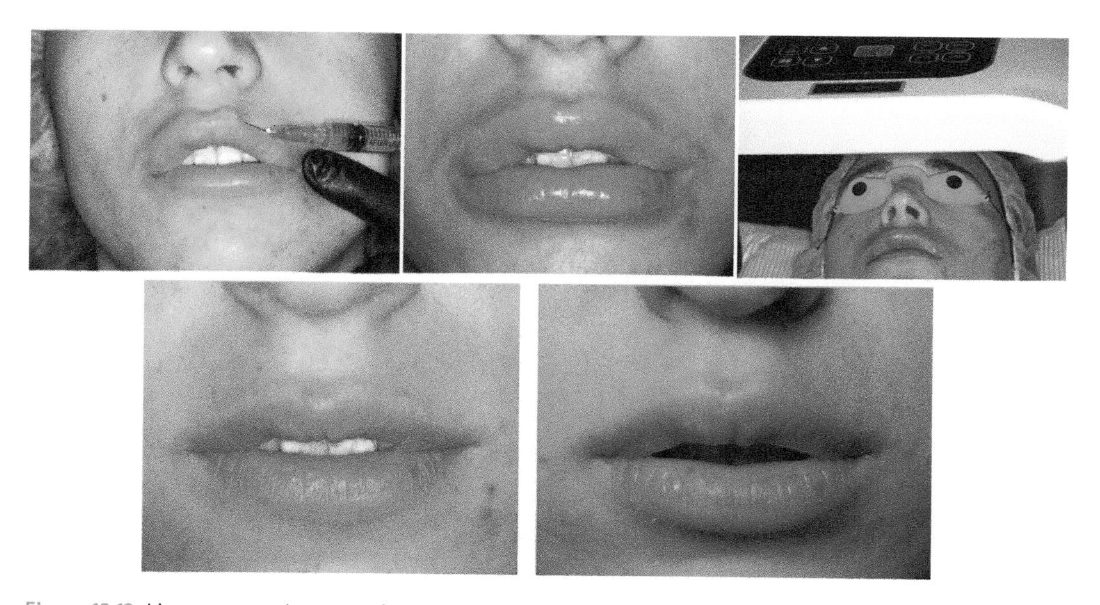

Figure 13.12 Lip augmentation procedure with before and after photos following injections with i-PRF.

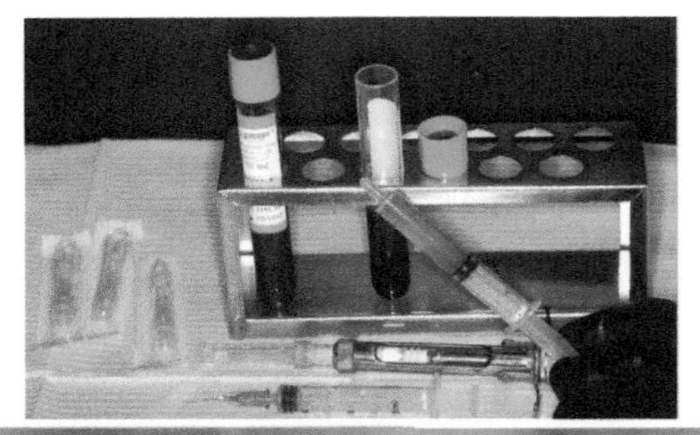

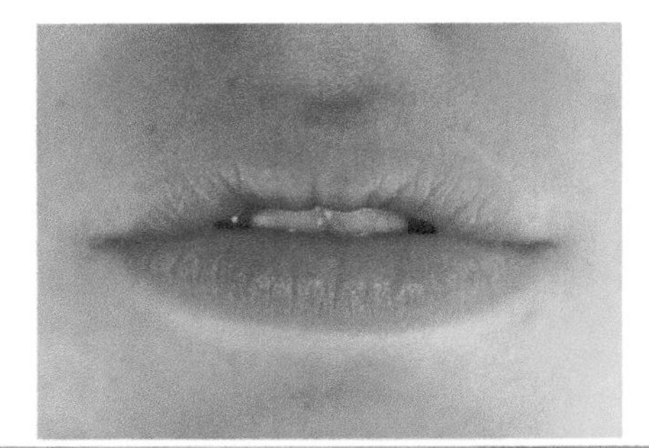

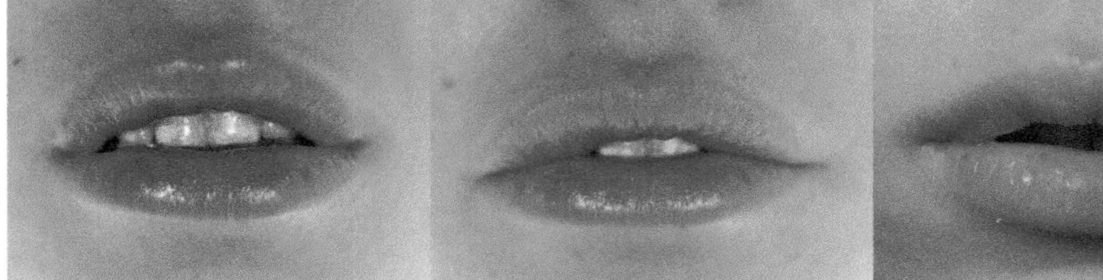

Figure 13.13 Lip augmentation procedure with outer injections performed to augment soft-tissue volume of the lip.

for mature and damaged skin. Small quantities of PRF are injected under the epidermis, creating small papules where PRF and i-PRF can be used to rejuvenate the epidermis skin layer. While the skin may appear red and inflamed at the end of this procedure, these papules disappear within 1 to 2 hours. The second method is the Multipuncture technique, which consists of superficial injections of rapid and regular movements. The punctures are applied evenly throughout the facial skin with an inter distance space between injections of 3 to 5 mm. This technique is utilized to rejuvenate the skin of the face,

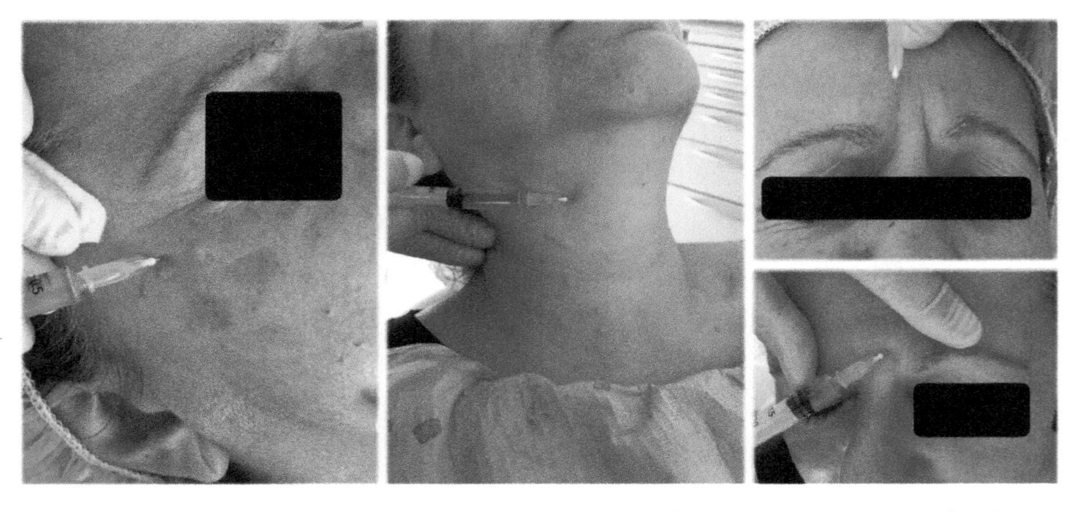

Figure 13.14 Example of various uses of injectable-PRF to augment soft tissues in various regions of the face.

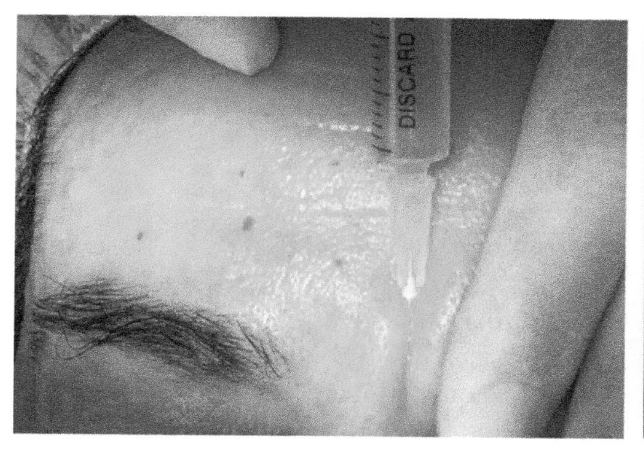

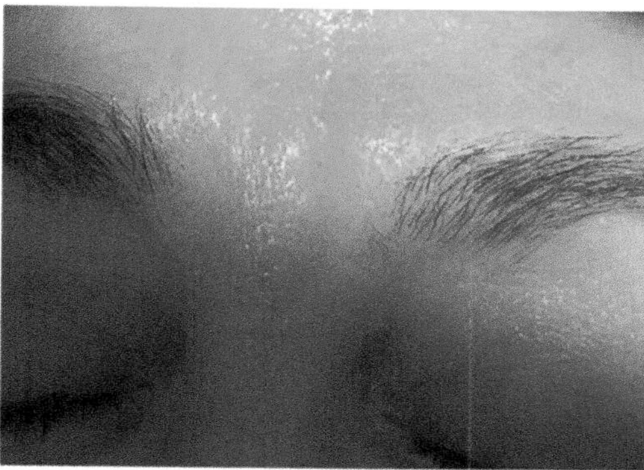

Figure 13.15 Example of injectable-PRF utilized to reduce forehead frowns.

decoletage, hands, and so on. The procedure can be repeated every 15 days and typically is utilized four times over a 60-day period. Maintenance can be done in relation to the condition of the skin. This second procedures is performed with i-PRF, whereas the mesotherapy can be utilized with both a PRF matrix (1300 rpm for 8 min) and a i-PRF (700 rpm for 3 min). With derma pen, the use of only i-PRF is required, whereas with the micropapular technique, both i-PRF and PRF scaffolds are required.

13.9 i-PRF injections with a derma rollers

When using the derma roller, examination of the needle stratum holes must first be performed without damaging the epidermis [31].

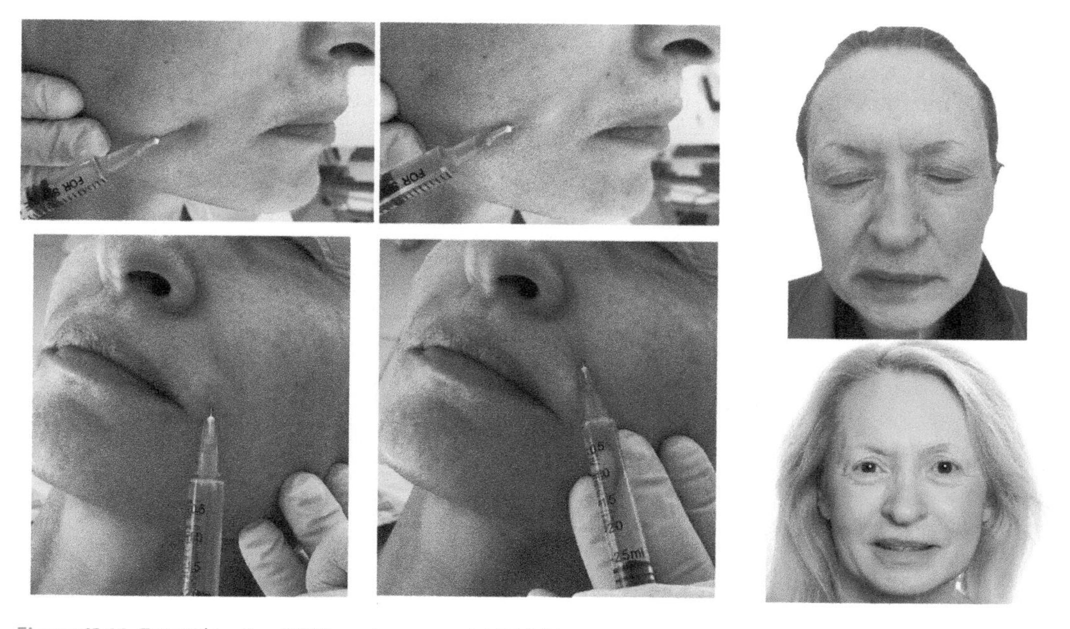

Figure 13.16 Example using PRF to reduce naso-labial folds.

There are multiple options for derma rollers depending on the needs of the skin. Macro needling leads to the release of growth factors that stimulate the formation of natural collagen and elastin in the papillary dermis. During this procedure, induction of neovascularization and neocollagenesis is performed. This procedure is often termed the "percutaneous collagen induction therapy." It is the ideal choice of therapy for skin rejuvenation of photo-aging skin. The procedure begins with the use of micro needles in the horizontal, vertical, and diagonal movements. New collagen synthesis is formed and may be increased and evenly spread resulting in a smoother texture, smaller pore sizes, reduction in scars, and finer visible lines in wrinkles by applying this procedure. It is typically repeated a minimum of four times with an increase in frequency if the skin is highly damaged. A follow-up every 3 to 6 months is recommended.

13.10 i-PRF injections with a derma pen

Another procedure where i-PRF has been frequently utilized is with a derma pen to create skin perforations for better absorption of i-PRF into host skin tissues in order to stimulate the healing process through growth factor release. This naturally increases the healing process of skin. This procedure in general is considered a mechanical skin stimulation and the total time lasts roughly 20 to 30 minutes. Maintenance is highly recommended in order to prolong clinical results. This procedure is used often at the beginning of treatment where the use of derma pen in horizontal, perpendicular, and diagonal movements is performed for approximately 20 to 30 minutes. Thereafter, blood is drawn to prepare PRF, and derma pen procedures can be applied simultaneously with application of PRF.

13.11 i-PRF and PRF for mesotherapy by syringe injections

In this procedure, a 4 mm needle is perforated underneath the epidermis where i-PRF can be injected more deeply into the skin (Figure 13.17 and 13.18) [32]. This has been shown to further result in a more radical change in skin rejuvenation. This procedure can be performed with both i-PRF but also with a PRF matrix utilizing a 4 mm × 32-30 g needle and a 12.7 mm × 27 g needle respectively. While this procedure is

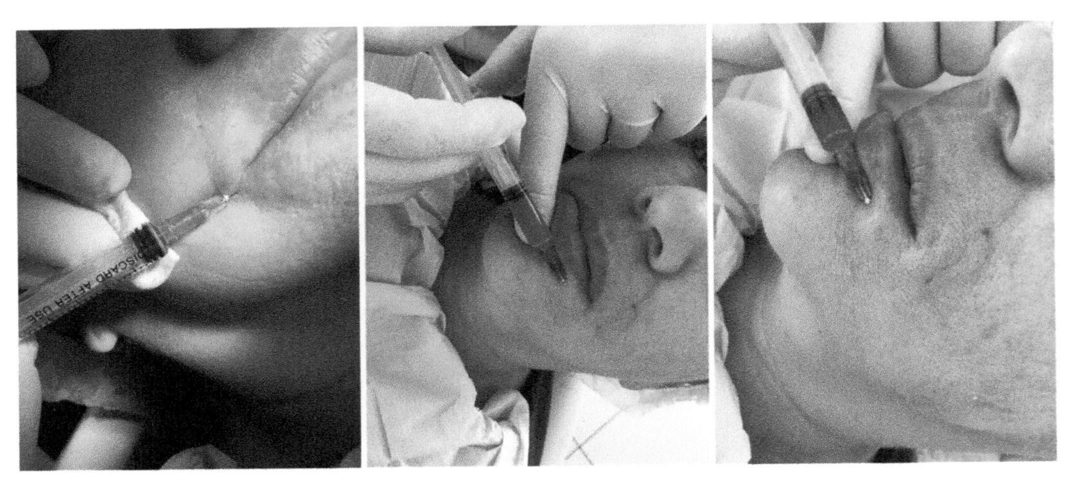

Figure 13.17 Use of PRF for deep injections of various facial folds to increase soft-tissue volume.

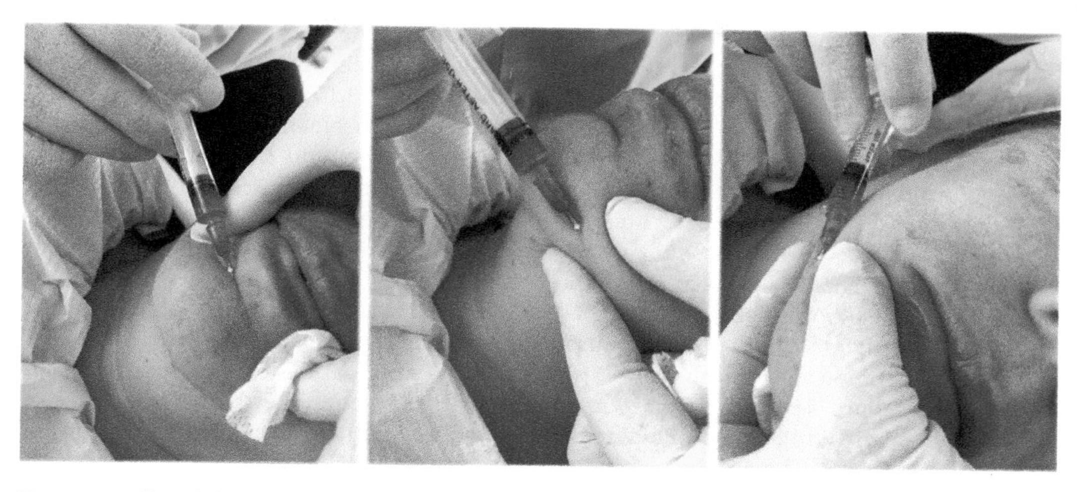

Figure 13.18 Deep injections with PRF to increase soft-tissue volume (same case as presented in Figure 13.16).

considered more invasive causing more skin damage, the results are more altering and superior to less invasive procedure. Maintenance is highly recommended to preserve the acquired results.

13.12 Platelet concentrate during the vampire technique

With aging, the skin becomes more yellow in color due to less vascularization and when this is encountered, a "Vampire Facelift" procedure by Charles Runels is recommended, which involves withdrawing a patient's blood, processing it to isolate blood derivatives with other added biomaterial, then re-injecting it into host tissues to reduce wrinkles and create a more youthful look.

13.13 Augmentation techniques with PRF matrix and i-PRF—combination Therapies

One commonly reported question is when to utilize i-PRF alone versus PRF matrix with i-PRF. To answer this question, it is important to note that while PRF matrix is produced with a three-dimensional fibrin scaffold necessary to increase tissue thickness, interestingly, advancements that have been made with the low-speed centrifugation concept has allowed the development of a liquid-PRF (i-PRF) that contains a higher concentration of leukocytes, growth factors, and therefore an ability to increase tissue wound healing and regeneration.

When both PRF and i-PRF are used in combination during augmentation procedures, greater tissue augmentation is expected. While platelets release their growth factors only after clotting, by using PRF matrix simultaneously, liquid fibrinogen may be converted to fibrin within the skin serving as a reservoir of growth factors producing a slow release. In such procedures, maintenance is also highly recommended in order to sustain the initial results from therapy as addressed below.

13.14 Nasolabial fold rejuvenation with PRF and i-PRF

Nasolabial folds, commonly known as "smile lines" or "laugh lines," are facial features that commonly result with age [33]. They represent the two skin folds that run from each side of the nose to the corners of the mouth. They are defined by facial structures that support the buccal fat pad and separate the cheeks from the upper lip.

By using a combination approach with PRF (1300 rpm for 8 min) and i-PRF (700 rpm for 3 min), 12.7 mm needles (27G × $\frac{1}{2}$ inches) can be utilized to penetrate the skin into the deep dermis by using the linear technique. Afterward, a 32G × 4 mm needle can be used to perform small papules with i-PRF alone—rich in leukocytes—in order to initiate the physiologic inflammatory response for skin augmentation and rejuvenation. Typically, this procedure is performed four times with an interval of 15 to 30 days to maintain ideal aesthetic results. The procedure can be repeated at 3 or 6 months should additional rejuvenation be required.

13.15 Use of PRF and i-PRF for lip augmentation

Due to the increased popularity of celebrity lip augmentations performed annually, a number of patients request lip augmentation procedures. The most natural way to achieve this is by utilizing blood derived PRF and i-PRF (Figure 13.19). Efficient lip augmentation and enhancement procedure can replace the lost volume and the contouring of the aging lips. Furthermore, it can be utilized to create balance between the upper and lower lip as well as loss of shape due to trauma or asymmetries.

For contouring of the lip, a 12.7 mm × 27 G needle size is also utilized with PRF and a 4 mm × 32 G or 30 G for i-PRF for lip enhancement. The derma pen can also be utilized with a setting at 1 mm depth of the needles utilizing i-PRF. This procedure is performed every 15 to 30 days as indicated. The results are long lasting and very natural looking.

13.16 PDO threads using PRF and i-PRF

PDO threads are one of the most popular and highly effective non-surgical means to lift

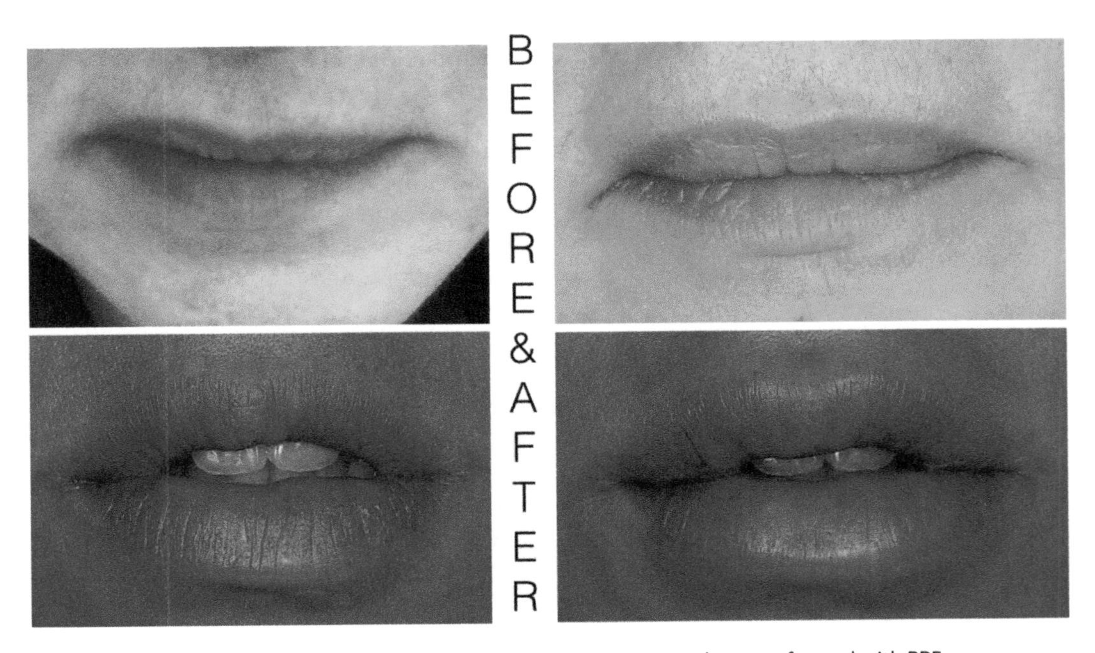

Figure 13.19 Before and after photos following lip augmentation procedures performed with PRF.

and tighten loose and sagging skin tissues as well dissolve small areas of fat on the lower face. PDO (polydioxanone) is a synthetic fiber that dissolves naturally in the body over time, which is widely used in areas of medicine such as general surgery and cardiology.

PDO threads have been utilized to enhance and improve the appearance of sagging necks, sagging cheeks, or jowls, as well as droopy eyebrows. A thread lift is suited to men and women between the ages of 40 and 70. The procedure is most effective on skin that has minimal sagging. Once the threads are in place the body starts to produce new bundles of collagen around each thread and this in turn creates a subtle and yet effective lift. While the results vary significantly between each individual, the final results are natural by nature giving a rejuvenated and refreshed look. There is no scarring and recovery times are much less in duration when compared to those associated with traditional invasive surgery.

Interestingly, more recent research has shown that this procedure may be enhanced when PDO threads are combined with naturally derived i-PRF. Mesotherapy treatment is typically performed first with i-PRF followed by PDO threads. This entire procedure takes roughly 30 minutes for mesotherapy and another 30 minutes for the insertion of the PDO threads and therefore can be accomplished within 1 hour. Figures 13.20, 13.21, 13.22, 13.23, and 13.24 demonstrate some before and after clinical photos of treatments accomplished with i-PRF.

13.17 Conclusion

Facial aesthetics is a rapidly growing field. With over 16 million procedures performed each year in the United States alone, it becomes obvious that patient demands and expectations will continue to rise. By utilizing naturally derived blood concentrates without having to use anti-coagulants, PRF can be utilized as a substitute to enhance tissue regeneration, speed wound healing and enhance collagen synthesis. While the use of PRF is still in its infancy in the facial aesthetic world, future research will further elucidate the beneficial aspects of utilizing PRF for facial procedures highlighted in this chapter.

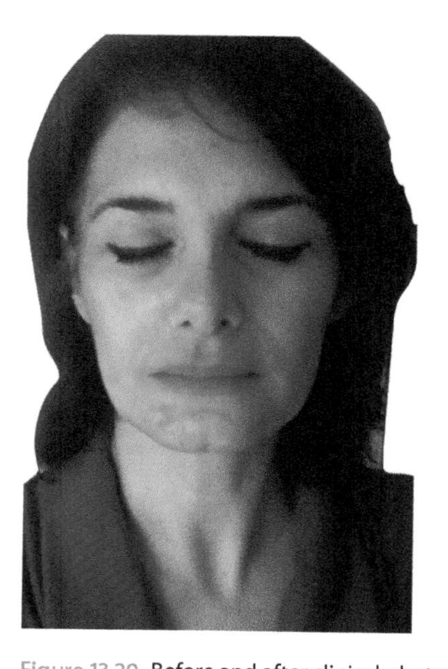

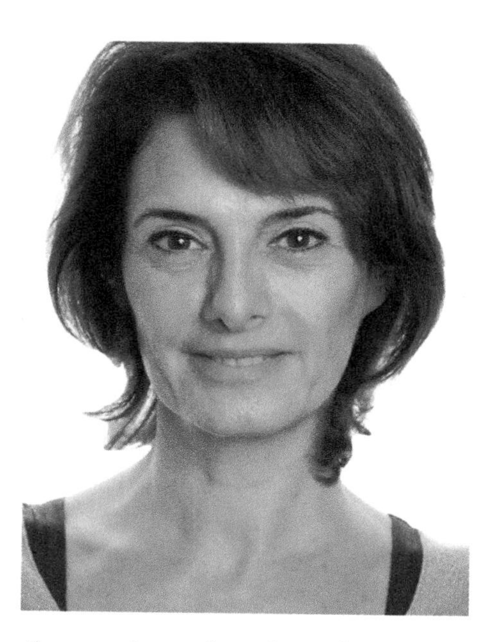

Figure 13.20 Before and after clinical photos of a facial rejuvenation procedure performed naturally with PRF.

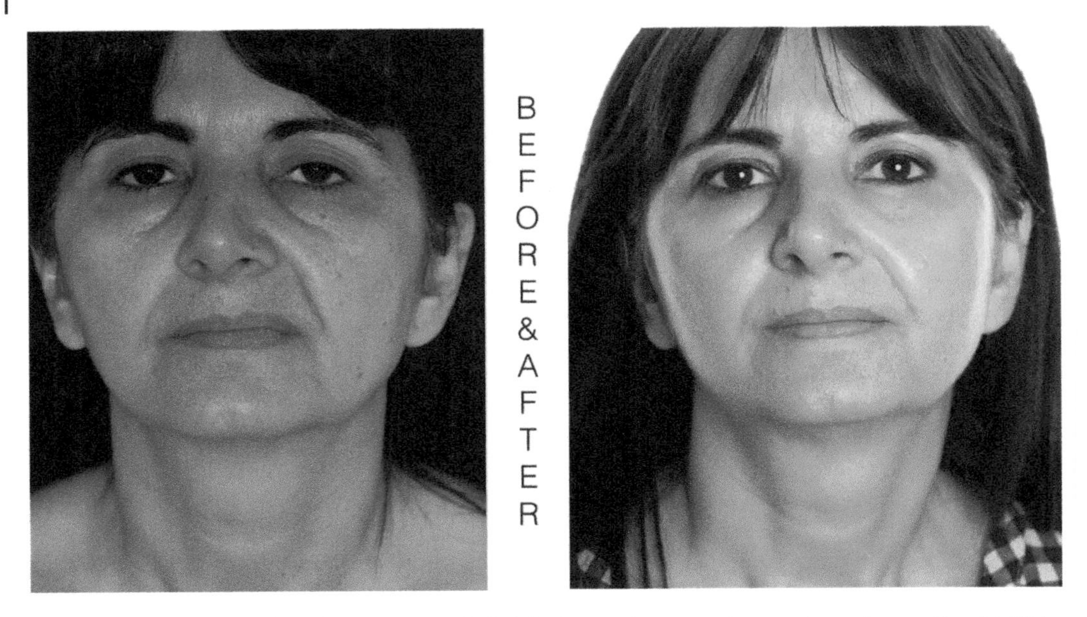

Figure 13.21 Before and after clinical photos of a facial rejuvenation procedure performed naturally with PRF.

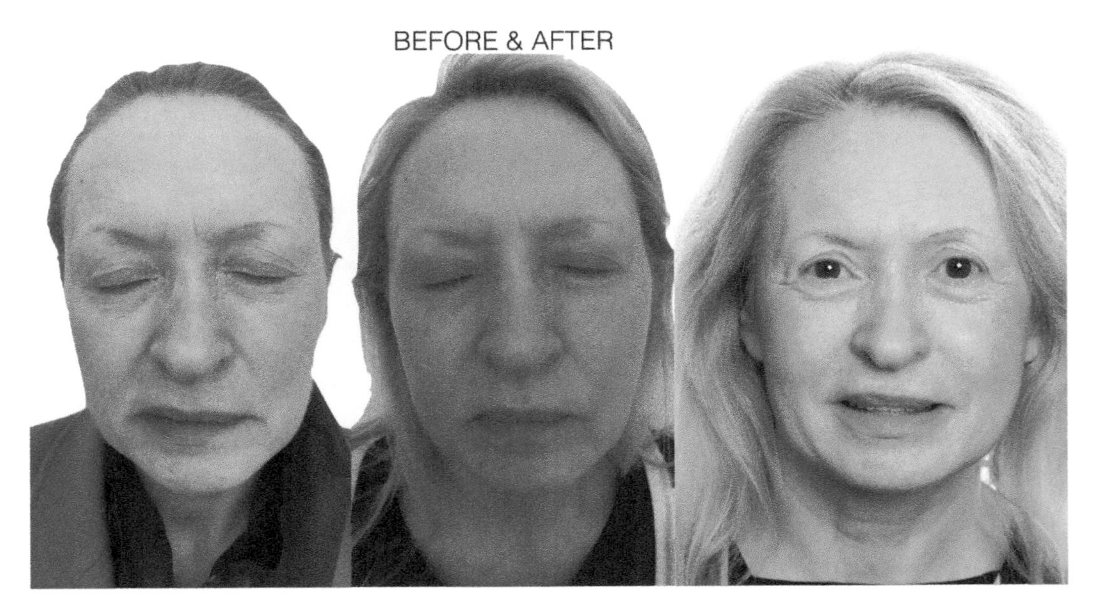

Figure 13.22 Before and after clinical photos of a facial rejuvenation procedure performed naturally with PRF.

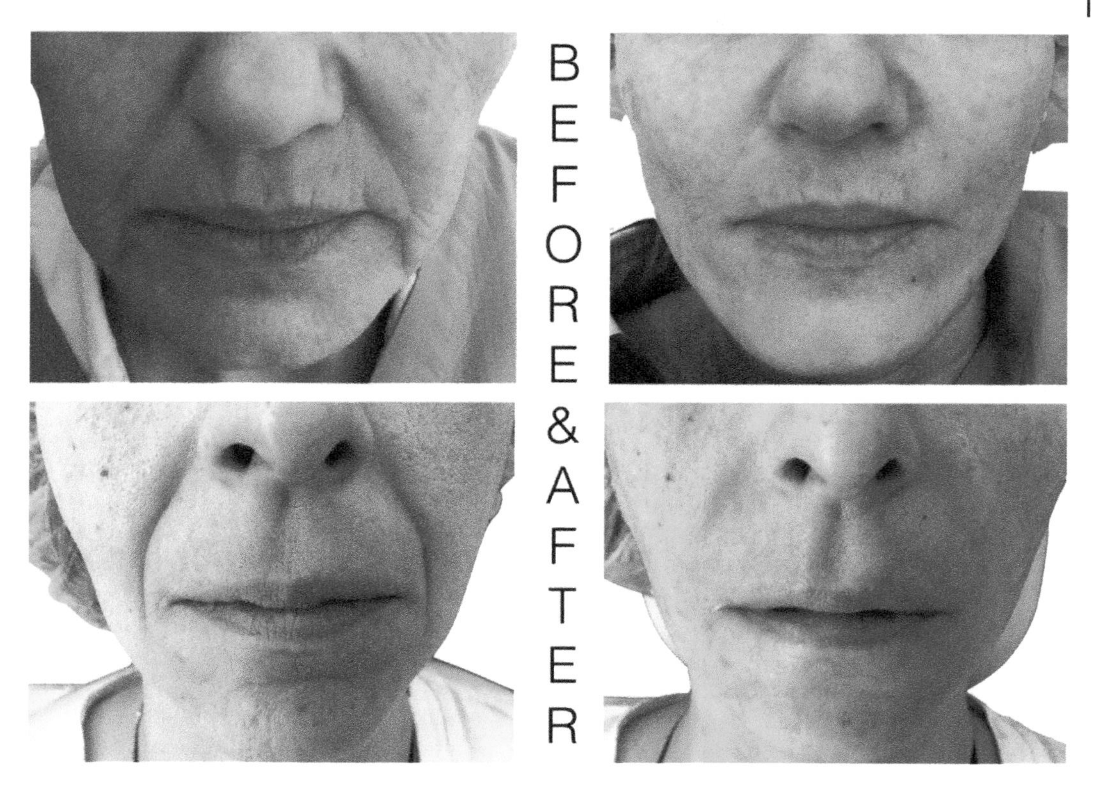

Figure 13.23 Before and after clinical photos of a facial rejuvenation procedure performed naturally with PRF.

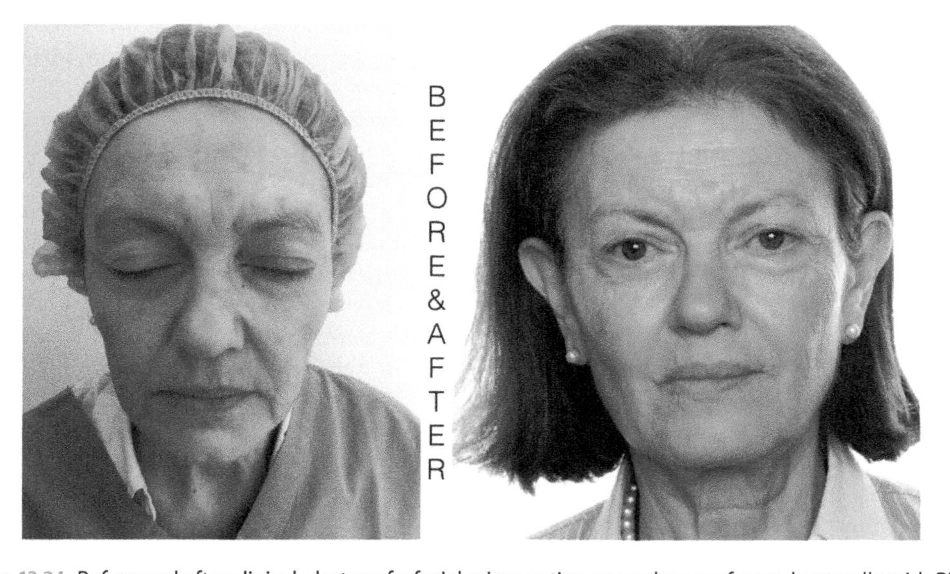

Figure 13.24 Before and after clinical photos of a facial rejuvenation procedure performed naturally with PRF.

References

1. Branchet M, Boisnic S, Frances C, Robert A. Skin thickness changes in normal aging skin. Gerontology. 1990;36(1):28–35.
2. Helfrich YR, Sachs DL, Voorhees JJ. Overview of skin aging and photoaging. Dermatology Nursing. 2008;20(3):177.
3. Herbig U, Ferreira M, Condel L, Carey D, Sedivy JM. Cellular senescence in aging primates. Science. 2006;311(5765): 1257.
4. Puizina-Ivi N. Skin aging. Acta Dermatoven APA. 2008;17(2):47.
5. Friedman O. Changes associated with the aging face. Facial plastic surgery clinics of North America. 2005;13(3):371–80.
6. Barrett JB. Acupuncture and facial rejuvenation. Aesthetic Surgery Journal. 2005;25(4):419–24.
7. Ramirez OM, Maillard GF, Musolas A. The extended subperiosteal face lift: a definitive soft-tissue remodeling for facial rejuvenation. Plastic and reconstructive surgery. 1991;88(2):227–36.
8. Rohrich RJ, Ghavami A, Lemmon JA, Brown SA. The individualized component face lift: developing a systematic approach to facial rejuvenation. Plastic and reconstructive surgery. 2009;123(3): 1050–63.
9. El-Domyati M, Medhat W. Minimally invasive facial rejuvenation: current concepts and future expectations. Expert Review of Dermatology. 2013;8(5):565–80.
10. Cooke G. Effacing the face: Botox and the anarchivic archive. Body and Society. 2008;14(2):23–38.
11. Park MY, Ahn KY, Jung DS. Botulinum toxin type A treatment for contouring of the lower face. Dermatologic surgery. 2003;29(5):477–83.
12. Carruthers JD, Glogau RG, Blitzer A. Advances in Facial Rejuvenation: Botulinum Toxin Type A, Hyaluronic Acid Dermal Fillers, and Combination Therapies—Consensus Recommendations. Plastic and reconstructive surgery. 2008; 121(5):5S–30S.
13. Trouba KJ, Hamadeh HK, Amin RP, Germolec DR. Oxidative stress and its role in skin disease. Antioxidants and Redox Signaling. 2002;4(4):665–73.
14. Martin P. Wound healing–aiming for perfect skin regeneration. Science. 1997; 276(5309):75–81.
15. Cumberbatch M, Dearman RJ, Griffiths CE, Kimber I. Epidermal Langerhans cell migration and sensitisation to chemical allergens. Apmis. 2003;111(7-8):797–804.
16. Lorencini M, Brohem CA, Dieamant GC, Zanchin NI, Maibach HI. Active ingredients against human epidermal aging. Ageing research reviews. 2014;15: 100–15.
17. Dimri GP, Lee X, Basile G, Acosta M, Scott G, Roskelley C, et al. A biomarker that identifies senescent human cells in culture and in aging skin in vivo. Proceedings of the National Academy of Sciences. 1995; 92(20):9363–7.
18. Majid O. Clinical use of botulinum toxins in oral and maxillofacial surgery. International journal of oral and maxillofacial surgery. 2010;39(3):197–207.
19. Johl SS, Burgett RA. Dermal filler agents: a practical review. Current opinion in ophthalmology. 2006;17(5):471–9.
20. Dayan SH. Complications from toxins and fillers in the dermatology clinic: recognition, prevention, and treatment. Facial plastic surgery clinics of North America. 2013;21(4):663–73.
21. Sadick NS, Manhas-Bhutani S, Krueger N. A novel approach to structural facial volume replacement. Aesthetic plastic surgery. 2013;37(2):266–76.
22. El-Domyati M, Attia SK, El-Sawy AE, Moftah NH, Nasif GA, Medhat W, et al. The use of Botulinum toxin-A injection for facial wrinkles: a histological and immunohistochemical evaluation. Journal of cosmetic dermatology. 2015;14(2): 140–4.
23. Li Y, Hsieh S-T, Chien H-F, Zhang X, McArthur JC, Griffin JW. Sensory and motor denervation influence epidermal thickness in rat foot glabrous skin.

Experimental neurology. 1997;147(2): 452–62.

24 Wang L, Sun Y, Yang W, Lindo P, Singh BR. Type A botulinum neurotoxin complex proteins differentially modulate host response of neuronal cells. Toxicon. 2014; 82:52–60.

25 Allemann IB, Kaufman J. Fractional photothermolysis—an update. Lasers in medical science. 2010;25(1):137–44.

26 Trelles MA, Allones I, Luna R. Facial rejuvenation with a nonablative 1320 nm Nd: YAG laser. Dermatologic surgery. 2001;27(2):111–6.

27 Alster TS, West TB. Resurfacing of atrophic facial acne scars with a high-energy, pulsed carbon dioxide laser. Dermatologic Surgery. 1996;22(2):151–5.

28 Kim DH, Je YJ, Kim CD, Lee YH, Seo YJ, Lee JH, et al. Can platelet-rich plasma be used for skin rejuvenation? Evaluation of effects of platelet-rich plasma on human dermal fibroblast. Annals of dermatology. 2011;23(4):424–31.

29 Redaelli A. Face and neck revitalization with Platelet-rich plasma (PRP): clinical outcome in a series of 23 consecutively treated patients. (ORIGINAL ARTICLES) (Clinical report). Journal of Drugs in Dermatology. 2010.

30 NA JI, CHOI JW, CHOI HR, JEONG JB, PARK KC, YOUN SW, et al. Rapid healing and reduced erythema after ablative fractional carbon dioxide laser resurfacing combined with the application of autologous platelet-rich plasma. Dermatologic Surgery. 2011;37(4): 463–8.

31 Doddaballapur S. Microneedling with dermaroller. Journal of cutaneous and aesthetic surgery. 2009;2(2):110.

32 El-Domyati M, El-Ammawi TS, Moawad O, El-Fakahany H, Medhat W, Mahoney MG, et al. Efficacy of mesotherapy in facial rejuvenation: a histological and immunohistochemical evaluation. International journal of dermatology. 2012;51(8):913–9.

33 Sclafani AP. Platelet-rich fibrin matrix for improvement of deep nasolabial folds. Journal of cosmetic dermatology. 2010; 9(1):66–71.

14

Use of Platelet Rich Fibrin in Other Areas of Medicine

Richard J. Miron and Joseph Choukroun

Abstract

Platelet rich fibrin (PRF) has extensively been utilized in dental medicine but many practitioners may be surprised to learn that it has far more often been applied in general medicine for a variety of indications highlighted in this chapter. While PRF was first utilized for the treatment of hard-to-heal leg ulcers, it remains interesting to point out that PRF has also been shown to improve a variety of leg and hand ulcers, utilized for facial soft-tissue defects, chronic rotator cuff tears, acute traumatic ear drum perforations, orthopedics, tendon injuries, management of knee osteoarthritis laparoscopic cholecystectomy, plastic surgery, superficial rhytids, acne scars, vaginal prolapse repair, urethracutaneous fistula repair, and lipostructure surgical procedures. This chapter provides an overview of the many indications of PRF for regeneration extended through various fields of medicine outside the dental field.

Highlights

- PRF for regeneration of chronic leg ulcers
- PRF as an adjunct to chondrocyte regeneration
- PRF for regeneration of ligaments and tendons
- PRF in orthopedic medicine
- PRF for improved facial and soft-tissue regeneration

14.1 Introduction

One key feature during the regeneration of tissues is the necessity for a constant source of blood supply supported by ingrowth of a vascular network [1]. Although most tissue engineering scaffolds are avascular by nature, platelet rich fibrin (PRF) was first introduced in 2001 with the potential to markedly improve angiogenesis through its accumulation of growth factors derived specifically from autogenous blood [2]. It has since been utilized for a variety of procedures in medicine and dentistry due to its ability to promote angiogenesis [1].

Equally important during the events leading to tissue regeneration is the ability for a wound to form a stable blood clot during the healing process. Typically regeneration occurs in a well-defined and well-ordered cascade of complex events in four overlapping phases including hemostasis, inflammation, proliferation, and remodeling [3–5]. These occur via the secretion of soluble mediators and signals capable of influencing the homing of circulating progenitor cells to damaged tissues [6]. Platelets are well-known cells that are responsible for the activation and release of important biomolecules including platelet-derived growth factor (PDGF), transforming growth factor beta (TGF-beta), vascular endothelial

Platelet Rich Fibrin in Regenerative Dentistry: Biological Background and Clinical Indications, First Edition.
Edited by Richard J. Miron and Joseph Choukroun.

growth factor (VEGF), as well as other coagulation factors, adhesion molecules, cytokines/chemokines, and angiogenic factors [7]. Furthermore, PRF is composed of a fibrin network known to improve blood clot stability responsible for tissue regeneration. In this chapter, we describe the uses of PRF in medicine (outside dentistry) to provide further insight that PRF supports regeneration of various tissues. We focus briefly on in vitro and in vivo studies and then present the numerous indications for which PRF has been utilized to improve the regeneration of various tissues in clinical medicine.

14.2 Effects of PRF on cell activity in vitro

PRF has been shown to effect primarily two cell types: endothelial cells and progenitor cells of the mesenchymal lineage. The effect of PRF has most commonly been observed in fibroblasts through numerous studies [8–11]. PRF stimulates dermal fibroblast proliferation, as well as production of extracellular matrix collagen1, a pro-fibrotic molecule response for wound healing of connective tissues [8]. It has further been shown that PRF not only supports the mitogenic activity of fibroblasts, but also acts to increase cell survival and migration favoring more rapid soft-tissue regeneration [9,10].

Similarly, PRF promotes angiogenesis by demonstrating a marked effect on endothelial cells. It was first shown that PRF induces the proliferation of endothelial cells via extracellular signal-regulated protein kinase activation pathway [12]. Furthermore, PRF induces the local release of VEGF within its fibrin scaffold; a known growth factor responsible for inducing angiogenesis [12]. It remains interesting to point out that PRF has also been shown to decrease the rate of infection as highlighted in previous chapters. Bayer *et al.* was one of the first to investigate the anti-inflammatory and anti-microbial activities of PRF in human keratinocytes [13]. Their research team found that PRF led to an increase in hBD-2 expression, a known gene responsible for its anti-microbial activity necessary for the treatment of chronic wounds [13]. Future research further investigating these pathways will provide much more support for the beneficial effects of PRF on soft-tissue wound healing and reveal the mechanism of action leading to its antibacterial effects.

14.3 Evidence that PRF improves soft-tissue wound healing/regeneration in vivo

Several studies have now shown that PRF induces soft-tissue regeneration in various animal models in the medical field. These include primarily studies that have focused on its wound healing capabilities during skin regeneration but are also extended to plastic and reconstructive surgery, urethral repair, and myocardial ventricular remodeling/regeneration.

Most notably, PRF has been shown to increase angiogenesis and soft-tissue regeneration in vivo. Roy *et al.* was one of the first to show that after 14 days of healing in a porcine ischemic excision model (8mm circular defects), PRF led to improvements in wound healing when compared to a collagen matrix (Figure 14.1) [12]. Other investigators have also found similar findings investigating dorsal tissue regeneration in various animal models [14–16]. PRF has also been shown to promote the regeneration of the parotid gland following irradiation [17] and increased type 1 collagen formation in full- and split-thickness flaps during skin grafting procedures in a porcine model [18].

More recent research has investigated the use of PRF in combination with adipose tissue for fat pad grafting in the ear's auricular [19]. This therapeutic adjuvant showed histologically that PRF could enhance

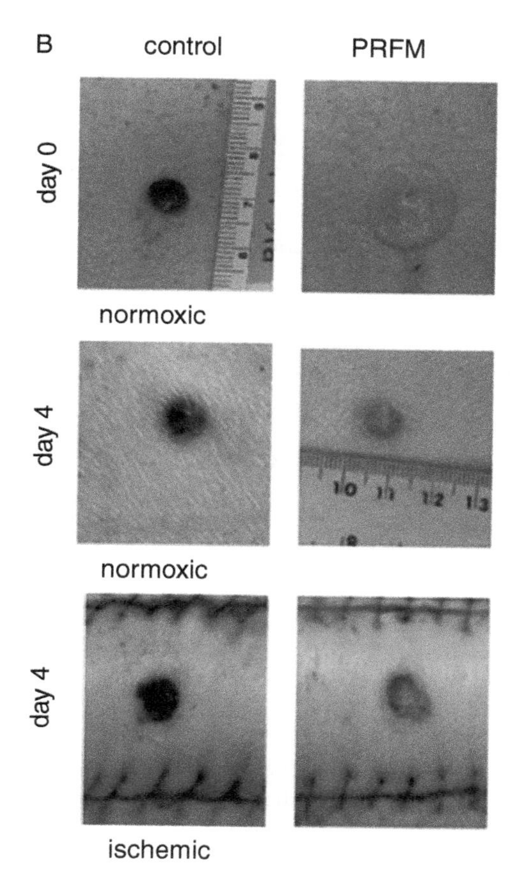

Figure 14.1 Treatment of porcine ischemic wound with PRF. Representative digital images of excisional wounds treated or not with PRFM on days 0 and 4 post-wounding. Adapted from Roy *et al.* 2011 [12].

microvesssel density at 4 weeks and improved the resorption rates of implanted tissues at 24 weeks [19]. The results from this study supports the concept that PRF facilitates angiogenesis when combined with adipose tissue with a clinically translatable strategy for soft-tissue augmentation and reconstruction of the ear or other defects requiring fat tissue grafting.

Lastly, one area of research limited to animals to date has been the effectiveness of PRF for the repair of myocardial ischemia and ventricular remodeling of the heart. In two studies, it has been shown that the combination of PRF with adipose-derived mesenchymal stem cells could be utilized to preserve left ventricular function in a rat model that induced regional myocardial ischemia by left coronary artery ligation [20]. Furthermore, in a second study, adipose-derived mesenchymal stem cells were embedded in PRF scaffolds to investigate its ability to promote angiogenesis in heart tissues [21]. It was found that this combination preserved heart function when compared to controls (Figure 14.2) [21]. While these results are still preliminary, ongoing research utilizing PRF for the treatment of various major defects of the heart could potentially lead to major breakthroughs in the medical field.

In summary, animal research has now convincingly shown that PRF can promote soft-tissue wound healing in various wound healing animal models and these reports show that this is primarily due to an increase in angiogenesis to defect sites.

14.4 Clinical studies evaluating the use of PRF in medicine

Many clinical studies have now shown that PRF is able to promote wound healing in the medical field. Recently our group showed in a systematic review that PRF was able to promote soft-tissue regeneration in 20 different clinical indications; 7 from the dental field, whereas the other 13 derived specifically from the medical field [22]. As highlighted throughout this textbook, PRF has been utilized successfully in dentistry and the maxillofacial region for the treatment of extraction sockets [23–26], gingival recessions [27–29], palatal wound closures [30–32], repair of potentially malignant lesions [33], regeneration of periodontal defects [34], hyperplastic gingival tissues [35], among other indications in oral surgery and periodontology [36]. In general medicine, PRF has also been utilized for a variety of treatments including hard-to-heal

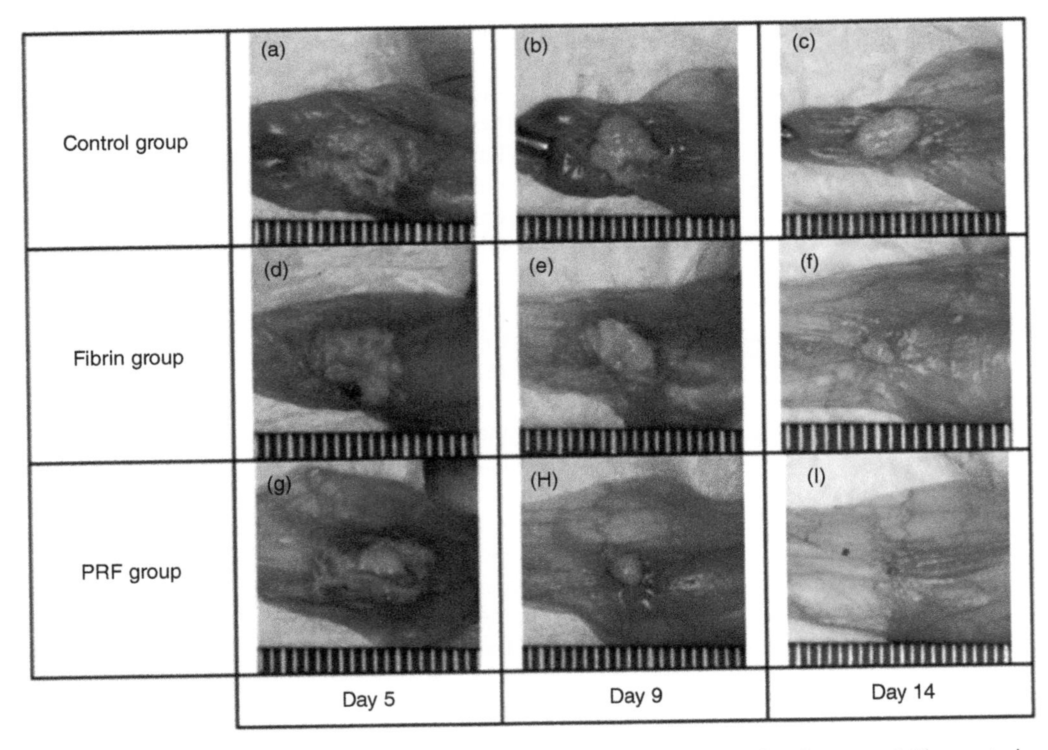

Figure 14.2 Macroscopic aspects of the cheek pouches of hamsters injected with 5-fluorouracil. The control group (A-C), the fibrin group (D-F), and the PRF group (G-I) are shown. Notice the significantly faster wound healing associated with the PRF group. Source: Horii *et al.* 2014 [16]. Reproduced with permission of Elsevier.

leg and hand ulcers [37–42], facial soft-tissue defects [43], laparoscopic cholecystectomy [44], deep nasolabial folds, volume-depleted midfacial regions, superficial rhytids, acne scars [45], induction of dermal collagenesis [46], vaginal prolapse repair [47], urethracutaneous fistula repair [48,49], lipostructure surgical procedures [50], chronic rotator cuff tears [51], and acute traumatic ear drum perforations [52]. In total, 27 of the 31 studies (87%) investigated from this systematic review reported having a positive outcome when PRF was combined with standard regenerative procedures for soft tissues [22]. Specifically, the remainder of this chapter focuses on the use of PRF for five clinical indications, including 1) regeneration of chronic leg ulcers, 2) chondrocyte regeneration, 3) ligament and tendon regeneration, 4) orthopedic medical regeneration, and 5) skin regeneration.

14.5 PRF for regeneration of chronic leg ulcers

As expressed in the first chapter of this textbook, PRF was first utilized for the treatment of hard to heal-leg ulcers in the early 2000s. For hard-to heal leg ulcers, it became common knowledge that infection was not only caused by bacterial pathogens, but also secondary to a lack of blood supply to wounds, thereby limiting entrance to infiltrating host immune cells to fight infection. As such, the use of PRF was first studied for the treatment of these patients to help support new blood angiogenesis, thereby bringing both immune cells from the PRF scaffolds as well as immune cells from the host via an increase in tissue angiogenesis, to fight infection (Figure 14.3). This strategy has since been adopted in many publications and this

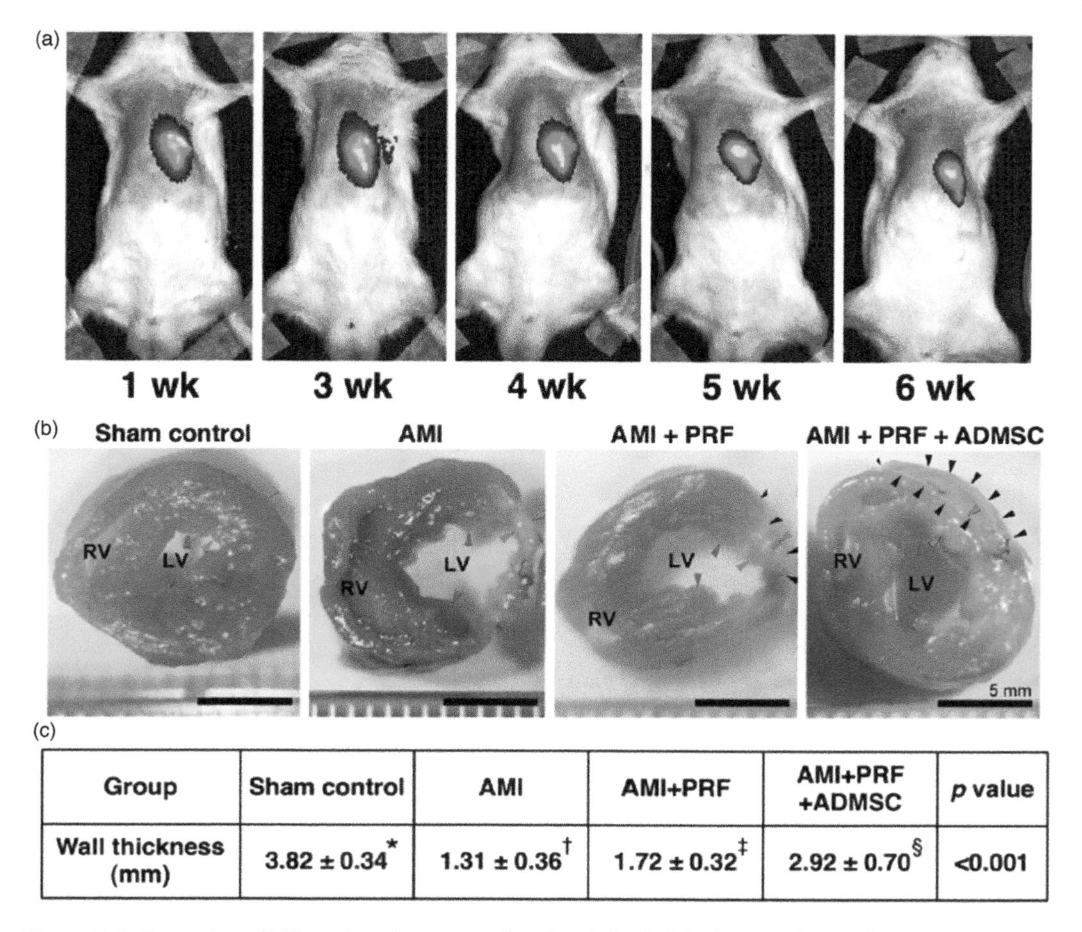

Group	Sham control	AMI	AMI+PRF	AMI+PRF +ADMSC	*p* value
Wall thickness (mm)	3.82 ± 0.34*	1.31 ± 0.36†	1.72 ± 0.32‡	2.92 ± 0.70§	<0.001

Figure 14.3 Illustration of IVIS study and anatomical and pathological findings on day 42 after AMI induction (n = 8). A. Serial assessments of living imaging by *In Vivo* Imaging System (IVIS) after acute myocardial infarction (AMI). B. The anatomical findings showed the cross-section area of the heart at the papillary muscle (blue arrows) among the four groups. The left ventricular (LV) chamber size was highest in AMI group, lowest in sham-control group, and notably higher in AMI + platelet rich fibrin (PRF) group than in AMI + PRF + adipose-derived mesenchymal stem cell (ADMSC); Conversely, the infarct size showed an apposite pattern of LV chamber size.The black arrows indicated PRF scaffold tissue in AMI + PRF group and ADMSC-embedded PRF scaffold (AMI + PRF + ADMSC) (i.e., engineered ADMSC grafts) group, whereas the green arrow shows the wall thickness in the infarct area. Scale bars in right lower corners represent 5 mm. C. *vs. other groups with different symbols (*, †, ‡, §), $p < 0.001$. Statistical analysis using one-way ANOVA, followed by Bonferroni multiple comparison post hoc test. Symbols (*, †, ‡, §) indicate significance (at 0.05 level). Adapted from Chen *et al.* 2015 [21].

field of research has continued to flourish. It remains of interest to note up to what point the human body can heal in entirely autogenous fashions by using naturally derived PRF scaffolds for the treatment of these hard to heal leg ulcers from various etiologies.

14.6 PRF for cartilage (knee) regeneration

One area of research that is rising in popularity has been the use of platelet derivatives for the regeneration of cartilage. Cartilage is one of the most avascular tissues found in the human body and therefore, has extremely low potential for regeneration. From this point of view, it makes logical sense to introduce blood flow via platelet derivatives to defective/damaged cartilage. This concept has been utilized for a variety of procedures in medicine as well as sports medicine where platelet rich plasma (PRP) has been utilized for knee regeneration for a wide range of patients including professional athletes [53–57]. The more recent introduction of an injectable-PRF that does not utilize additional anti-coagulants (such as PRP) and includes the potential to form a fibrin clot several minutes following injection has been a proposed method to further regenerate cartilage, particularly in the knee (Figures 14.4 and 14.5). The ability for i-PRF to form a fibrin clot would theoretically act to further improve regeneration by providing a fibrin network/space capable of diminishing pain felt from bone-to-bone contact commonly reported in osteoarthritic patients. Further research in this field is prominent.

14.7 PRF for the regeneration of ligaments and tendons

In a similar fashion, platelet concentrates have also been heavily utilized for the repair of ligaments and tendons such as rotator cuffs found in the shoulder and various forms of tendinopathy [58–61]. These studies have utilized PRP as an adjunct to conventional therapy to improve blood flow and regeneration to these defects. Therefore, with the development of injectable-PRF, it is theoretically hypothesized that i-PRF can also replace conventional therapies utilizing PRP without necessitating the use of additives including anti-coagulants, known inhibitors of wound healing. Future research in this field is also eminently needed.

14.8 PRF in orthopedic medicine

Recently, PRF has also been utilized in orthopedic medicine for the repair of large bone defects. While this field is very early in its

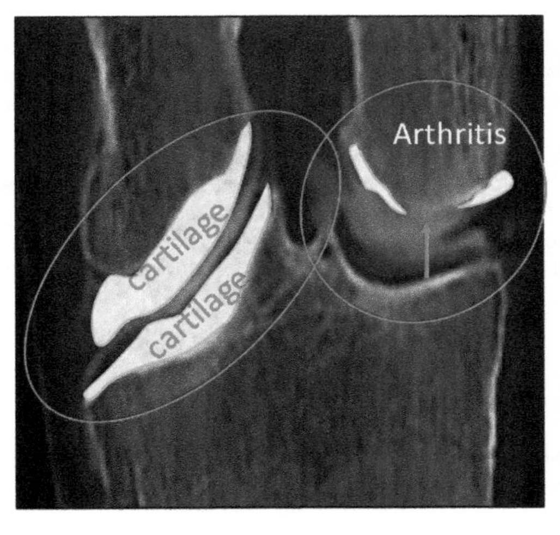

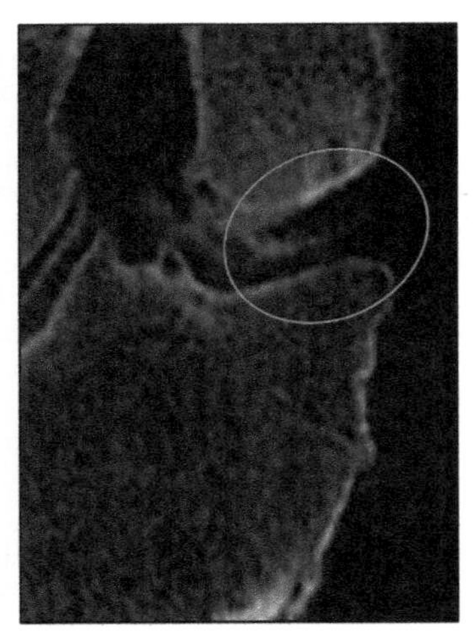

Figure 14.4 Various cases of osteoarthritis of the knee treated with an injectable-PRF (i-PRF). Notice the region of calcification between the knee and the bone-to-bone contact that may be regenerated with i-PRF. Case performed by Dr. Joseph Choukroun.

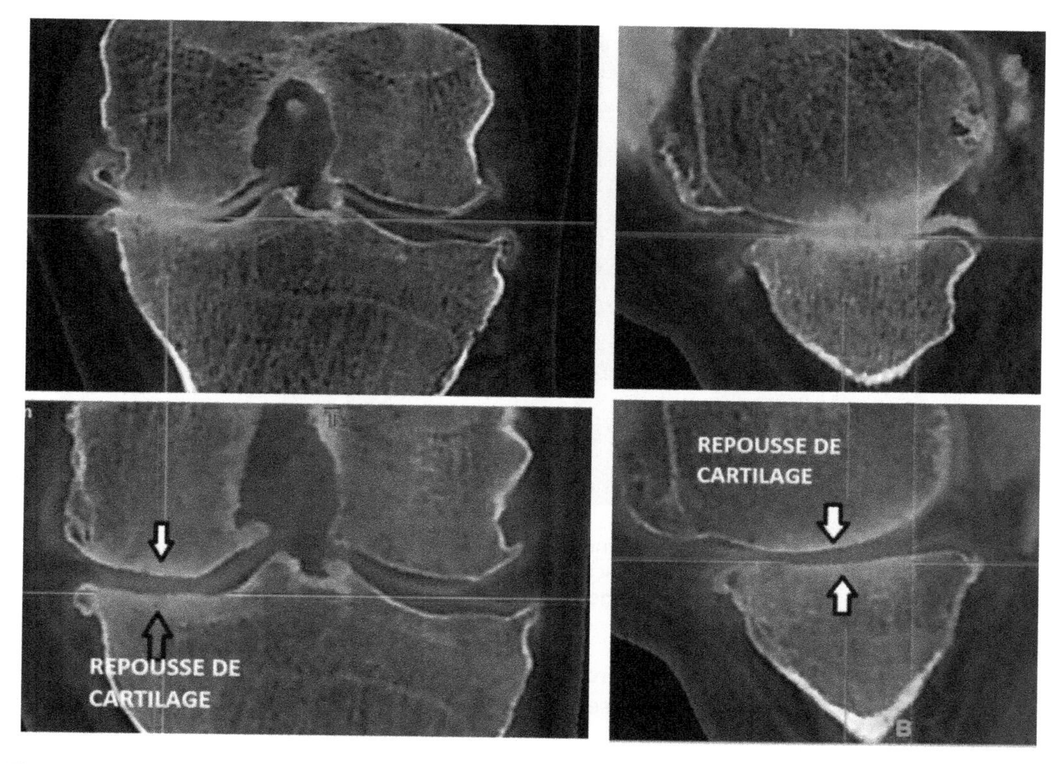

Figure 14.5 Regeneration of osteoarthritis of the knee with an injectable-PRF (i-PRF). Notice the region of calcification between the knee and the communication and bone-to-bone contact that may be regenerated with i-PRF. Case performed by Dr. Joseph Choukroun.

attempts to characterize the potential benefit of utilizing PRF for such surgeries, it remains an area of future research that may provide superior and shorter healing periods for major bone/hip defects by favoring angiogenesis and wound healing in such cases. Figure 14.6 illustrates an orthopedic case treated with PRF.

14.9 PRF for skin regeneration

Lastly and briefly mentioned in the previous chapter, an array of research is currently investigating the use of PRF for either facial/soft-tissue regeneration. Despite its common use in aesthetic facial dentistry, further research could benefit from the regenerative potential of PRF for the rejuvenation of soft tissues following medical removal of various skin cancers such as basal cell carcinomas and other soft-tissue defects that require healing. Although this field of research is extremely premature, it certainly represents an area of future research worth further investigation.

14.10 Discussion and future perspectives

This chapter was included in this textbook to highlight the many other uses of PRF for regenerative procedures in medicine outside the dental field. These include various uses in reconstructive surgery, plastic surgery, and dermatology. One of the advantages of PRF is that it can be utilized and tested in a safe and efficient way to deliver supra-physiological doses of autologous growth factors to host

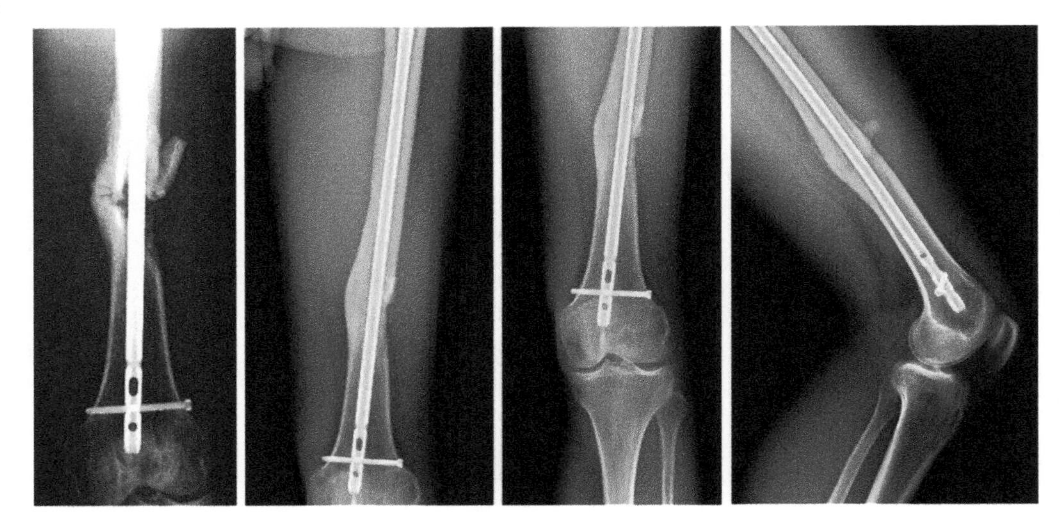

Figure 14.6 Use of PRF used in conjunction in the field of orthopeadic medicine fort he regeneration of both soft and hard tissues. By introduction growth factors capable of stimulating angiogenesis and new blood vessel formation, the use of PRF can achieve regeneration of various tissues across many fields of medicine.

tissues without fearing a foreign body reaction or tissue rejection. While the use of PRP has seen widespread use due to its liquid composition, it remains of interest to determine which clinical indications could i-PRF be utilized as a substitute material to PRP without having to utilize anti-coagulants found in PRP [58,62–65]. It is obvious that further research remains to further characterize the regenerative potential of either i-PRF in comparison to PRP for the variety of regenerative procedures proposed in this chapter. Future research is ongoing.

Two key advantages of utilizing PRF for regeneration of defects found in the medical field are its ability to deliver leukocytes (host immune cells capable of fighting infection and controlling inflammation) as well as the ability for a fibrin network to act to support tissue regeneration and limit bone/bone contact in space-limiting defects such as osteoarthritis or temporomandibular joint disorders. Furthermore, chronic non-healing wounds are a significant and constant medical challenge resulting in amputation and the pathogenesis of non-healing wounds thereby requires new treatment options to improve clinical outcomes. One main advantage of PRF over PRP is the fact it contains leukocytes that fight infection as well as its ability to release a significantly higher concentrations of growth factors over a 10-day period [66].

Another area of research that remains ongoing is to determine if the strength, stiffness, or toughness of PRF scaffolds should be modified via centrifugation protocols for the different clinical indications proposed in this chapter. For instance, should a PRF membrane be different for regeneration of a tendon versus that of cartilage or bone? It remains of interest to better characterize PRF scaffolds for future research across various fields of medicine and for various biomedical applications. Experts across many fields of medicine need to gather more frequently to discuss protocols, which may lead to further clinical improvements.

While the next wave of research is expected to address in a more systematic way the use of PRF for the variety of controlled randomized clinical trials the effective of PRF in medicine, reports from this chapter highlight numerous clinical reports having investigated its effectiveness. Future randomized clinical trials are necessary.

References

1 Upputuri PK, Sivasubramanian K, Mark CS, Pramanik M. Recent developments in vascular imaging techniques in tissue engineering and regenerative medicine. BioMed research international. 2015; 2015:783983.
2 Choukroun J, Adda F, Schoeffler C, Vervelle A. Une opportunité en paro-implantologie: le PRF. Implantodontie. 2001;42(55):e62.
3 Gosain A, DiPietro LA. Aging and wound healing. World journal of surgery. 2004; 28(3):321–6.
4 Eming SA, Brachvogel B, Odorisio T, Koch M. Regulation of angiogenesis: wound healing as a model. Progress in histochemistry and cytochemistry. 2007; 42(3):115–70.
5 Eming SA, Kaufmann J, Lohrer R, Krieg T. [Chronic wounds. Novel approaches in research and therapy]. Der Hautarzt; Zeitschrift fur Dermatologie, Venerologie, und verwandte Gebiete. 2007;58(11): 939–44.
6 Guo S, Dipietro LA. Factors affecting wound healing. J Dent Res. 2010;89(3): 219–29.
7 Nurden AT. Platelets, inflammation and tissue regeneration. Thrombosis and haemostasis. 2011;105 Suppl 1: S13–33.
8 Lundquist R, Dziegiel MH, Agren MS. Bioactivity and stability of endogenous fibrogenic factors in platelet-rich fibrin. Wound repair and regeneration : official publication of the Wound Healing Society [and] the European Tissue Repair Society. 2008;16(3):356–63.
9 Lundquist R, Holmstrom K, Clausen C, Jorgensen B, Karlsmark T. Characteristics of an autologous leukocyte and platelet-rich fibrin patch intended for the treatment of recalcitrant wounds. Wound repair and regeneration : official publication of the Wound Healing Society [and] the European Tissue Repair Society. 2013;21(1):66–76.
10 Clipet F, Tricot S, Alno N, Massot M, Solhi H, Cathelineau G, et al. In vitro effects of Choukroun's platelet-rich fibrin conditioned medium on 3 different cell lines implicated in dental implantology. Implant dentistry. 2012;21(1):51–6.
11 Vahabi S, Vaziri S, Torshabi M, Rezaei Esfahrood Z. Effects of Plasma Rich in Growth Factors and Platelet-Rich Fibrin on Proliferation and Viability of Human Gingival Fibroblasts. Journal of dentistry (Tehran, Iran). 2015;12(7):504–12.
12 Roy S, Driggs J, Elgharably H, Biswas S, Findley M, Khanna S, et al. Platelet-rich fibrin matrix improves wound angiogenesis via inducing endothelial cell proliferation. Wound repair and regeneration : official publication of the Wound Healing Society [and] the European Tissue Repair Society. 2011;19(6):753–66.
13 Bayer A, Lammel J, Rademacher F, Gross J, Siggelkow M, Lippross S, et al. Platelet-released growth factors induce the antimicrobial peptide human beta-defensin-2 in primary keratinocytes. Experimental dermatology. 2016.
14 Suzuki S, Morimoto N, Ikada Y. Gelatin gel as a carrier of platelet-derived growth factors. Journal of biomaterials applications. 2013;28(4):595–606.
15 Li Q, Pan S, Dangaria SJ, Gopinathan G, Kolokythas A, Chu S, et al. Platelet-rich fibrin promotes periodontal regeneration and enhances alveolar bone augmentation. BioMed research international. 2013; 2013:638043.
16 Horii K, Kanayama T, Miyamoto H, Kohgo T, Tsuchimochi T, Shigetomi T, et al. Platelet-rich fibrin has a healing effect on chemotherapy-induced mucositis in hamsters. Oral surgery, oral medicine, oral pathology and oral radiology. 2014;117(4): 445–53.
17 Chen Y, Niu Z, Xue Y, Yuan F, Fu Y, Bai N. Improvement in the repair of defects in maxillofacial soft tissue in irradiated minipigs by a mixture of adipose-derived

stem cells and platelet-rich fibrin. The British journal of oral & maxillofacial surgery. 2014;52(8):740–5.
18 Reksodiputro M, Widodo D, Bashiruddin J, Siregar N, Malik S. PRFM enhance wound healing process in skin graft. Facial plastic surgery : FPS. 2014;30(6):670–5.
19 Liu B, Tan XY, Liu YP, Xu XF, Li L, Xu HY, et al. The adjuvant use of stromal vascular fraction and platelet-rich fibrin for autologous adipose tissue transplantation. Tissue engineering Part C, Methods. 2013; 19(1):1–14.
20 Sun CK, Zhen YY, Leu S, Tsai TH, Chang LT, Sheu JJ, et al. Direct implantation versus platelet-rich fibrin-embedded adipose-derived mesenchymal stem cells in treating rat acute myocardial infarction. International journal of cardiology. 2014; 173(3):410–23.
21 Chen YL, Sun CK, Tsai TH, Chang LT, Leu S, Zhen YY, et al. Adipose-derived mesenchymal stem cells embedded in platelet-rich fibrin scaffolds promote angiogenesis, preserve heart function, and reduce left ventricular remodeling in rat acute myocardial infarction. American journal of translational research. 2015;7(5): 781–803.
22 Miron RJ, Fujioka-Kobayashi M, Bishara M, Zhang Y, Hernandez M, Choukroun J. Platelet-Rich Fibrin and Soft Tissue Wound Healing: A Systematic Review. Tissue engineering Part B, Reviews. 2016.
23 Sammartino G, Dohan Ehrenfest DM, Carile F, Tia M, Bucci P. Prevention of hemorrhagic complications after dental extractions into open heart surgery patients under anticoagulant therapy: the use of leukocyte- and platelet-rich fibrin. The Journal of oral implantology. 2011; 37(6):681–90.
24 Hoaglin DR, Lines GK. Prevention of localized osteitis in mandibular third-molar sites using platelet-rich fibrin. International journal of dentistry. 2013; 2013:875380.
25 Suttapreyasri S, Leepong N. Influence of platelet-rich fibrin on alveolar ridge preservation. The Journal of craniofacial surgery. 2013;24(4):1088–94.
26 Yelamali T, Saikrishna D. Role of platelet rich fibrin and platelet rich plasma in wound healing of extracted third molar sockets: a comparative study. Journal of maxillofacial and oral surgery. 2015;14(2): 410–6.
27 Anilkumar K, Geetha A, Umasudhakar, Ramakrishnan T, Vijayalakshmi R, Pameela E. Platelet-rich-fibrin: A novel root coverage approach. Journal of Indian Society of Periodontology. 2009;13(1): 50–4.
28 Jankovic S, Aleksic Z, Klokkevold P, Lekovic V, Dimitrijevic B, Kenney EB, et al. Use of platelet-rich fibrin membrane following treatment of gingival recession: a randomized clinical trial. The International journal of periodontics & restorative dentistry. 2012;32(2):e41–50.
29 Eren G, Tervahartiala T, Sorsa T, Atilla G. Cytokine (interleukin-1beta) and MMP levels in gingival crevicular fluid after use of platelet-rich fibrin or connective tissue graft in the treatment of localized gingival recessions. Journal of periodontal research. 2015.
30 Jain V, Triveni MG, Kumar AB, Mehta DS. Role of platelet-rich-fibrin in enhancing palatal wound healing after free graft. Contemporary clinical dentistry. 2012; 3(Suppl 2):S240–3.
31 Kulkarni MR, Thomas BS, Varghese JM, Bhat GS. Platelet-rich fibrin as an adjunct to palatal wound healing after harvesting a free gingival graft: A case series. Journal of Indian Society of Periodontology. 2014; 18(3):399–402.
32 Femminella B, Iaconi MC, Di Tullio M, Romano L, Sinjari B, D'Arcangelo C, et al. Clinical Comparison of Platelet-Rich Fibrin and a Gelatin Sponge in the Management of Palatal Wounds After Epithelialized Free Gingival Graft Harvest: A Randomized Clinical Trial. Journal of periodontology. 2016;87(2):103–13.
33 Pathak H, Mohanty S, Urs AB, Dabas J. Treatment of Oral Mucosal Lesions by

Scalpel Excision and Platelet-Rich Fibrin Membrane Grafting: A Review of 26 Sites. Journal of oral and maxillofacial surgery : official journal of the American Association of Oral and Maxillofacial Surgeons. 2015;73(9):1865–74.
34 Ajwani H, Shetty S, Gopalakrishnan D, Kathariya R, Kulloli A, Dolas RS, et al. Comparative evaluation of platelet-rich fibrin biomaterial and open flap debridement in the treatment of two and three wall intrabony defects. Journal of international oral health : JIOH. 2015; 7(4):32–7.
35 di Lauro AE, Abbate D, Dell'Angelo B, Iannaccone GA, Scotto F, Sammartino G. Soft tissue regeneration using leukocyte-platelet rich fibrin after exeresis of hyperplastic gingival lesions: two case reports. Journal of medical case reports. 2015;9:252.
36 Munoz F, Jimenez C, Espinoza D, Vervelle A, Beugnet J, Haidar Z. Use of leukocyte and platelet-rich fibrin (L-PRF) in periodontally accelerated osteogenic orthodontics (PAOO): Clinical effects on edema and pain. Journal of clinical and experimental dentistry. 2016;8(2): e119–24.
37 Danielsen P, Jorgensen B, Karlsmark T, Jorgensen LN, Agren MS. Effect of topical autologous platelet-rich fibrin versus no intervention on epithelialization of donor sites and meshed split-thickness skin autografts: a randomized clinical trial. Plastic and reconstructive surgery. 2008; 122(5):1431–40.
38 O'Connell SM, Impeduglia T, Hessler K, Wang XJ, Carroll RJ, Dardik H. Autologous platelet-rich fibrin matrix as cell therapy in the healing of chronic lower-extremity ulcers. Wound repair and regeneration : official publication of the Wound Healing Society [and] the European Tissue Repair Society. 2008;16(6):749–56.
39 Steenvoorde P, van Doorn LP, Naves C, Oskam J. Use of autologous platelet-rich fibrin on hard-to-heal wounds. Journal of wound care. 2008;17(2):60–3.
40 Jorgensen B, Karlsmark T, Vogensen H, Haase L, Lundquist R. A pilot study to evaluate the safety and clinical performance of Leucopatch, an autologous, additive-free, platelet-rich fibrin for the treatment of recalcitrant chronic wounds. The international journal of lower extremity wounds. 2011;10(4):218–23.
41 Londahl M, Tarnow L, Karlsmark T, Lundquist R, Nielsen AM, Michelsen M, et al. Use of an autologous leucocyte and platelet-rich fibrin patch on hard-to-heal DFUs: a pilot study. Journal of wound care. 2015;24(4):172–4, 6–8.
42 Chignon-Sicard B, Georgiou CA, Fontas E, David S, Dumas P, Ihrai T, et al. Efficacy of leukocyte- and platelet-rich fibrin in wound healing: a randomized controlled clinical trial. Plastic and reconstructive surgery. 2012;130(6):819e–29e.
43 Desai CB, Mahindra UR, Kini YK, Bakshi MK. Use of Platelet-Rich Fibrin over Skin Wounds: Modified Secondary Intention Healing. Journal of cutaneous and aesthetic surgery. 2013;6(1):35–7.
44 Danielsen PL, Agren MS, Jorgensen LN. Platelet-rich fibrin versus albumin in surgical wound repair: a randomized trial with paired design. Annals of surgery. 2010;251(5):825–31.
45 Sclafani AP. Safety, efficacy, and utility of platelet-rich fibrin matrix in facial plastic surgery. Archives of facial plastic surgery. 2011;13(4):247–51.
46 Sclafani AP, McCormick SA. Induction of dermal collagenesis, angiogenesis, and adipogenesis in human skin by injection of platelet-rich fibrin matrix. Archives of facial plastic surgery. 2012;14(2):132–6.
47 Gorlero F, Glorio M, Lorenzi P, Bruno-Franco M, Mazzei C. New approach in vaginal prolapse repair: mini-invasive surgery associated with application of platelet-rich fibrin. International urogynecology journal. 2012;23(6): 715–22.
48 Soyer T, Cakmak M, Aslan MK, Senyucel MF, Kisa U. Use of autologous platelet rich fibrin in urethracutaneous fistula repair:

preliminary report. International wound journal. 2013;10(3):345–7.

49 Guinot A, Arnaud A, Azzis O, Habonimana E, Jasienski S, Fremond B. Preliminary experience with the use of an autologous platelet-rich fibrin membrane for urethroplasty coverage in distal hypospadias surgery. Journal of pediatric urology. 2014;10(2):300–5.

50 Braccini F, Chignon-Sicard B, Volpei C, Choukroun J. Modern lipostructure: the use of platelet rich fibrin (PRF). Revue de laryngologie - otologie - rhinologie. 2013; 134(4-5):231–5.

51 Zumstein MA, Rumian A, Lesbats V, Schaer M, Boileau P. Increased vascularization during early healing after biologic augmentation in repair of chronic rotator cuff tears using autologous leukocyte- and platelet-rich fibrin (L-PRF): a prospective randomized controlled pilot trial. Journal of shoulder and elbow surgery / American Shoulder and Elbow Surgeons [et al]. 2014;23(1):3–12.

52 Habesoglu M, Oysu C, Sahin S, Sahin-Yilmaz A, Korkmaz D, Tosun A, et al. Platelet-rich fibrin plays a role on healing of acute-traumatic ear drum perforation. The Journal of craniofacial surgery. 2014;25(6): 2056–8.

53 Campbell KA, Saltzman BM, Mascarenhas R, Khair MM, Verma NN, Bach BR, Jr., et al. Does Intra-articular Platelet-Rich Plasma Injection Provide Clinically Superior Outcomes Compared With Other Therapies in the Treatment of Knee Osteoarthritis? A Systematic Review of Overlapping Meta-analyses. Arthroscopy : the journal of arthroscopic & related surgery : official publication of the Arthroscopy Association of North America and the International Arthroscopy Association. 2015;31(11):2213–21.

54 Kanchanatawan W, Arirachakaran A, Chaijenkij K, Prasathaporn N, Boonard M, Piyapittayanun P, et al. Short-term outcomes of platelet-rich plasma injection for treatment of osteoarthritis of the knee. Knee surgery, sports traumatology, arthroscopy : official journal of the ESSKA. 2016;24(5):1665–77.

55 Meheux CJ, McCulloch PC, Lintner DM, Varner KE, Harris JD. Efficacy of Intra-articular Platelet-Rich Plasma Injections in Knee Osteoarthritis: A Systematic Review. Arthroscopy : the journal of arthroscopic & related surgery : official publication of the Arthroscopy Association of North America and the International Arthroscopy Association. 2016;32(3):495–505.

56 Nguyen C, Lefevre-Colau MM, Poiraudeau S, Rannou F. Evidence and recommendations for use of intra-articular injections for knee osteoarthritis. Annals of physical and rehabilitation medicine. 2016;59(3):184–9.

57 Sanchez M, Anitua E, Delgado D, Sanchez P, Prado R, Goiriena JJ, et al. A new strategy to tackle severe knee osteoarthritis: Combination of intra-articular and intraosseous injections of Platelet Rich Plasma. Expert opinion on biological therapy. 2016;16(5):627–43.

58 Cai YZ, Zhang C, Lin XJ. Efficacy of platelet-rich plasma in arthroscopic repair of full-thickness rotator cuff tears: a meta-analysis. Journal of shoulder and elbow surgery / American Shoulder and Elbow Surgeons [et al]. 2015;24(12): 1852–9.

59 Nourissat G, Ornetti P, Berenbaum F, Sellam J, Richette P, Chevalier X. Does platelet-rich plasma deserve a role in the treatment of tendinopathy? Joint, bone, spine : revue du rhumatisme. 2015;82(4): 230–4.

60 Saltzman BM, Jain A, Campbell KA, Mascarenhas R, Romeo AA, Verma NN, et al. Does the Use of Platelet-Rich Plasma at the Time of Surgery Improve Clinical Outcomes in Arthroscopic Rotator Cuff Repair When Compared With Control Cohorts? A Systematic Review of Meta-analyses. Arthroscopy : the journal of arthroscopic & related surgery : official publication of the Arthroscopy Association of North America and the International

Arthroscopy Association. 2016;32(5): 906–18.

61 Warth RJ, Dornan GJ, James EW, Horan MP, Millett PJ. Clinical and structural outcomes after arthroscopic repair of full-thickness rotator cuff tears with and without platelet-rich product supplementation: a meta-analysis and meta-regression. Arthroscopy : the journal of arthroscopic & related surgery : official publication of the Arthroscopy Association of North America and the International Arthroscopy Association. 2015;31(2): 306–20.

62 Andia I, Abate M. Platelet-rich plasma in the treatment of skeletal muscle injuries. Expert opinion on biological therapy. 2015;15(7):987–99.

63 Figueroa D, Figueroa F, Calvo R, Vaisman A, Ahumada X, Arellano S. Platelet-rich plasma use in anterior cruciate ligament surgery: systematic review of the literature. Arthroscopy : the journal of arthroscopic & related surgery : official publication of the Arthroscopy Association of North America and the International Arthroscopy Association. 2015;31(5):981–8.

64 Zhao JG, Zhao L, Jiang YX, Wang ZL, Wang J, Zhang P. Platelet-rich plasma in arthroscopic rotator cuff repair: a meta-analysis of randomized controlled trials. Arthroscopy : the journal of arthroscopic & related surgery : official publication of the Arthroscopy Association of North America and the International Arthroscopy Association. 2015;31(1): 125–35.

65 Hudgens JL, Sugg KB, Grekin JA, Gumucio JP, Bedi A, Mendias CL. Platelet-Rich Plasma Activates Proinflammatory Signaling Pathways and Induces Oxidative Stress in Tendon Fibroblasts. The American journal of sports medicine. 2016.

66 Kobayashi E, Fluckiger L, Fujioka-Kobayashi M, Sawada K, Sculean A, Schaller B, et al. Comparative release of growth factors from PRP, PRF, and advanced-PRF. Clinical oral investigations. 2016.

15

Future Research with Platelet Rich Fibrin

Richard J. Miron and Joseph Choukroun

Abstract

One constantly evolving field demanding much research has been dedicated to the use of platelet rich fibrin (PRF) in regenerative dentistry. Over the past half-decade, the number of publications listed on Medline has exponentially increased and this trend is only expected to continue. In the early stages of its use, attempts were made to determine where and how PRF could be utilized in various procedures in periodontology, oral surgery, and implant dentistry. More recently, specific indications have been recommended as outlined in this textbook. This final chapter outlines the 10 fields of research of most interest moving forward. These include the influence of blood hematocrit and centrifugation speeds on final PRF scaffolds. It also includes the use of PRF for various new procedures in dentistry including its investigation for treatments of osteonecrosis of the jaw, temporo-mandibular joint disorders, and pulp regeneration. Lastly, the influence of whether leukocytes or fibrin plays a more prominent role in PRF scaffolds is discussed as potential avenues for future research.

Highlights

- The effect of hematocrit/centrifugation speeds on PRF size, density, and cell counts
- Regeneration or repair during periodontal regeneration
- PRF for temporomandibular joint disorders
- PRF and osteonecrosis
- PRF and leukocyte/fibrin biology
- PRF and bone regeneration/osteoinduction

15.1 PRF and centrifugation speeds

As highlighted in Chapters 2 and 3, the influence of centrifugation speed has been shown to affect leukocyte number, scaffold length, and fibrin network density. Furthermore, lower speeds of approximately 60 G (700 RPM) for a mere 3 minutes has been shown to produce a liquid PRF that may be utilized as an injectable biomaterial (i-PRF). Despite these findings, the low-speed centrifugation concept is very early in its use and clinical reports investigating its ability to further improve wound healing are limited. Nevertheless, it has now been confirmed that lower centrifugation speed leads to higher leukocyte numbers more evenly distributed throughout the PRF scaffolds [1] and further improves growth factor release from these matrixes [2].

It is also known that despite lower centrifugation speeds containing more cells and higher release of growth factors, it has been demonstrated that higher centrifugation

Platelet Rich Fibrin in Regenerative Dentistry: Biological Background and Clinical Indications, First Edition.
Edited by Richard J. Miron and Joseph Choukroun.

speed leads to longer and more densely packed PRF membranes with less cells. Despite this, it remains interesting to point out that in some indications, it might be advantageous to produce a more densely packed and longer PRF membrane for indications such as Schneiderian membrane repair, whereas lower centrifugation speeds might be advantageous when an increased number of leukocytes and growth factor release may be necessary such as for the treatment of extraction sockets by secondary intension and when mixed with biomaterials. By bringing the concept that different centrifugation speeds may lead to differences in PRF scaffolds, it therefore opens the possibility that perhaps not one centrifugation speed may serve the purpose for all dental procedures much in the same way that not one bone-grafting material should be utilized for all bone-grafting procedures.

15.2 Effect of hematocrit count on PRF scaffolds

Along the same lines as "PRF and centrifugation speeds," one very interesting observation recently has been the effect of hematocrit count on PRF scaffolds. It was specifically found that the formation of PRF is not only dependent on the centrifugal preparation method, but also related to the composition of peripheral blood cells. The precise mechanism by which platelet/fibrin clots affects wound healing and bone formation remains unclear. Many clinicians have now observed that while utilizing PRF during routine clinical practice, drastic differences in the macroscopic morphology of PRF has been reported between patients. A group in Netherlands recently prepared PRF membranes utilizing different centrifugation protocols and thereafter the composition of PRF was analyzed with light and scanning electron microscopy. In order to study the effect of blood cell composition on the PRF membrane, a total of 93 patients were included in their study.

The authors report that a decrease in centrifugal G-force as well as a decrease in time of centrifugation resulted in an enormous increase of platelet yield in PRF. Furthermore, it was found that increased G-force and time of centrifugation were associated with increased PRF membrane length. However, and most interestingly, the membrane length was significantly inversely correlated to patient's hemoglobin, hematocrit, and erythrocyte count, while leucocyte count was not associated with the membrane length. In conclusion, it was found that the preparation of PRF membranes is largely dependent on the centrifugation conditions and it was further suggested that the traditional methods of preparing PRF could be improved. These authors point to the fact that the composition of PRF membrane is not only dependent on the centrifugation method/speed, but also significantly correlates with the composition of donor blood (Brouwards *et al.* 2016, conference abstract).

Therefore, it remains to be investigated how hematocrit count may affect PRF composition and whether specific protocols should further be provided for patients with certain hematocrit values. Future research in this area is prominently needed. Furthermore, certain clinicians have also reported that fat dietary intake prior to blood collection leads to a "milky" consistency of PRF clots (Figure 15.1). Therefore, it is likely that food intake, time of day, and other factors such as hematocrit count and/or various blood disorders may affect final PRF scaffold architecture although little study to date has been performed on these topics.

15.3 The influence of PRF for the treatment of osteonecrosis of the jaw

Osteonecrosis of the jaw is a major clinical challenge encountered, whereby bone tissues with limited vascularization results in bone exposure commonly associated with high

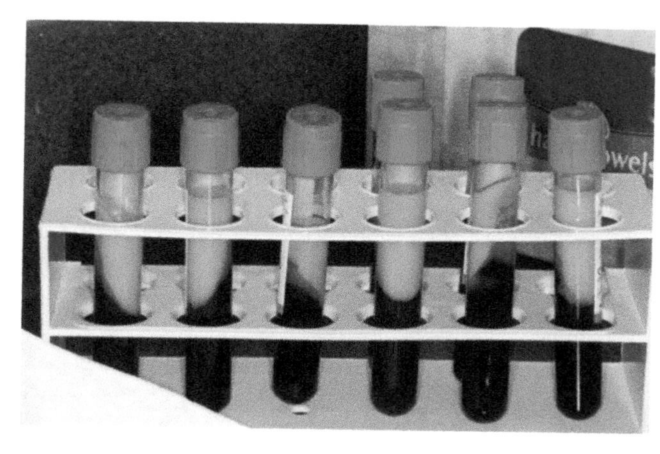

Figure 15.1 Pink PRF obtained following a centrifugation cycle with a patient who had just consumed a fatty diet high in chylomicrons an hour prior to surgery. The clots can be observed entirely differently formulated with a milky consistency. Courtesy of Dr. Michael Zidile.

radiation therapy or bisphosphonate use. Interestingly, the use of PRF has been shown to enhance new blood vessel formation and angiogenesis to defect tissues. Recently a few case reports or case series have investigated the use of PRF for the management of osteonecrosis of the jaw [3–11]. The clinical case presented in Figure 15.2 demonstrated a typical ONJ patient requiring surgical intervention. Due to the decrease in vascularization to defective tissues caused by ONJ, PRF has been investigated as a potential surgical intervention modality. While the aim of these studies is to assess the feasibility of using PRF for the treatment of bisphosphonate-/radiation-related osteonecrosis of the jaw, the effectiveness cannot be fully judged by most of these study designs and randomized prospective clinical trials are therefore still needed. Future studies investigating its use in randomized clinical trials are necessary to further characterize its full beneficial potential.

15.4 Injectable platelet rich fibrin as a potential therapy for temporomandibular joint disorders

Platelet concentrates including primarily platelet rich plasma (PRP) has been previously investigated as a modality for TMJ disorders [12–20]. In comparative studies with other available standard treatment options such as with hyaluronic acid (HA), PRP was shown to perform better than HA for the management of TMJ-osteoarthritis [12]. During long-term follow-up, improvements in pain reduction and increased inter-incisal distance were noted. Therefore, and in light of these findings, it is clear that the management of TMJ-osteoarthritis can theoretically be treated also with an injectable-PRF. Advantages of this technique are that i-PRF does not contain any additional anti-coagulants such as those found in PRP and therefore, wound healing of these tissues should (at least theoretically) be superior. Furthermore, since i-PRF forms a fibrin clot shortly after injection, it therefore provides the potential added benefit of forming a superficial fibrin pad within the interdiscal cartilageous space where osteoarthritis and bone-to-bone contact may be the source of the disorder (Figure 15.3). Future research in this area is consequently needed to elicit the beneficial advantages with much future randomized clinical studies needed prior to recommending this procedure for routine clinical practice.

15.5 Potential use of platelet rich fibrin for pulp regeneration

In theory, pulp regeneration which requires an agent capable of 1) inducing

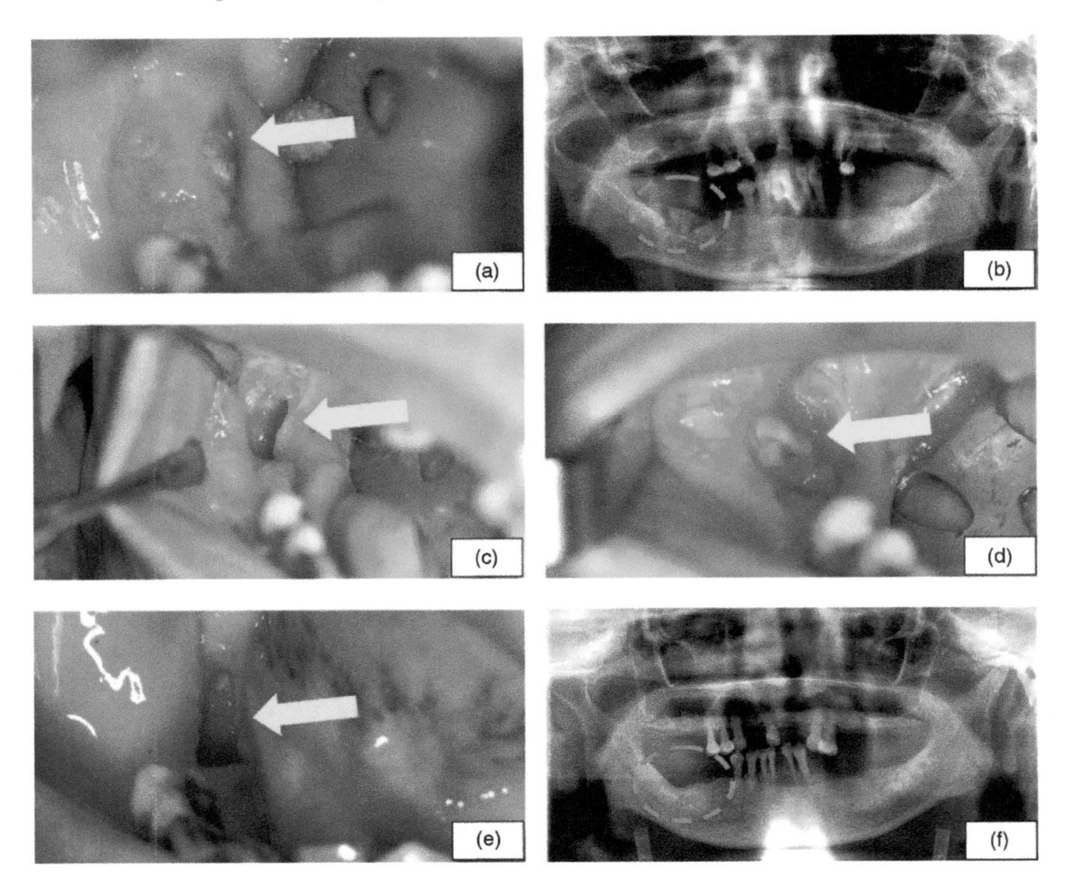

Figure 15.2 Clinical and radiographic photographs of the affected area. (A) Initial intraoral view showing the exposed necrotic bone and pronounced mucosal ulceration over the right posterior mandibular edentulous area caused by BRONJ. (B) Sequestration was obvious in the right posterior mandibular edentulous area shown on an initial panoramic tomographic scan. (C) The sequestrum was removed by surgical sequestrectomy and saucerization. (D) Clinical application of PRF as the sole grafting material in bony lesion. (E) Clinical photograph of the lesion with PRF coverage after 10 days. (F) Postoperative panoramic radiograph revealed dense bonelike tissues over the right posterior mandibular edentulous area 10 months after the surgery.
BRONJ = bisphosphonate-related osteonecrosis of the jaw; PRF = platelet rich fibrin. Source: Tsai *et al.* 2016 [11]. Reproduced with permission of Elsevier.

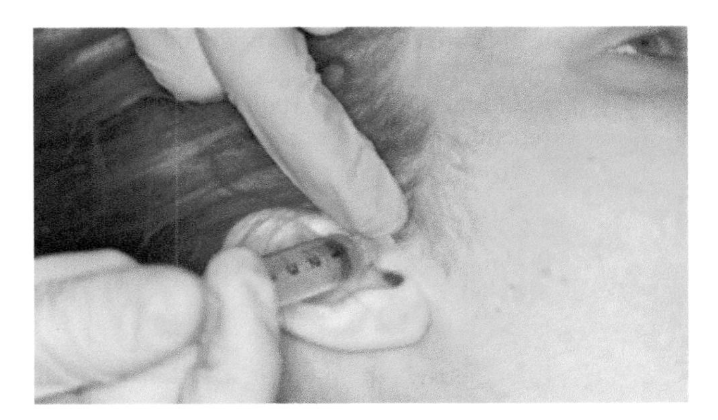

Figure 15.3 Clinical demonstration of i-PRF being injected into the temporo-mandibular joint (TMJ). Case performed by Dr. Joseph Choukroun.

re-vascularization of damaged/necrotic tissue, 2) fighting off bacterial infection and 3) secreting a wide-range of growth factors capable of inducing pulp cell proliferation and differentiation. In this context, PRF displays strong potential in all these categories. An early in vitro study utilizing PRF as a potential agent for pulp regeneration concluded that PRF stimulates the proliferation and differentiation of cells found in the dental pulp [21]. Indeed, significant increases in levels of osteoprotegrins and alkaline phosphatase, essential for biomineralization was observed, suggesting that PRF may promote reparative dentin in damaged pulps [21]. Two later clinical case studies report that after removal of the necrotic pulp in two traumatized permanent central incisors, PRF could be added to the level of the cemento-enamel junction and restored in a conventional manner [22,23]. In both cases, teeth responded positively to electrical testing, cold testing, and complete apical closure as visualized radiographically after 15 months (Figure 15.4, 15.5, and 15.6) [22,23]. While these results are also extremely preliminary, these case studies demonstrate in theory the potential of PRF, however, such studies are both a) difficult to perform ethically and b) require a larger

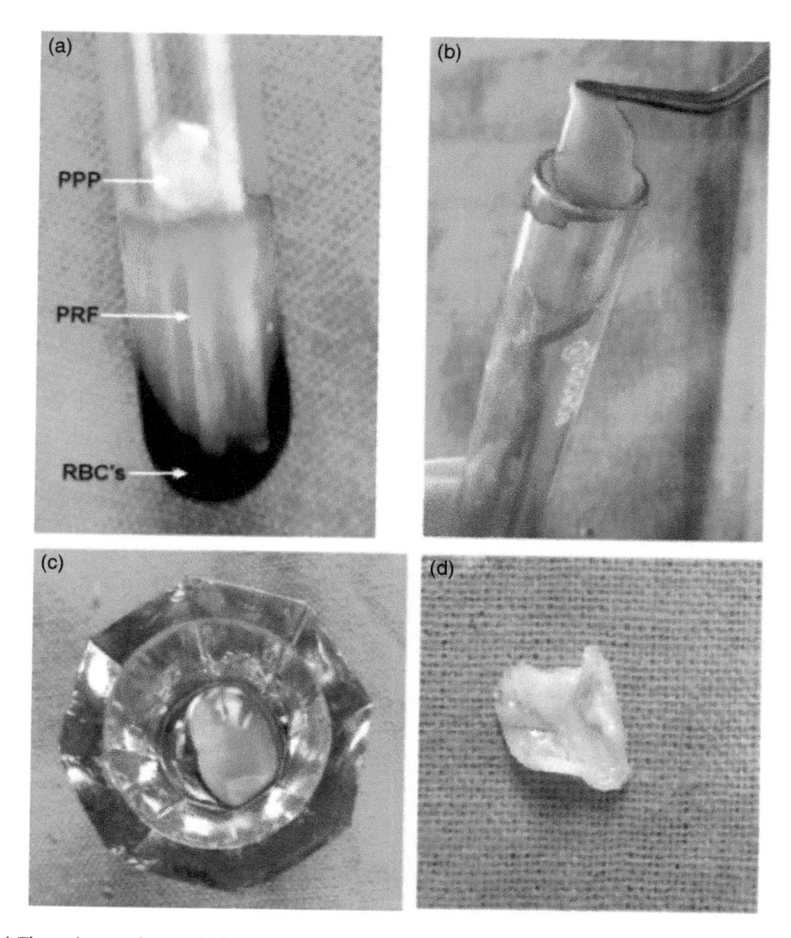

Figure 15.4 (a) Three layers formed after centrifugation: platelet-poor plasma at the top, platelet rich fibrin in middle and base layer of red blood cells (RBCs). (b) Sterile tweezers inserted into the tube to gently retrieve the fibrin clot. (c) platelet rich fibrin clot. (d) platelet rich fibrin membrane. Source: Keswani & Pandey 2013 [22]. Reproduced with permission of John Wiley & Sons.

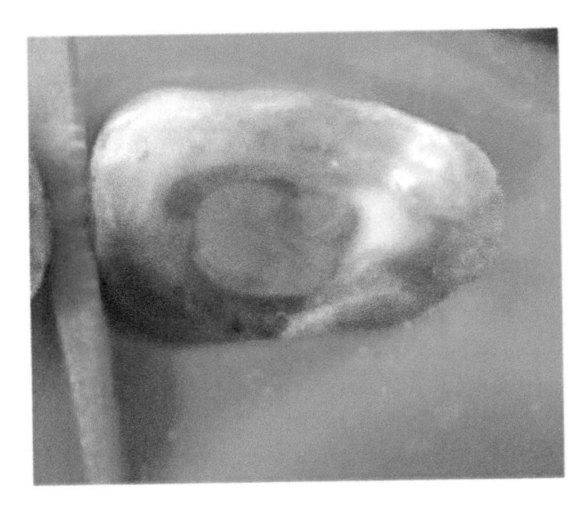

Figure 15.5 Platelet rich fibrin placed into the root canal space of tooth. Source: Keswani & Pandey 2013 [22]. Reproduced with permission of John Wiley & Sons.

number of patients to better determine their effectiveness.

Recently, a systematic review performed by Lolata *et al.* (2016) was conducted investigating the effects of platelet concentrates on pulp regeneration/revitalization of necrotic pulps [24]. Only three randomized parallel studies and one split-mouth case series were included (61 immature necrotic teeth treated in 56 patients with a mean follow-up ranging between 12 and 18 months). All studies used PRP with one using PRF. Periapical healing and apical closure were found to be improved in the treated groups using PRP although no statistical significance was achieved ($P = 0.08$ and $P = 0.06$, respectively). These authors report that the outcomes were most probably due to the limited sample size [24]. The authors further conclude that despite the potential effectiveness of either PRP or PRF in promoting root development of necrotic immature teeth, scarce evidence exists regarding this subject. Future research is therefore necessary.

15.6 Platelet rich fibrin and periodontal regeneration

True periodontal regeneration is defined by regeneration of the periodontal ligament with attachment of Sharpey's fibers spanning the alveolar bone and cementum. As mentioned earlier in Chapter 8, PRF has now been utilized in 11 randomized clinical trials investigating its use in regeneration of periodontal intrabony defects [25–35]. While the collected randomized clinical studies have demonstrated that the use of PRF leads to statistically superior periodontal repair by demonstrating improvements in periodontal pocket depths and clinical attachment level gains, no histological findings have revealed to date whether the observed clinical gains are simply improved connective tissue attachment or may be characterized as true periodontal regeneration. Future research is therefore necessary to investigate histologically the effects of PRF on intrabony/furcation defect regeneration in humans.

15.7 Potential use of stem cells derived from blood

It is well known that blood contains an abundance of cell types including leukocytes, monocytes, platelets, and to a certain extent, progenitor stem cells. While it is known that the stem cell numbers found in blood remains extremely low (certainly less than 1% of total cells), it remains interesting to point out that certain labs are focused on isolating these cells with the aim of further utilizing them later as specialized cells such as osteoblasts, fibroblasts, or chondrocytes for tissue regenerative strategies. While this strategy remains but a future potential hopeful avenue, it remains of interest to further survey upcoming research studies on this topic.

15.8 PRF: regeneration by growth factors, leukocytes, or fibrin?

It has been shown that both leukocytes and fibrin affect new bone formation. The role of leukocytes act not only to defend against incoming pathogens but also to act locally

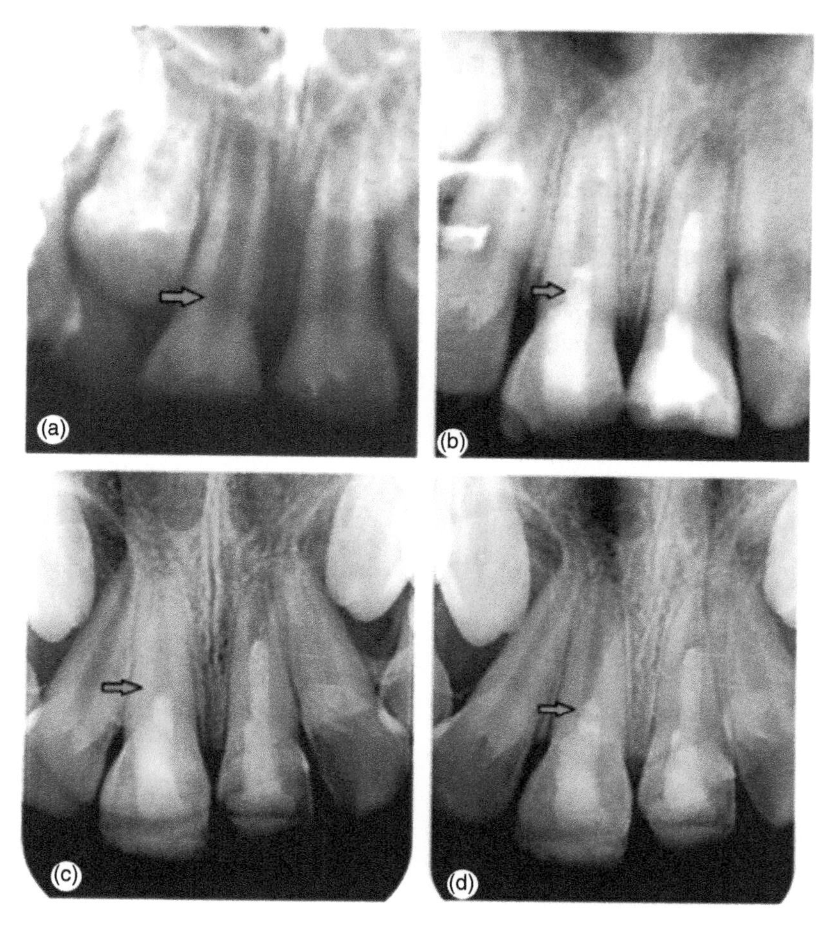

Figure 15.6 (a) Pre-operative intraoral periapical radiograph showing wide root canal with open apex in maxillary central incisor tooth. (b) At 7-month follow-up, tooth showing noticeably increased thickness of root canal. (c) At 12-month follow-up, tooth showing continued root development (d) At 15-month follow-up, tooth showing apical closure with normal periradicular architecture. *Right maxillary central incisor (red arrow). Source: Keswani & Pandey 2013 [22]. Reproduced with permission of John Wiley & Sons.

on tissue homeostasis and regeneration in a positive manner [36–38]. It has furthermore been shown that a fibrin matrix enhances the osteogenic differentiation of progenitor cells and increases the expression of vascular endothelial growth factor (VEGF) [39]. Despite the multi-factorial facet of PRF scaffolds, it remains of interest to investigate which component of PRF (cells, growth factors versus fibrin scaffold) plays the greatest role in influencing the wound healing properties of PRF. Therefore, investigators are interested to determine each of their individual roles in wound healing (potential by blocking certain factors/cells) to determine what influence each component has on tissue regeneration.

15.9 PRF and its degradation properties

Very little research to date has thus far investigated the degradation properties of various PRF membranes. While it is known that PRF typically has a degradation rate of 10 to 14 days, certain studies have further shown that healing of PRF scaffolds can significantly be extended should heat treatment be utilized (such as using an iron). One reported drawback for utilizing PRF for certain dental procedures including its use during guided bone regeneration (GBR), has been its fast resorption time. Typically, collagen membranes with a resorption time of 4 to 8 weeks has been recommended. Therefore, some investigators suggest using two PRF membranes simultaneously in thickness or attempt to modify the properties of PRF membranes through heating or other procedures. Little is known what effect these various alterations or double layering techniques will cause on tissue regeneration, growth factor release, or cell survival/behavior. When adjustments to standardized protocols are modified, future research is also subsequently needed.

15.10 PRF and osteoinduction

Lastly, a misconception exists thus far stating that PRF is osteoinductive. PRF is not osteoinductive, as characterized by the ability for a material to induce ectopic bone formation (Figure 15.7) [40,41]. Nevertheless, while PRF is not osteoinductive, interestingly it may be combined with osteoblasts for instance and injected subcutaneously and show signs of ectopic bone formation (osteoinduction) [42]. In combination with the low evidence that PRF induced guided bone regenerative (GBR) procedures, it remains to be further characterized exactly how PRF influences bone regeneration and if certain centrifugation spin cycles could be modified to improve previous results. Future research is therefore still needed investigating the low-speed centrifugation concept.

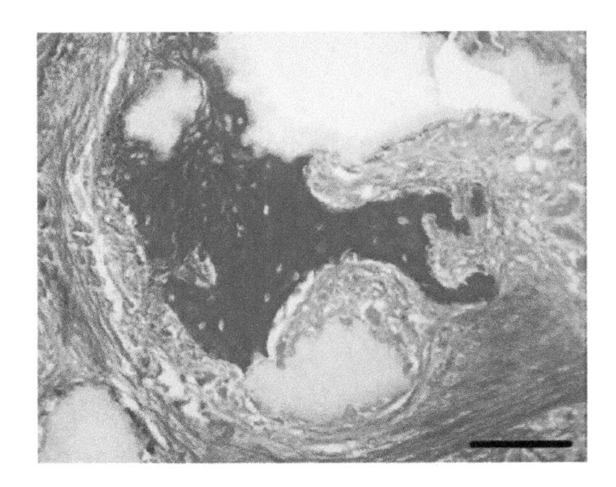

Figure 15.7 Mason staining demonstrating ectopic bone formation (blue) of a bone grafting material (white) when implanted in the muscle of beagle dogs at 60 days. It remains to be investigated under which situations i-PRF may help promote ectopic bone formation. Adapted from Miron *et al.* 2016 [41].

References

1 Ghanaati S, Booms P, Orlowska A, Kubesch A, Lorenz J, Rutkowski J, et al. Advanced platelet-rich fibrin: a new concept for cell-based tissue engineering by means of inflammatory cells. The Journal of oral implantology. 2014;40(6):679–89.

2 Fujioka-Kobayashi M, Miron RJ, Hernandez M, Kandalam U, Zhang Y, Choukroun J. Optimized Platelet Rich Fibrin With the Low Speed Concept: Growth Factor Release, Biocompatibility and Cellular Response. Journal of periodontology. 2016:1–17.

3 Gonen ZB, Yilmaz Asan C. Treatment of bisphosphonate-related osteonecrosis of the jaw using platelet-rich fibrin. Cranio : the journal of craniomandibular practice. 2016:1–5.

4 Kim JW, Kim SJ, Kim MR. Leucocyte-rich and platelet-rich fibrin for the treatment of bisphosphonate-related osteonecrosis of the jaw: a prospective feasibility study. The British journal of oral & maxillofacial surgery. 2014;52(9):854–9.

5 Asaka T, Ohga N, Yamazaki Y, Sato J, Satoh C, Kitagawa Y. Platelet-rich fibrin may

reduce the risk of delayed recovery in tooth-extracted patients undergoing oral bisphosphonate therapy: a trial study. Clinical oral investigations. 2016.

6 Dinca O, Zurac S, Staniceanu F, Bucur MB, Bodnar DC, Vladan C, et al. Clinical and histopathological studies using fibrin-rich plasma in the treatment of bisphosphonate-related osteonecrosis of the jaw. Romanian journal of morphology and embryology = Revue roumaine de morphologie et embryologie. 2014;55(3): 961–4.

7 Kim JW, Kim SJ, Kim MR. Simultaneous Application of Bone Morphogenetic Protein-2 and Platelet-Rich Fibrin for the Treatment of Bisphosphonate-Related Osteonecrosis of Jaw. The Journal of oral implantology. 2016;42(2):205–8.

8 Maluf G, Pinho MC, Cunha SR, Santos PS, Fregnani ER. Surgery Combined with LPRF in Denosumab Osteonecrosis of the Jaw: Case Report. Brazilian dental journal. 2016;27(3):353–8.

9 Norholt SE, Hartlev J. Surgical treatment of osteonecrosis of the jaw with the use of platelet-rich fibrin: a prospective study of 15 patients. Int J Oral Maxillofac Surg. 2016;45(10):1256–60.

10 Soydan SS, Uckan S. Management of bisphosphonate-related osteonecrosis of the jaw with a platelet-rich fibrin membrane: technical report. Journal of oral and maxillofacial surgery : official journal of the American Association of Oral and Maxillofacial Surgeons. 2014;72(2):322–6.

11 Tsai LL, Huang YF, Chang YC. Treatment of bisphosphonate-related osteonecrosis of the jaw with platelet-rich fibrin. Journal of the Formosan Medical Association = Taiwan yi zhi. 2016;115(7):585–6.

12 Hegab AF, Ali HE, Elmasry M, Khallaf MG. Platelet-Rich Plasma Injection as an Effective Treatment for Temporomandibular Joint Osteoarthritis. Journal of oral and maxillofacial surgery : official journal of the American Association of Oral and Maxillofacial Surgeons. 2015;73(9):1706–13.

13 Comert Kilic S, Gungormus M. Is arthrocentesis plus platelet-rich plasma superior to arthrocentesis plus hyaluronic acid for the treatment of temporomandibular joint osteoarthritis: a randomized clinical trial. Int J Oral Maxillofac Surg. 2016;45(12):1538–44.

14 Comert Kilic S, Gungormus M, Sumbullu MA. Is Arthrocentesis Plus Platelet-Rich Plasma Superior to Arthrocentesis Alone in the Treatment of Temporomandibular Joint Osteoarthritis? A Randomized Clinical Trial. Journal of oral and maxillofacial surgery : official journal of the American Association of Oral and Maxillofacial Surgeons. 2015;73(8):1473–83.

15 Hanci M, Karamese M, Tosun Z, Aktan TM, Duman S, Savaci N. Intra-articular platelet-rich plasma injection for the treatment of temporomandibular disorders and a comparison with arthrocentesis. Journal of cranio-maxillo-facial surgery : official publication of the European Association for Cranio-Maxillo-Facial Surgery. 2015;43(1):162–6.

16 Kim SG. Necessity of standardized protocol for platelet-rich plasma therapy in temporomandibular joint osteoarthritis. Journal of the Korean Association of Oral and Maxillofacial Surgeons. 2016;42(2): 65–6.

17 Kutuk N, Bas B, Soylu E, Gonen ZB, Yilmaz C, Balcioglu E, et al. Effect of platelet-rich plasma on fibrocartilage, cartilage, and bone repair in temporomandibular joint. Journal of oral and maxillofacial surgery : official journal of the American Association of Oral and Maxillofacial Surgeons. 2014;72(2):277–84.

18 Marty P, Louvrier A, Weber E, Dubreuil PA, Chatelain B, Meyer C. [Arthrocentesis of the temporomandibular joint and intra-articular injections : An update]. Revue de stomatologie, de chirurgie maxillo-faciale et de chirurgie orale. 2016;117(4):266–72.

19 Mehrotra D, Kumar S, Dhasmana S. Hydroxyapatite/collagen block with platelet rich plasma in temporomandibular

joint ankylosis: a pilot study in children and adolescents. The British journal of oral & maxillofacial surgery. 2012;50(8):774–8.
20 Pihut M, Szuta M, Ferendiuk E, Zenczak-Wieckiewicz D. Evaluation of pain regression in patients with temporomandibular dysfunction treated by intra-articular platelet-rich plasma injections: a preliminary report. BioMed research international. 2014;2014:132369.
21 Huang FM, Yang SF, Zhao JH, Chang YC. Platelet-rich fibrin increases proliferation and differentiation of human dental pulp cells. Journal of endodontics. 2010;36(10): 1628–32.
22 Keswani D, Pandey RK. Revascularization of an immature tooth with a necrotic pulp using platelet-rich fibrin: a case report. International endodontic journal. 2013.
23 Shivashankar VY, Johns DA, Vidyanath S, Sam G. Combination of platelet rich fibrin, hydroxyapatite and PRF membrane in the management of large inflammatory periapical lesion. Journal of conservative dentistry : JCD. 2013;16(3):261–4.
24 Lolato A, Bucchi C, Taschieri S, El Kabbaney A, Del Fabbro M. Platelet concentrates for revitalization of immature necrotic teeth: a systematic review of the clinical studies. Platelets. 2016:1–10.
25 Agarwal A, Gupta ND, Jain A. Platelet rich fibrin combined with decalcified freeze-dried bone allograft for the treatment of human intrabony periodontal defects: a randomized split mouth clinical trail. Acta odontologica Scandinavica. 2016;74(1):36–43.
26 Ajwani H, Shetty S, Gopalakrishnan D, Kathariya R, Kulloli A, Dolas RS, et al. Comparative evaluation of platelet-rich fibrin biomaterial and open flap debridement in the treatment of two and three wall intrabony defects. Journal of international oral health : JIOH. 2015; 7(4):32–7.
27 Elgendy EA, Abo Shady TE. Clinical and radiographic evaluation of nanocrystalline hydroxyapatite with or without platelet-rich fibrin membrane in the treatment of periodontal intrabony defects. Journal of Indian Society of Periodontology. 2015;19(1):61–5.
28 Joseph VR, Sam G, Amol NV. Clinical evaluation of autologous platelet rich fibrin in horizontal alveolar bony defects. Journal of clinical and diagnostic research : JCDR. 2014;8(11):Zc43–7.
29 Panda S, Sankari M, Satpathy A, Jayakumar D, Mozzati M, Mortellaro C, et al. Adjunctive Effect of Autologus Platelet-Rich Fibrin to Barrier Membrane in the Treatment of Periodontal Intrabony Defects. The Journal of craniofacial surgery. 2016;27(3):691–6.
30 Pradeep AR, Nagpal K, Karvekar S, Patnaik K, Naik SB, Guruprasad CN. Platelet-rich fibrin with 1% metformin for the treatment of intrabony defects in chronic periodontitis: a randomized controlled clinical trial. Journal of periodontology. 2015;86(6):729–37.
31 Pradeep AR, Rao NS, Agarwal E, Bajaj P, Kumari M, Naik SB. Comparative evaluation of autologous platelet-rich fibrin and platelet-rich plasma in the treatment of 3-wall intrabony defects in chronic periodontitis: a randomized controlled clinical trial. Journal of periodontology. 2012;83(12):1499–507.
32 Shah M, Patel J, Dave D, Shah S. Comparative evaluation of platelet-rich fibrin with demineralized freeze-dried bone allograft in periodontal infrabony defects: A randomized controlled clinical study. Journal of Indian Society of Periodontology. 2015;19(1):56–60.
33 Thorat M, Pradeep AR, Pallavi B. Clinical effect of autologous platelet-rich fibrin in the treatment of intra-bony defects: a controlled clinical trial. J Clin Periodontol. 2011;38(10):925–32.
34 Pradeep AR, Bajaj P, Rao NS, Agarwal E, Naik SB. Platelet-Rich Fibrin Combined With a Porous Hydroxyapatite Graft for the Treatment of Three-Wall Intrabony Defects in Chronic Periodontitis: A Randomized Controlled Clinical Trial. J Periodontol. 2012.

35 Sharma A, Pradeep AR. Treatment of 3-wall intrabony defects in patients with chronic periodontitis with autologous platelet-rich fibrin: a randomized controlled clinical trial. Journal of periodontology. 2011;82(12): 1705–12.

36 Kawazoe T, Kim HH. Tissue augmentation by white blood cell-containing platelet-rich plasma. Cell transplantation. 2012;21(2-3): 601–7.

37 Perut F, Filardo G, Mariani E, Cenacchi A, Pratelli L, Devescovi V, et al. Preparation method and growth factor content of platelet concentrate influence the osteogenic differentiation of bone marrow stromal cells. Cytotherapy. 2013;15(7): 830–9.

38 Pirraco RP, Reis RL, Marques AP. Effect of monocytes/macrophages on the early osteogenic differentiation of hBMSCs. Journal of tissue engineering and regenerative medicine. 2013;7(5): 392–400.

39 Lohse N, Schulz J, Schliephake H. Effect of fibrin on osteogenic differentiation and VEGF expression of bone marrow stromal cells in mineralised scaffolds: a three-dimensional analysis. European cells & materials. 2012;23:413–23; discussion 24.

40 Miron RJ, Zhang YF. Osteoinduction: a review of old concepts with new standards. Journal of dental research. 2012;91(8): 736–44.

41 Miron RJ, Sculean A, Shuang Y, Bosshardt DD, Gruber R, Buser D, et al. Osteoinductive potential of a novel biphasic calcium phosphate bone graft in comparison with autographs, xenografts, and DFDBA. Clinical oral implants research. 2016;27(6):668–75.

42 Wang Z, Weng Y, Lu S, Zong C, Qiu J, Liu Y, et al. Osteoblastic mesenchymal stem cell sheet combined with Choukroun platelet-rich fibrin induces bone formation at an ectopic site. Journal of biomedical materials research Part B, Applied biomaterials. 2015;103(6):1204–16.

Index

Platelet Rich Fibrin in Regenerative Dentistry: Biological Background and Clinical Indications, First Edition.
Edited by Richard J. Miron and Joseph Choukroun.